CANCER ETIOLOGY, DIAGNOSIS AND TREATMENTS

GASTRIC CANCER

RISK FACTORS, TREATMENT AND CLINICAL OUTCOMES

CANCER ETIOLOGY, DIAGNOSIS AND TREATMENTS

Additional books in this series can be found on Nova's website under the Series tab.

Additional e-books in this series can be found on Nova's website under the e-book tab.

CANCER ETIOLOGY, DIAGNOSIS AND TREATMENTS

GASTRIC CANCER

RISK FACTORS, TREATMENT AND CLINICAL OUTCOMES

JASNEET SINGH BHULLAR, M.D.
EDITOR

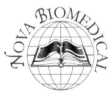

New York

Copyright © 2014 by Nova Science Publishers, Inc.

All rights reserved. No part of this book may be reproduced, stored in a retrieval system or transmitted in any form or by any means: electronic, electrostatic, magnetic, tape, mechanical photocopying, recording or otherwise without the written permission of the Publisher.

For permission to use material from this book please contact us:
Telephone 631-231-7269; Fax 631-231-8175
Web Site: http://www.novapublishers.com

NOTICE TO THE READER

The Publisher has taken reasonable care in the preparation of this book, but makes no expressed or implied warranty of any kind and assumes no responsibility for any errors or omissions. No liability is assumed for incidental or consequential damages in connection with or arising out of information contained in this book. The Publisher shall not be liable for any special, consequential, or exemplary damages resulting, in whole or in part, from the readers' use of, or reliance upon, this material. Any parts of this book based on government reports are so indicated and copyright is claimed for those parts to the extent applicable to compilations of such works.

Independent verification should be sought for any data, advice or recommendations contained in this book. In addition, no responsibility is assumed by the publisher for any injury and/or damage to persons or property arising from any methods, products, instructions, ideas or otherwise contained in this publication.

This publication is designed to provide accurate and authoritative information with regard to the subject matter covered herein. It is sold with the clear understanding that the Publisher is not engaged in rendering legal or any other professional services. If legal or any other expert assistance is required, the services of a competent person should be sought. FROM A DECLARATION OF PARTICIPANTS JOINTLY ADOPTED BY A COMMITTEE OF THE AMERICAN BAR ASSOCIATION AND A COMMITTEE OF PUBLISHERS.

Additional color graphics may be available in the e-book version of this book.

Library of Congress Cataloging-in-Publication Data

ISBN: 978-1-63117-983-9

Published by Nova Science Publishers, Inc. † New York

Contents

Preface		**vii**
Editor Contact Information		**xi**
Chapter 1	Geographical Differences in Risk Factors, Systems and Outcomes in Gastric Cancer *Omar M. Rashid, M.D., J.D., Sangeetha Prabhakaran, M.D., Kyo-young Song, M.D., Ph.D. and Joyce Wong, M.D.*	**1**
Chapter 2	Gastric Cancer: Focus on Epidemiology, Pathology, Diagnosis and Treatment - A Global Overview *Lan Mo, M.D., Jafar Al-Mondhiry, M.S. and Jennifer Wu, M.D.*	**23**
Chapter 3	Gastric Cancer Staging *Matthew Dixon, Abraham El-Sedfy and Natalie Coburn*	**57**
Chapter 4	Early Gastric Cancer: A Comprehensive View of Management *Wenbo Meng, Xun Li, M.D., Ph.D., Wence Zhou, Yan Li, Kiyohito Tanaka, M.D., Ph.D. and Liang Qiao*	**89**
Chapter 5	Advancements in Murine Models of Human Gastric Cancer *Jasneet Singh Bhullar, M.D., M.S., Neha Varshney, M.D. and Vijay K. Mittal, M.D., FACS*	**125**
Chapter 6	Adjuvant Treatment Modalities for Gastric Cancer *Leyla Kilic, M.D. and Cetin Ordu, M.D.*	**141**
Chapter 7	Surgical Evaluation of Lymph Node Involvement in Gastric Cancer - Maruyama Computer Program and the Sentinel Lymph Node Biopsy *Dezső Tóth, M.D., Ph.D. and Miklós Török, M.D.*	**157**
Chapter 8	Clinical and Surgical Management of Gastric Cancer: Principles of Treatment *Stefano Rausei, M.D., Ph.D., Sebastiano Spampatti, M.D., Federica Galli, M.D., Laura Ruspi, M.D., Francesca Rovera, M.D., Luigi Boni, M.D., FACS and Gianlorenzo Dionigi, M.D., FACS*	**171**

Chapter 9	Bursectomy in Gastric Cancer Surgery *Konstantinos Blouhos, M.D., MSc, Ph.D.,* *Konstantinos Tsalis, M.D., Ph.D.,* *Konstantinos A. Boulas, M.D., MSc.* *and Anestis Hatzigeorgiadis, M.D., MSc.*	**195**
Index		**209**

Preface

Gastric cancer is one of the leading causes of malignancy-related deaths worldwide with differences in incidence and treatment patterns geographically. There is extensive ongoing research for a better understanding of the cancer pathology and finding newer treatments. Though some advancements in basic science research are being translated for improving gastric cancer patient care, but improving the overall outcome of such patients still remains a cherished goal. This book discusses an extensive array of different topics on gastric cancer in which strides of improvement have been achieved. The current statuses, debates and ongoing controversies in addition to the advancements on different aspects of gastric cancer research, diagnosis, staging and treatment are discussed.

Chapter 1 - This review focuses on the etiologies, treatment, national systems, and outcomes of gastric cancer, particularly as it relates to global differences seen in the approach to treating gastric cancer. Demographic, incidence and pathologic patterns differ widely between Asian and western patients. It is apparent that distal tumors of a favorable histologic subtype are more common in Asian patients, with a tendency towards a mixed or diffuse histology. Western patients, on the contrary, tend to have more advanced disease with more proximal tumors. The role of *Helicobacter pylori*, in addition to other etiologies, perhaps diet-related or genetic, may also contribute to the disparities seen. Treatment strategies also demonstrate geographic differences, with western countries often favoring a neoadjuvant chemotherapy approach, prior to surgical resection, while surgical resection remains the mainstay of therapy for gastric cancer in Asian countries, with an emphasis on the extent of lymphadenectomy. Often, lymph node dissection and examination occur intraoperatively, according to the Japanese classification system. This is unlike the western technique that tends towards *en bloc* submission of the gastric specimen with the lymphadenectomy to pathology for examination. Although much debate has historically centered on the extent of lymphadenectomy, D2 lymphadenectomy is now widely considered standard for resection for gastric cancer. Despite the American Joint Committee on Cancer (AJCC) staging system being widely referenced, Asian countries demonstrate an improved survival, even when matched stage for stage with patients in western countries. Demographic factors, prevalence of obesity, location of tumor, and other contributing factors may impact the differences seen in outcome.

Chapter 2 - Discusses the global overview of gastric cancer with focus on epidemiology, pathology, diagnosis and treatment. Risk factors for gastric cancer are highly dependent on dietary habits, *H. pylori* infections and less frequently, genetic syndromes. The chapter describes the pathogenesis of gastric cancer from these three risk factors. Various histology of gastric cancer and their potential implications in prognosis are also discussed. Certain endemic areas with high incidence of gastric cancer have instituted effective screening program to detect early stage gastric cancer, a strategy worth exploring in the future where gastric cancer incidence is amongst the fastest growing cancer in the world. For local or superficial disease (Stage IA), surgery alone is curative, and the treatment may involve endoscopic mucosal resection, although subtotal or total gastrectomy is still a common choice depending on tumor location. For more advanced disease (Stage IB-III), surgery is the main modality to achieve cure. The various techniques of gastrectomies are discussed, especially the differences and controversies of D1 and D2 lymph node dissection. In addition, adjuvant treatment including either chemoradiation with (5-FU) or chemotherapy alone using capecitabine and oxaliplatin are options of standard care in various parts of the world. A combination of triplet in the perioperative setting, which includes fluoropyramidine, anthracycline and platinum, has also been widely adapted as an effective therapy that improves patient outcome. Treatment options for metastatic disease along with the newer treatment options like ramucirumab are also discussed. It thus provides insights into the careful selection of anti-angiogenesis treatments in gastric cancer, suggesting that the overexpression of angiogenesis in gastric cancer is just the beginning of an exciting journey in our understanding of this disease.

Chapter 3 - Discusses the different gastric cancer staging reported. Accurate staging forms the basis for which treatments for gastric cancer are selected. An understanding of the staging systems commonly used is important for physicians involved in the treatment of gastric cancer. In addition, several staging modalities are routinely prescribed in an attempt to accurately stage the patient with gastric cancer. Each of these staging modalities has their own benefits and drawbacks with varying degrees of accuracy, sensitivity and specificity. The following staging modalities are reviewed in detail: computed tomography, magnetic resonance imaging, abdominal ultrasound, Fluorodeoxyglucose-positron emission tomography, esophagogastroduodenoscopy, endoscopic ultrasound, staging laparoscopy, peritoneal cytology and sentinel lymph node biopsy. The ultimate goal is correlation between staging modalities and pathology findings such that accurate staging is performed with delivery of the most appropriate stage-specific treatment.

Chapter 4 - Describes a comprehensive review of early gastric cancer (EGC), including the recent development in the endoscopic diagnosis and treatment of EGC. Late diagnosis, lack of effective treatment with tumor invasion and distant metastasis, as well as the poor understanding of the molecular mechanisms involved in the development of gastric cancer are among the major factors responsible for poor prognosis and high mortality rate. The witnessed improvement in long-term survival rate of patients with gastric cancer over the past few decades is mainly attributable to improved early diagnosis and radical management. Apparently, early diagnosis and treatment are the key components of effective management of patients with gastric cancer. Pathologically, EGC refers to the carcinoma with invasion depth limited to mucosa or submucosa and can only be reliably diagnosed endoscopically. Over the recent years, many endoscopic diagnostic approaches have been developed, such as endoscopic ultrasound (EUS), chromoscopy, the narrowband imaging zoom endoscope (NBI), confocal laser endomicroscopy, magnifying chromoendoscopy, autoflourescent endoscopy and infrared endoscopy. Measurement of serum biochemical parameters such as pepsinogen and *Helicobacter Pylori* IgG (HP-IgG) coupled with intelligent dyeing endoscopy (i-scan) has also been shown to greatly improve the detection rates of EGC. These newly developed endoscopic procedures have remarkably improved the diagnostic accuracy and enhanced the resection rate of EGC. This has led to Endoscopic submucosl dissection (ESD) which has many advantages over conventional surgical resection in the management of EGC.

Chapter 5 - Murine models of gastric carcinogenesis are an in vivo tool essential in understanding the mechanisms of pathogenesis in search of better treatment. Over the years considerable changes in the understanding of the murine models of human gastric cancer have resulted in numerous models being reported in the literature. The chapter discusses the different human gastric cancer murine models, their background, the technique of creating them along with their advantages and limitations. The studies in which human gastric murine models are used are also briefly discussed. This extensive overview and details of an array of different resources in this field offer researchers a wide choice to choose a model which is more applicable to the type of study being planned.

Chapter 6 - Discusses the adjuvant treatment modalities available for treating gastric cancer. Discussion about the Intergroup trial and the subsequent update form the historical background for adjuvant treatment trials. The subsequent worldwide trials along with the two recently completed trials comparing different postoperative adjuvant regimens have been described. Also discussed is the ARTIST (Adjuvant Chemoradiation Therapy in Stomach Cancer) trial compared postoperative capecitabine and cisplatin (XP) to chemoradiotherapy (XP plus radiotherapy with capecitabine) in patients with curative gastrectomy with D2 dissection. Ultimately, beyond the primary objectives of these proposed and ongoing trials, research must continue to identify new prognostic and predictive factors, such as human epidermal growth factor receptor 2 overexpression or diffuse histology in adjuvant setting, that may serve for a tailored therapeutic approaches.

Chapter 7 - Lymphadenectomy as a part of gastric cancer treatment has remained an ongoing debate. Approximately, one-third of patients with gastric cancer undergo an unnecessary extended lymph node dissection resulting in a higher rate of morbidity and mortality so sentinel lymph node biopsy would be helpful in such cases. Unfortunately preoperative diagnostic tools have a low sensitivity and specificity in determining lymph node involvement. The chapter discusses the Maruyama computer program (MCP), used for estimating the lymph node involvement preoperatively and the sentinel lymph node (SLN) biopsy and may help to reduce the number of redundant lymphadenectomy intraoperatively. The Maruyama computer program had a sensitivity of 90.2%, specificity of 63.3% and an accuracy of 78.4 %. The accuracy of SLN mapping was 98.2%. The intraoperative sentinel lymph node examination was superior to the preoperative estimation by the Maruyama computer program. However, using these two methods in a parallel fashion could be useful in decision-making for determining the appropriate extent of lymphadenectomy. The individualized stage-adapted surgery can guarantee the best outcome for the patients with gastric cancer.

Chapter 8 - This chapter gives an overview on risk factors, staging and principles of treating gastric cancer. Open issues in the surgical management of gastric malignancies alongwith the validity and usefulness of the 7th edition of the AJCC/UICC tumor node metastases classification in the context of clinical management of gastric cancer are discussed. Additionally, the hot topic of the role of laparoscopy in gastric cancer treatment debate is described. While the laparoscopic approach is strongly recommended for staging, but the use of minimally invasive surgery for resection and lymphadenectomy is yet to be established. Multimodal treatment strategies, including adjuvant chemotherapy and/or radiotherapy options, are analyzed in order to clarify its indications and results.

Chapter 9 - Discusses role of bursectomy in gastric cancer surgery. The continued practice of bursectomy stems from its utility in facilitating: (a) elimination of microscopic tumor deposits in the greater omentum and lesser sac; (b) complete resection of disease from the head of the pancreas; (c) complete clearance of the high-risk subpyloric station lymph nodes (LNs); (d) an aesthetic, clean, celiac based node dissection; and (e) direct access to the "difficult" LNs. D2 gastrectomy plus bursectomy can be safely performed in high volume experience centers or by experienced surgeons with mortality rates of <1 % and morbidity rates of around 14–24 %. The Japanese gastric cancer treatment guidelines suggest performance of bursectomy for tumors penetrating the serosa of the posterior gastric wall. This chapter discusses in detail the surgical aspects of bursectomy and its other details.

Editor Contact Information

Dr. Jasneet Singh Bhullar, M.D., M.S.
3684 Lexington Dr, Auburn Hills
MI 48326, USA
Cell: 248-701-4321
drjsbhullar@gmail.com

In: Gastric Cancer
Editor: Jasneet Singh Bhullar

ISBN: 978-1-63117-983-9
© 2014 Nova Science Publishers, Inc.

Chapter 1

Geographical Differences in Risk Factors, Systems and Outcomes in Gastric Cancer[*]

Omar M. Rashid, M.D., J.D.[1], Sangeetha Prabhakaran, M.D.[1], Kyo-young Song, M.D., Ph.D.[2] and Joyce Wong, M.D.[3]

[1]Department of Surgical Oncology, Moffitt Cancer Center, Tampa, FL, US
[2]Department of Surgery, The Catholic University of Korea, Seoul, Korea
[3]Department of Surgical Oncology, Penn State Hershey Medical Center, Hershey, PA, US

Abstract

Gastric cancer is one of the leading causes of malignancy-related death worldwide; however, a unique demographic distribution exists. Global differences are seen with an increased incidence noted in Asia as compared to Western countries. Demographic and pathologic patterns also differ widely between Asian and Western patients. It is apparent that distal tumors of a favorable histologic subtype are more common in Asian patients, with a tendency towards a mixed or diffuse histology. Western patients, on the contrary, tend to have more advanced disease with more proximal tumors. It still remains unclear what the exact etiology is behind this demographic difference. The role of *Helicobacter pylori*, in addition to other etiologies, perhaps diet-related or genetic, may also contribute to the disparities seen.

Treatment strategies also demonstrate geographic differences, with Western countries often favoring a neoadjuvant chemotherapy approach, prior to surgical resection. Surgical resection remains the mainstay of therapy for gastric cancer in Asian countries, with an emphasis on the extent of lymphadenectomy. Often, lymph node dissection and examination occur intraoperatively, according to the Japanese classification system. This is unlike the Western technique that tends towards *en bloc* submission of the gastric specimen with the lymphadenectomy to pathology for

---

[*] Edited by Khaldoun Almhanna, MD MPH. Assistant Member of the Department of Gastrointestinal Oncology. Moffitt Cancer Center, Tampa, FL.

examination. Although much debate has historically centered on the extent of lymphadenectomy, D2 lymphadenectomy is now widely considered standard for resection for gastric cancer.

Despite the American Joint Committee on Cancer (AJCC) staging system being widely referenced, Asian countries demonstrate an improved survival, even when matched stage for stage with patients in Western countries. Demographic factors, prevalence of obesity, location of tumor, and other contributing factors may impact the differences seen in outcome. This review focuses on the etiologies, treatment, national systems, and outcomes of gastric cancer, particularly as it relates to global differences seen in the approach to treating gastric cancer.

Introduction

Gastric cancer is a unique malignancy, with a known geographical distribution, with a far greater incidence in Eastern countries such as Korea, Japan, and China. While gastric cancer is not in the top ten highest-incident cancers in the United States (U.S.), it is number one and four amongst males and females, respectively, according to the Korea National Cancer Incidence Database [1, 2]. The U.S. still sees an estimated 21,600 new cases of gastric cancer per year.

The age-adjusted death rate, however, has been steadily declining [1]. Korea, a much smaller country geographically and far more homogeneous in terms of its population, has the highest worldwide rate of gastric cancer [2, 3]. The incidence of gastric cancer is over 33,000 per year, with an estimated 8,200 deaths. Mongolia, Japan and China have the second, third and fourth highest rates of gastric cancer globally [3]. Gastric cancer is so prevalent in the East that countries such as Korea have implemented mandatory endoscopic or radiographic screening for its citizens under its National Cancer Screening Program. Not only did implementation of a screening program improve survival from gastric cancer, but it was also a cost-effective strategy in countries of high-prevalence [4]. On the contrary, the U.S. and Europe have not adopted routine screening strategies since the incidence of gastric cancer is significantly lower, and there is no proven cost-effective benefit. The exception to this would be endoscopic screening for esophageal cancer, in the setting of Barrett's esophagus, a condition with increasing prevalence in the U.S. While gastroesophageal junction tumors are considered as esophageal lesions in the West, there are groups in Asia that advocate treating these lesions as gastric cancers. This remains controversial, however, and will not be addressed in this chapter.

While the systematic approach to gastric cancer differs markedly between the East and West, the typical patient profile seen in these regions also differs. This undoubtedly relates to epidemiology and unique risk factors inherent either in the environment or within the composition of the population. Indeed, even patients in the U.S. of Asian descent have an improved overall survival compared with white, black, and Hispanic patients, seen in large studies using California cancer registries as well as the National Cancer Data Base [5-7]. This chapter reviews the clinical presentation, demographic and etiologic differences and treatment strategies seen in both the East and West as related to gastric adenocarcinoma.

Patient Characteristics/Pathology

Gastric cancer comprises a heterogeneous group of tumors with different morphologies, molecular backgrounds, and histogenesis [8]. The main histologic classifications are the Lauren system and World Health Organization (WHO) histologic system [9, 10]. The Lauren system classifies gastric cancer as intestinal, diffuse or mixed type. Intestinal-type cancers range from well to poorly differentiated, and have expanding, rather than infiltrative, patterns. They exhibit gland formation and are associated with intestinal metaplasia, chronic atrophic gastritis and *Helicobacter pylori (H. pylori)* infection. The diffuse-type tumors have non-cohesive tumor cells diffusely infiltrating the stroma of the stomach and often exhibit deep infiltration of the stomach wall with little or no gland formation. They may have pronounced desmoplasia and associated inflammation, with relative sparing of the overlying mucosa. They occur more often in young patients and are associated with worse prognosis. In an analysis of 805 resectable patients with gastric adenocarcinoma, the diffuse-type comprised 48.7% of the cohort and showed worse prognosis than intestinal-type. Multivariate analysis revealed that independent prognostic factors were T stage, N stage, tumor size and Lauren classification [11].

In the WHO classification (2010), gastric cancer is categorized primarily into papillary, tubular, mucinous, and poorly cohesive variants, including signet ring cell carcinoma (SRC). The main histology of the tumor is determined by the cell type that comprises more than 50% of the total [12]. Tubular adenocarcinoma is the most common histologic type and grossly tends to form polypoid or fungating masses. The papillary type is another common histologic variant and tends to affect older people, occur in the proximal stomach, and is frequently associated with liver metastasis and a higher rate of lymph node involvement. Mucinous adenocarcinoma accounts for 10% of gastric cancer and is characterized by extracellular mucinous pools which constitute at least 50% of tumor volume.

Signet ring cell (SRC) carcinoma has different microscopic and biologic characteristics compared with other types of gastric adenocarcinoma. The incidence of SRC carcinoma has been reported to vary between 8.7% and 23.4%. Signet ring cell, and other poorly cohesive carcinomas, have a propensity to invade the duodenum via submucosal and subserosal routes. In early gastric cancer, SRC histology has been reported to have a better prognosis than non-SRC because of less lymph node metastasis. However, in advanced gastric cancer, SRC has been characterized to be more grossly infiltrative, with a greater likelihood of peritoneal dissemination and a similar or worse prognosis than non-SRC cancers. In a group of 2208 patients with early gastric cancer who underwent surgery in Seoul, Korea, the SRC group was associated with younger age, female gender, mid-body location, mucosal location, depressed type, fewer lymph node metastasis, less lymphovascular invasion, and a better survival rate than the mixed-SRC and adenocarcinoma groups. Interestingly, the mixed-SRC group showed more submucosal invasion, were larger in size, and had a higher lymph node metastasis rate than other groups, indicating a more aggressive behavior [13].

Other studies refute these observations. Piessen, et al. [14] performed an intention-to-treat, case matched analysis of 180 patients with gastric carcinoma, 59 of whom had SRC, and observed that median survival was significantly lower for SRC patients (21 vs. 44 months, P = 0.004). Resected patients with signet ring cell histology exhibited higher rates of peritoneal carcinomatosis and lymph node involvement at diagnosis, a lower R0 resection rate, and earlier tumor relapse, which was generally seen as peritoneal carcinomatosis. Based on multivariate analysis, the authors concluded that SRC histology was independently associated with a dismal prognosis after adjustment for confounding variables. In a review of 10,246 cases of patients with gastric cancer from the U.S. National Cancer Institute Surveillance, Epidemiology, and End Results (SEER) database, SRC was found in younger patients and most often in men. Signet ring cell carcinoma was more likely to be of a more advanced AJCC stage, with a greater proportion having T3-4 (45.8% vs. 33.3%) tumors and lymph node spread (59.7% vs. 51.8%), compared with adenocarcinoma. Signet ring cell carcinoma was more likely to be found in the distal stomach and more likely to be stage IV, compared with adenocarcinoma (50% vs. 42.8%, p<0.001) [15]. However, when survival was adjusted for stage, SRC did not confer a worse prognosis and was not found to be a predictor of worse survival on multivariate analysis [15]. Despite presentation with more advanced disease, the SRC histology does not appear to portend worse survival as previously thought, although this must also be balanced against the change in treatment and operative approaches.

The HER2 protein is a 185-kDa transmembrane tyrosine kinase (TK) receptor and a member of the epidermal growth factor receptor (EGFR) family. This receptor consists of an extracellular ligand-binding domain, a short transmembrane domain, and an intracellular domain with TK activity (except HER3). The binding of a ligand to the extracellular domain initiates a signal transduction cascade that can influence many aspects of tumor cell biology, including cell proliferation, apoptosis, adhesion, migration, and differentiation. In carcinomas, *HER2* acts as an oncogene; high-level amplification of the gene induces protein overexpression in the cellular membrane and subsequent acquisition of advantageous properties for a malignant cell. Overexpression of HER2 and amplification of HER2/c-erbB2 are seen in gastric adenocarcinomas, among which HER2 is dysregulated in 7–34% of primary tumors [16]. It has been correlated with poor outcomes and more aggressive disease; research efforts continue to work on characterizing tumors at a molecular level to help individualize treatment and determine prognosis [17]. In a prospective analysis of 63 patients with resectable gastric carcinomas, high levels of EGFR and HER2 were significantly associated with a shorter overall survival period [18]. A retrospective review of 1,006 consecutive patients with gastric cancer who underwent surgery in Japan found HER2 overexpression detected in 118 (11.7 %) patients [19]. HER2 overexpression was correlated with older age, gender, well differentiated tumors, expanding growth pattern, and nodal status. In the survival analysis, HER2 overexpression was not found to be correlated with either disease-specific survival or recurrence-free survival.

Approximately 1–3% of gastric cancers arise as a result of inherited gastric cancer syndromes. These may be of the diffuse or intestinal type, and linkage analysis has recently implicated E-cadherin (CDH1) mutations in an estimated 25% of families with an autosomal dominant predisposition to diffuse type gastric cancers. This subset of gastric cancer has been termed hereditary diffuse gastric cancer (HDGC) [20]. There are 2 main criteria to qualify for a diagnosis of HDGC: 1) 2 or more documented cases of diffuse gastric cancer in a first or second degree relative, with at least one diagnosed before the age of 50 years and 2) 3 or more cases of documented diffuse gastric cancer in first or second degree relatives, independent of age of onset. Preliminary data suggest that the penetrance of CDH-1 gene mutations is high, with an estimated range of 70–80%. Women from these families also have a 40% lifetime risk of lobular breast cancer.

Pathologic Differences, East vs. West

Location of tumor differs between the Western and Eastern populations. In the West, there is a higher incidence of tumors located in the proximal third of the stomach, and these are known to be associated with worse outcomes while pathology in Eastern countries tends to be more prevalent in the distal stomach [21]. The incidence of adenocarcinoma of the lower esophagus and gastric cardia has been increasing in the U.S. and Europe, but this pattern has not been observed in Japan and may be related to the lower incidence of reflux esophagitis and Barrett's metaplasia. There is a higher prevalence of diffuse histology in Western patients as well. The poor prognosis of diffuse and signet ring histology and the prevalence of more advanced disease seen in the West could explain the worse outcomes. Patients in the U.S. generally develop gastric cancer later in life and have higher body mass index. Obesity has been linked to perioperative complications and this, in turn, could account for some of the differences in outcome, although survival was not shown to be affected by obesity [22].

Significant differences exist not only in the intraoperative assessment of resected gastrectomies, but also in the histologic interpretation of neoplasms of the GI tract between Japanese and Western pathologists. Intraoperatively, both the Korean and Japanese surgeons dissect out lymph node packets by lymph node station and submit this to pathology as separate specimens, whereas the U.S. and European surgeons tend towards submitting the specimen *en bloc* with associated lymph nodes [23]. To test the hypothesis regarding histologic interpretation, a group of Japanese and Western pathologists collaborated on a number of studies in GI tract pathologic correlation. A group of investigators reviewed pathologic slides encompassing the range of changes seen in progression from benign mucosal lesions to carcinoma. The gastric neoplasia study was performed on slides obtained from 19 gastric lesions: 17 biopsy specimens and 18 endoscopic mucosal resections from patients treated at one institution in Japan, with all submitted carcinomas being of the intestinal type. Of the total diagnoses made by the Western pathologists, 38% were classified as suspected or definite carcinoma, compared to 87% of Japanese pathologists. Japanese pathologists relied heavily on nuclear cytologic and glandular architectural abnormalities to diagnose carcinoma. In the view of Western pathologists, the term carcinoma is synonymous with invasive carcinoma, leaving a potentially considerable overlap between high-grade dysplasia and early invasive gastric cancer [24]. This may lead to geographical treatment bias and ultimately differences in outcome for gastric cancer.

Schempler, et. al also postulated that the differences in pathologic review may contribute to the relatively high incidence and good prognosis of gastric carcinoma in Japan when compared with Western countries [24]. Even among Japanese and Chinese patients, there were differences in clinicopathological behaviors and prognosis in gastric cancer [25]. Compared to Japan, the occurrence of gastric cancer was more common in the younger Chinese population, and these patients demonstrated higher degrees of pathologic invasion and metastasis. Intestinal and mixed types of carcinomas were more frequently observed in Japanese patients. The cumulative survival rate of Chinese patients was significantly higher compared to Japanese in stratified groups based on depth of invasion, stage, or Lauren histology. While pathologic variances have been traditionally thought to be between Eastern and Western countries, there are also subtle differences even amongst Asian countries. Further study is needed to elucidate these differences and determine their impact on outcome.

Etiology and *Helicobacter pylori*

Although the precise etiology of gastric cancer has yet to be conclusively demonstrated, there are several known risk factors that have been well described (Table 1) [26-29]. In the United States, where the gastric cancer incidence is 14th among major malignancies, risk factors include advanced age, male gender, family history of gastric cancer, and familial adenomatous polyposis [26-29]. Certain sociological factors have been associated with gastric cancer as well, such as a diet low in fruits and vegetables, diet high in salted, smoked, or preserved food, and cigarette smoking, which has also been implicated in the formation of gastric ulcers [26-29]. Associated medical conditions include *H. pylori* gastric infection, chronic atrophic gastritis, intestinal metaplasia, pernicious anemia, gastric adenomatous polyps, and giant hypertrophic gastritis (Menetrier disease) [26-28]. In the United States, male gender, African American race, low socioeconomic status, obesity, occupational hazards in metal and rubber work, mining, wood and asbestos dust exposure, and cigarette smoking are associated with gastric cancer; whereas in Asia, chronic *H. pylori* exposure and diet have been associated with gastric cancer [26-29]. There may also be an association between Epstein-Barr virus infection and gastric cancer in Caucasian and Hispanic patients [29]. High salt diet, smoked foods, nitrates, nitrites, poorly preserved foods and secondary amines are thought to alter the gastric milieu, resulting in production of *N*-nitroso compounds which are carcinogenic [26-29]. The correlation between *H. pylori* and gastric cancer has been so strong that it deserves special mention.

Table 1. Common etiologies contributing to the development of gastric cancer, as seen in the West (U.S and Europe) vs. the East (Japan, Korea, and China)

West	East
Cigarette smoking	Chronic H. pylori infection
Ethnicity (e.g., African American)	High salt foods
Low socioeconomic status	Smoked foods
Obesity	Nitrates
Occupational exposures to carcinogens	Nitrites
Chronic gastritis	Poorly preserved foods
Age	Chronic gastritis
Male gender	
Family history of gastric cancer	
FAP	

Although *H. pylori* infection has historically been emphasized in the pathogenesis of peptic ulcer disease, it has also been linked to the development of chronic gastritis in patients who are chronically infected, which in turn leads to the development of both epithelial and lymphoid malignancies of the stomach [30]. In fact, the International Agency for Research on Cancer has classified this organism as a class I carcinogen and as a definite cause of human gastric cancer [31]. Because of the prevalence of gastric cancer worldwide, there are some who advocate the eradication of this organism as a public health measure, especially considering the low cost breath tests available to detect it [30]. Considering the significance of this prognostic factor, it is worthwhile to discuss the evidence supporting the link between *H. pylori* and gastric cancer.

The strongest earliest evidence suggesting the link between chronic *H. pylori* infection and gastric cancer was based on nested case-control seroepidemiologic studies in the United States and Britain, which compared the serum of patients with and without gastric cancer, evaluating for IgG antibodies to *H. pylori*, with a subsequent meta-analysis suggesting a relative risk of 9 [32-35]. A study evaluating *H. pylori* seropositivity in 17 populations in Europe, Japan and the United states demonstrated a direct correlation between infection and high incidence of gastric cancer [36]. The strongest link for pathogenesis was demonstrated in gastric-mucosa-associated lymphoid tissue in multiple clinical studies, showing both the development of mucosa-associated lymphoid tissue, as well as regression by *H. pylori* eradication; however, the exact mechanism remains under investigation [37, 38]. The correlation between *H. pylori* and gastric cancer is thought to be as a causative factor to the development of chronic atrophic gastritis, a precursor to adenocarcinoma [27].

Retrospective reviews have demonstrated that 80 – 90% of patients with gastric cancer had atrophic gastritis, a condition present in nearly all those at risk of developing gastric cancer. On the contrary, patients with normal gastric mucosa, or only superficial gastritis, were not found to develop cancer [39-43]. *H. pylori* infection causes a chronic active gastritis with superficial inflammation spreading from the antrum, a subsequent reduction in the inflammatory infiltrate and mucosal atrophy, with as many as half of infected patients progressing to atrophic gastritis [44]. While the presence of *H. pylori* infection appears to explain the high prevalence of gastric cancer, especially when considering that *H. pylori* is endemic at an early age in citizens of Japan, China and South America where gastric cancer rates are high [45-47], infection alone remains only one of the causative factors. Interestingly, gastric cancer rates are low in early-age *H. pylori* endemic areas like Africa and Costa Rica [48, 49], and there is a <1% gastric cancer rate in *H. pylori*-infected North American patients [50]. Similarly, although there has been a link described between pickled food consumption and gastric cancer as mentioned previously, epidemiologic studies have demonstrated a greater association within populations in Korea and China, once again emphasizing the importance of host factors in addition to environmental factors in carcinogenesis [51].

Characterizing the additional elements needed to truly establish the link between *H. pylori* infection and carcinogenesis has been the subject of much inquiry. The current theory focuses on the multifactorial combination of bacterial virulence, e.g., genetic mutations determining carcinogenic toxin production, and host factors, e.g., immunologic and repair responses [27]. Multiple biological, molecular and genetic mechanisms are currently being tested, from ammonia production, cytokine release, reactive oxygen metabolites, induced hypergastrinemia, to aquired genetic mutations including adenomatosis polyposis coli; however, there is no proven overarching mechanism [27].

Although there have been some reports that *H. pylori* eradication reversed pre-neoplastic changes and prevented secondary gastric cancer [52-56], there have been multiple other studies which have failed to demonstrate similar results [57-60]. In addition, there remains a theory pertaining to the survival benefit of *H. pylori* [27]. Recent advances in the understanding of gastric cancer carcinogenesis, such as copy-number variations implicating chromosomal instability, exome-sequencing identifying specific somatic mutations of interest, genetic profiling of gastric tumors to further subcategorize gastric cancer subtypes, specific DNA methylation events, and novel putative tumor suppressors [61], raise the possibility for more targeted approaches to both treatment and prevention of gastric cancer. All these factors are important to consider when evaluating appropriate public health programs to gastric cancer prevention, especially via *H. pylori* surveillance and eradication. As more data emerge in the future, there is promise to further guide such efforts in a more targeted and cost-effective fashion; however, the current data in multiple studies demonstrate conflicting results [52-60].

Cancer Care Systems Approach

At the end of the 1800's to the early 1900's, multiple commissions in Europe and North America were charged with improving the understanding and treatment of cancer. Over the course of the 20th century, as the understanding of cancer biology and treatment improved, and as health care delivery evolved into more complex systems, efforts to measure and improve the quality of cancer care have also been developed. The main mechanisms to address quality have been through promotion of best practice guidelines and evaluating 1) the structural capabilities of institutions to provide complex cancer care (e.g., having access to endoscopic ultrasound for adequate staging), 2) the compliance of institutions with processes of care which are thought to improve outcomes (e.g., appropriate adjuvant therapy administered within a specific timeframe after surgical resection), and 3) outcomes of patients undergoing treatment (e.g., overall survival). However, there remains a great deal of debate as to how each of these mechanisms may improve outcomes as well as how each of these mechanisms should be evaluated (i.e., should these data be publicly reported? Should only designated centers be allowed to treat cancer patients?). Because of the increasing focus on cancer-treatment outcomes by all parties interested in cancer care, it is important to review the major initiatives to systematically improve cancer care worldwide, with an emphasis on gastric cancer.

The systematic approach to improving outcomes and the quality of care provided to patients with gastric cancer has varied across the world. In the United States, the approach has been characterized by partnerships among various institutions and organizations. In September, 2013, the Institute of Medicine of the National Academies issued its updated report on the quality of cancer care in the U.S., over a decade after its initial report. It framed a six-pronged approach to improving quality, including patient engagement, workforce development and coordination, evidence-based care, information technology, evidenced-based practice and quality improvement, and accessible and affordable care [62]. The Institute of Medicine's initial report, along with collaborative efforts of the American Society of Clinical Oncology (ASCO), the National Cancer Institute (NCI), the National Comprehensive Cancer Network (NCCN), and the American College of Surgeons (ACS), facilitated by the National Quality Forum, has produced "accountability measures" for public reporting, payment incentive programs, and provider selection by consumers, health plans, or purchasers [63, 64]. In the U.S., with its mosaic of health care delivery systems for a diverse population across different states and territories, this approach has allowed for a mechanism of measuring and comparing the outcomes produced in such a large and complex environment.

As an example, the process measure quality indicators in breast cancer included radiation therapy administered within 1 year of diagnosis, hormonal therapy within 1 year, and adjuvant chemotherapy within 120 days of diagnosis when indicated; in colon cancer, examination of 12 lymph nodes at resection and adjuvant chemotherapy within 120 days of diagnosis for stage III disease [63, 64]were considered quality indicators. Compliance with these measures is only considered if at least 90% of cases meet these standards [63, 64]. These measures are part of a broader effort in the U.S. to more closely link payment to value in health care to theoretically improve outcomes and reduce costs simultaneously. However, there are currently no such mandated requirements in delivering quality gastric cancer care in the U.S. Although there are treatment guidelines for gastric cancer as outlined by the NCCN, and criteria for designated cancer centers accredited by the NCI, as well as licensing requirements for physicians and a legal tort system for patients to compensate for negligence, there are no specific gastric cancer focused measures implemented to evaluate, compare, and enforce quality across populations and health care systems. As initiatives continue to progress in the United States to improve quality, it is foreseeable that gastric cancer outcomes will also come under greater scrutiny, as third party payers in the private U.S. system increasingly seek to limit costs by payment based on outcomes rather than services.

In Japan, there is a strong tradition of investigating and promoting treatment guidelines for gastric cancers, particularly with regards to extent of resection and lymphadenectomy, with the Japan Gastric Cancer Association promoting such guidelines [65]. However, a review of 1,687 gastric cancer patients diagnosed in 2007 demonstrated an overall 68.3% compliance with quality indicators, with chemotherapy, pre-therapeutic care and diagnostics, and surgical and endoscopic compliance being 61%, 76%, 66%, and 71% respectively [66]. Because of the increasing incidence of cancer in Japan and a leveling off of reductions in cancer mortality, the Cancer Control Act was legislated into law in 2006, which included quality cancer care [67]. As of 2003, the Japanese government had already begun to designate which facilities had the structural resources to provide the level of care required, such as the availability of radiation therapy and multidisciplinary teams [67]. Beyond the logistical capabilities, in 2007 and 2008 the member facilities of the Japan Association of Clinical Cancer Centers publically reported their 5-year survival data for major malignancies with stage stratification [67-69]. How the media and public have been able to interpret and apply these results remain subjects of debate [67]. Japanese gastric cancer process-based quality indicators, akin to those mandated in the United States for breast and colorectal cancer, include 27 major areas, from diagnostic evaluation, medical records documentation, and deep vein thrombosis prophylaxis, to extent of surgical resection, pathologic evaluation, post-operative diet, appropriate follow up compliance, and patient counseling [66]. However, these measures are not mandated and are not publicly reported. Although there have been efforts to investigate how to incorporate these process-based quality indicators as recommended by the Japan Gastric Cancer Association, addressing the limitations of how well process compliance actually measures cancer care quality has delayed its implementation at this point [67]. As the Japanese experience continues to evolve, development of further mechanisms to measure and improve the quality of gastric cancer care will need to be implemented and may apply broadly to other international systems.

The European experience regarding the treatment of gastric cancer has historically been characterized by outcomes inferior to those in the East and substantial variability among the European communities [70-73]. To address these differences, the European Organization for

Research and Treatment of Cancer (EORTC) has promoted initiatives to improve gastric cancer care in medical and radiation oncology, and there are audits of surgical oncology institutions in the United Kingdom, Denmark and the Netherlands [74-78], and multiple reports on outcomes in gastric cancer from Spain and Italy [79, 80]. In fact, the European Society for Medical Oncology, the European Society for Surgical Oncology and the European Society of Radiotherapy and Oncology published clinical practice guidelines for the recommended treatment of gastric cancer, similar to that outlined by the U.S. NCCN guidelines [81]. However, there are no formally mandated quality indicators or publicly reported systems for gastric cancer in Europe, although a published review in 2013 has recommended such efforts [70].

In South Korea, the approach to gastric cancer, the leading malignancy in the country, has been characterized by centralized care, with over 50% of gastric cancer surgery performed at 5 hospitals and most surgeons performing over 100 radical gastric resections a year [82]. In addition, limiting oncologic gastric resections to academic institutions has further centralized gastric cancer care to select institutions. However, there is no standard uniform approach to extent of resection or to chemotherapeutic regimen implemented across these centers [82]. In 2003, the National Cancer Control Program of Korea Early Detection Program was initiated and gastrectomy with extended lymphadenectomy (D2 or D3) is considered the standard of care [82], but surgical resection has also included endoscopic, laparoscopic, and more recently robotic techniques, when indicated [83]. Although there is no consensus regarding chemotherapeutic regimen, there are multiple clinical trials taking place in Korea to determine the outcomes of those currently utilized [82, 83]. Public health efforts for gastric cancer in Korea have focused on prevention as well as investment in research, including in the emerging field of targeted and personalized therapy [83].

In China where gastric cancer has a high incidence (90.9 versus 6.5 per 100,000 in the U.S.),[84] the approach has also been characterized by centralized care, where only designated centers with academic surgeons functioning in multidisciplinary teams perform cancer gastric resections. The standard surgical resection entails a D2 lymphadenectomy, but when results were compared retrospectively with outcomes in Japan, they demonstrated curative resection, overall 5-year survival and rates of patients with early stage disease in the curative population of 67.5% versus 85.9%, 57.1% versus 77.2%, and 17.3% versus 57.2%, respectively [85]. To address these differences in outcomes, there have been efforts to improve early detection as well as participation in clinical trials. Although chemotherapy plays an important role in treatment, the use and type of chemotherapy is not as uniformly implemented in the treatment of gastric cancer as the use of gastric resection with D2 lymphadenectomy [86]. Again, public health efforts have focused on early detection and investment has been in research, with limited evaluation of the quality of care, compliance to recommended guidelines of treatment, and outcomes [86].

As knowledge regarding the appropriate approaches to gastric cancer have evolved, so too have international efforts developed to systematically improve the quality of services to treat this disease, as summarized in Table 2. In the U.S., while it has been mandated to publicly report process-based quality indicators in breast and colorectal cancer, which has been linked to how providers are paid, there has been no such focused effort on gastric cancer per se. In Japan, while survival data per institution have been publicly reported for gastric cancer, compliance with detailed process-based measures for gastric cancer have not been systematically tracked and reported. In Europe, while there are practice guidelines for gastric cancer, there are no process-based measures or publicly reported outcomes measures focused on gastric cancer. In South Korea, while oncologic gastric resection is centralized at select institutions and there are practice guidelines, there are also no process-based measures or outcomes that are publicly tracked or reported. There are currently efforts under way to evaluate how best to measure, report and improve the quality of gastric cancer care. To what degree process-based, outcome-based, or some combination of these measures shall play a role will depend on how strengths and weaknesses of these approaches are balanced.

Survival Outcomes and Perioperative Therapy Strategies

While the United States, European and Asian countries utilize the American Joint Committee on Cancer (AJCC) staging system for determination of prognosis, actual survival has been thought to differ markedly by geographical location, even when matched stage for stage. In a comparison of patients seen at high-volume centers in Korea and the U.S. who underwent margin-negative resection, disease specific survival was much improved in Korea versus the U.S., and the 5 year probability of death due to gastric cancer was only 17% in the Korean population, versus 32% in the U.S. [87]. However, a subset cohort analysis from these same institutions of T1N0 patients demonstrated similar recurrence-free survival and similar probabilities of death due to gastric cancer [88]. Markar, et al. published a meta-analysis of randomized, controlled trials comparing survival rates following gastrectomy between the East and West, concluding that overall, 5-year survival was improved in the East, with an adjusted odds ratio of 3.22 (95% Confidence Interval 1.85-5.58), adjusting for patient age, chemotherapy, gender, and tumor size [89]. The authors concluded that intangible factors, such as surgical technique, may attribute to the differences seen in survival.

Certainly, attention to the extent of lymphadenectomy has been a topic of great debate in considering the evolution of gastric cancer treatment and surgery. Historically, the Eastern countries have advocated a minimum of D2 lymphadenectomy, defined as removal of lymph nodes around the stomach as well as around the celiac axis and direct branches of the celiac trunk) [90]. A 15 year follow-up of the Dutch D1D2 trial, a prospective, randomized clinical trial, observed a lower locoregional recurrence and gastric-cancer-related death rate for those undergoing D2 lymphadenectomy versus D1 lymphadenectomy [91]. However, overall survival was similar between both groups, and the morbidity, mortality, and reoperation rate was much higher in the D2 lymphadenectomy group [91]. With growing experience in the U.S. and Europe in routinely performing D2 lymphadenectomy, the morbidity associated with this operation should improve.

Perioperative therapy is also utilized in different strategies, with the Western approach adopting neoadjuvant therapy as standard of care for any T2 or greater lesion or with any evidence of nodal involvement [92, 93], whereas most Eastern institutions prefer a surgery-first approach [90]. The British medical research council adjuvant gastric cancer infusional chemotherapy (MAGIC) trial was a landmark study, demonstrating improved survival in patients with operable gastric, esophageal and GE junction cancer that received preoperative and postoperative chemotherapy. Survival was increased from 23% in the surgery-alone arm to 36% in the surgery and chemotherapy arm, p=0.009, setting the standard for Europe and the U.S.; however, criticism of the trial included inclusion of esophageal cancers as well as suboptimal surgical resection, based on lymphadenectomy [94]. The Japanese, in particular, have investigated the utility of preoperative S-1 and cisplatin in phase II, and now phase III, trials to determine efficacy, demonstrating improved survival to historical survival rates with acceptable morbidity and mortality; however, there is currently no standard neoadjuvant regimen [95, 96]. Patients with bulky nodal or para-aortic nodal disease were also randomized to a similar neoadjuvant regimen, with S-1 and cisplatin, followed by D2 plus para-aortic nodal resection. An overall survival of 58.8% was observed, prompting further phase II/III trials [96, 97].

Adjuvant therapy has also stirred controversy internationally. The Intergroup 0116 (INT-0116) trial was a randomized phase III trial for patients with T3 and/or node-positive, margin-negative, resected gastric cancer, randomized to observation versus radiochemotherapy. With a ten year follow-up, the radiochemotherapy arm demonstrated improved overall and relapse-free survival, compared to observation, p=0.0046 and p<0.001, respectively [98]. A meta-analysis of randomized controlled trials in Asia comparing chemoradiotherapy versus chemotherapy following D2 lymphadenectomy and gastric resection found an improved disease-free survival; however, there was no difference in overall survival or the development of distant metastases [99]. In particular, the Adjuvant Chemoradiation Therapy in Stomach Cancer Trial (ARTIST), a phase III prospective randomized controlled study from Korea, investigating adjuvant chemotherapy versus chemotherapy and radiation, found no improvement in 3-year disease free survival [100], leaving the benefit of adjuvant radiation in question. While the standard practice in the U.S. is to continue adjuvant chemotherapy as per the MAGIC protocol, the Japanese have established monotherapy with S-1 as an acceptable standard treatment throughout East Asia, based on the 10.6% improvement in 5 year OS in the Adjuvant Chemotherapy Trial of S-1 for Gastric Cancer (ACTS-GC) study [101]. The Capecitabine and Oxaliplation Adjuvant Study in Stomach Cancer (CLASSIC) trial, a large phase III Korean trial, demonstrated a significant disease-free survival benefit with adjuvant capecitabine and oxaliplatin (XELOX) following D2 gastrectomy versus gastrectomy-alone [102]. Applicability of these regimens internationally, however, remains controversial, particularly in the setting of varying patient characteristics and disease biology.

Targeted therapy has contributed to the armamentarium available for gastric cancer treatment and has certainly allowed patient-specific, or pathology-specific, therapy in a way that was not feasible several decades ago. The Trastuzumab for Gastric Cancer (TOGA) study randomised patients with metastatic gastric or gastroesophageal junction cancers overexpressing human epidermal growth factor receptor 2 (HER2) to either chemotherapy with capecitabine plus cisplatin or cisplatin or fluorouracil plus cisplatin in combination with trastuzumab, a targeted monoclonal antibody against HER2. This trial demonstrated a significantly improved overall survival in the trastuzumab arm, expanding the treatment options available for patients [103]. Indeed, a subset analysis of Japanese patients included in the ToGA trial demonstrated an even greater length of survival in the trastuzumab arm, [104] suggesting that trastuzumab in combination with chemotherapy could be considered standard therapy in patients with HER2 positive tumors. Studies evaluating the effect of Trastuzumab in both the neoadjuvant and adjuvant setting are continuing.

Table 2. Summary of systems-based measures to improve gastric cancer care and outcomes, as instituted by country

	Cancer Center Accreditation	Centralized Gastric Cancer Treatment	Treatment Guidelines	Uniform Surgical Approach	Process Measures for Gastric Cancer	Public Reporting of Institutional Survival Outcomes	Public Health Early Detection Screening Efforts
U.S.	X		X				
Europe			X				
Japan	X		X	X	X	X	X
Korea		X		X			X
China		X		X			X

Table 3. Summary of trials evaluating surgical, chemotherapy and radiation therapy for treatment of gastric cancer. OS, overall survival. PFS, progression free survival. RCT, randomized controlled trial

Title	Country	Design	N	Comparison	OS	PFS	Outcome
Dutch D1 D2 Trial 15yr update	Holland	RCT	711	D2 v D1 lymphadenectomy	No difference	Improved with D2	D2 higher operative morbidity and mortality but lower recurrence and disease specific mortality than D1
MRC-STO2 (MAGIC)	UK	RCT	503	Chemo+surgery v surgery	36% v 23% 5yr.	Improved with chemo	Chemo improved OS and PFS
JCOG0210	Japan	Phase II	36	Neoadjuvant S-1+cisplantin	24.5% 3yr.	N/A	Promising results warrant phase 3 study
SWOG 0116	US	Phase III	559	surgery v surgery+chemoXRT	Improved	Improved	Adjuvant XRT for T3 or N+ improved outcomes

Table 3. (Continued)

Title	Country	Design	N	Comparison	OS	PFS	Outcome
Metanalysis for adjuvant s/p D2	China	Meta-analysis	895, 3RTC	D2+chemo v D2+chemoxrt	No difference	Improved locoregional PFS but not distant	Less benefit from adjuvant therapies in Asian patients
ARTIST	Korea	Phase III	458	D2+capecitibine+ cisplatin v. D2+capecitibine+ cisplatin+xrt	N/A	no difference	Possible benefit in lymph node positive patients
NCT00152217	Japan	RCT	1,059	D2 v D2+S-1	70% v 80% 3yr.	N/A	S-1 effective in stage II/III Asian patients
CLASSIC	Korea	Phase III	1,035	D2+capecitibine+ cisplatin v D2	74% v 59% 3yr.	N/A	Consider in stage II - IIIB
TOGA	Korea	Phase III	594	chemo v chemo+trastuzumab	11.1 v 13.8 mo.	N/A	Consider for advanced HER2 positive cancers
TOGA subgroup analysis	Japan	Subgroup analysis	101	Japanese patients in TOGA	17.7 v. 15.9 mo.	N/A	Survival improved in Japanese
AVAGAST	Japan	RCT	774	bevacizumab+chemo v chemo	No difference	6.7 mo. v 5.3 mo.	Improved PFS and response rate, but did not achieve goal of detecting OS difference

The addition of bevacizumab (Avastin) to chemotherapy was found to significantly increase progression free survival, as demonstrated in the Avastin in Gastric Cancer (AVAGAST) trial, a multi-center, international, placebo-controlled trial [105]. However, the primary endpoint of the AVAGAST study, improved overall survival, was not reached. Table 3 summarizes the trials mentioned in the above text. Ongoing studies are attempting to determine whether specific populations of patients may derive even greater survival benefit from these targeted therapies.

Conclusion

The pathogenesis of gastric cancer remains complex, a culmination of multiple factors, including genetic and environmental influences. While *H. pylori* remains a significant etiologic factor, with eradication improving the gastric cancer incidence worldwide, it remains a significant cause of cancer-related morbidity and mortality. The treatment strategies, as related to neoadjuvant and adjuvant therapy, differ widely between the East and West. However, with surgical technique becoming more uniform globally, and the era of personalized medicine promoting patient-directed therapy, observed geographic differences might soon be explained by more objective data. A systematic approach, with cancer-related outcomes linked to clinical care, may allow for an ability to develop uniform standards within countries and potentially globally, although this remains to be proved.

References

[1]   American Cancer Society. *Cancer Facts & Figures 2013.* Atlanta: American Cancer Society; 2013.

[2]   Jung KW, Won YJ, Kong HJ, et al. Prediction of Cancer Incidence and Mortality in Korea, 2013. *Cancer Research and Treatment,* 2013; 45(1): 15-21.

[3]   GLOBOCAN 2008 database (version 1.2). http://globocan.iarc.fr

[4]   Cho E, Kang MH, Choi KS, et al. Cost-effectiveness Outcomes of the National Gastric Cancer Screening Programs in South Korea. *Asian Pacific J Cancer Prevention,* 2013; 14(4): 2533-2540.

[5]   Kunz PL, Gubens M, Fisher GA, et al. Long-Term Survivors of Gastric Cancer: A California Population-Based Study. *Journal of Clinical Oncology,* 2012; 30(28): 3507-3515.

[6]   Kim J, Sun CL, Mailey B, et al. Race and ethnicity correlate with survival in patients with gastric adenocarcinoma. *Annals of Oncology,* 2010; 21(1): 152-160.

[7]   Al-Refaie WB, Tseng JF, Gay G, et al. The Impact of Ethnicity on the Presentation and Prognosis of Patients With Gastric Adenocarcinoma. Results from the National Cancer Data Base. *Cancer,* 2008; 13(3): 461-9.

[8]   Yakirevich E, Resnick MB. Pathology of gastric cancer and its precursor lesions. *Gastroenterol Clin N Am,* 2013; 42(2): 261–84.

[9] Lauren P. The two histologic main types of gastric carcinoma: Diffused and so-called intestinal type carcinoma. An attempt at a histo-clinical classification. *Acta Pathol Microbiol Scand,* 1965; 64: 31-49.

[10] Lauwers GY, Carneiro F, Graham DY. Gastric carcinoma. In: Bowman FT, Carneiro F, Hruban RH, eds. *Classification of Tumours of the Digestive System.* Lyon: IARC; 2010.

[11] Qiu MZ, Cai MY, Zhang DS, et al. Clinicopathological characteristics and prognostic analysis of Lauren classification in gastric adenocarcinoma in China. *Journal of Translational Medicine,* 2013; 11:58.

[12] Hu B, El Hajj N, Sittler S, et al. Gastric cancer: Classification, histology and application of molecular pathology. *J Gastrointest Oncol,* 2012; 3(3): 251–261.

[13] Huh CW, Jung DH, Kim J-H, et al. Signet ring cell mixed histology may show more aggressive behavior than other histologies in early gastric cancer. *J Surg Oncol,* 2013; 107(2):124–9.

[14] Piessen G, Messager M, Leteurtre E, et al. Signet ring cell histology is an independent predictor of poor prognosis in gastric adenocarcinoma regardless of tumoral clinical presentation. *Ann Surg,* 2009; 250:878–887.

[15] Taghavi S, Jayajaran S, Davey A, Willis A. Prognostic significance of signet ring gastric cancer. *J Clin Oncol,* 2012;30(28):3493–3498.

[16] Gravalos C, Jimeno A. HER2 in Gastric Cancer: A New Prognostic Factor and a Novel Therapeutic Target. *Ann Oncol,* 2008; 19(9):1523-1529.

[17] Wadhwa R, Taketa T, Sudo K, et al. Modern oncological approaches to gastric adenocarcinoma. *Gastroenterology clinics of North America,* 2013; 42(2): 359-69.

[18] García I, Vizoso F, Martín A, et al. Clinical significance of the epidermal growth factor receptor and HER2 receptor in resectable gastric cancer. *Ann Surg Oncol,* 2003; 10(3):234-41.

[19] Aizawa M, Nagatsuma AK, Kitada K, et al. Evaluation of HER2-based biology in 1,006 cases of gastric cancer in a Japanese population. *Gastric Cancer,* 2013; February 22 [Epub ahead of print].

[20] Fitzgerald RC, Caldas C. Clinical implications of E-cadherin associated hereditary diffuse gastric cancer. *Gut,* 2004; 53(6): 775-778.

[21] Davis PA, Sano T. The difference in gastric cancer between Japan, USA and Europe: What are the facts? What are the suggestions? *Critical Reviews in Oncology/Hematology,* 2001; 40: 77–94.

[22] Bickenbach KA, Denton B, Gonen M, et al. Impact of obesity on perioperative complications and long-term survival of patients with gastric cancer. *Ann Surg Oncol,* 2013; 20(3): 780-7.

[23] Kajitani T. The general rules for the gastric cancer study in surgery and pathology: parts I and II. *Jpn J Surg,* 1981; 11: 127-45.

[24] Schlemper RJ, Itabashi M, Kato Y, et al. Differences in diagnostic criteria for gastric carcinoma between Japanese and Western pathologists. *The Lancet,* 1997; 349(9067): 1725-1729.

[25] Yu M, Zheng H, Xia P, et al. Comparison in pathological behaviours & prognosis of gastric cancers from general hospitals between China & Japan. *Indian J Med Res,* 2010; 132: 295-302.

[26] Kurtz RC, Sherlock P. The diagnosis of gastric cancer. *Seminars in Oncology, 1985*; 12(1): 11-8.

[27] Scheiman JM, Cutler AF: Helicobacter pylori and gastric cancer. *Am J Med,* 1999: 106 (2): 222-6.

[28] Fenoglio-Preiser CM, Noffsinger AE, Belli J, et al.: Pathologic and phenotypic features of gastric cancer. *Semin Oncol,* 1996: 23 (3): 292-306.

[29] Siegel, Rebecca, Deepa Naishadham, and Ahmedin Jemal. Cancer statistics, 2013. CA: *A cancer journal for clinicians,* 2013: 63.1: 11-30.

[30] Scheiman JM, Cutler AF. Helicobacter pylori and gastric cancer. The American journal of medicine, 1999: 106(2): 222-226.

[31] IARC Working Group on the Evaluation of Carcinogenic Risks to Humans, Schistosomes, Liver Flukes and *Helicobacter pylori. Infection with Helicobacter pylori.* IARC monographs on the evaluation of carcinogenic risks to humans. Vol 61. Lyon, France: *International Agency for Research on Cancer,* 1994;177–240.

[32] Nomura A, Stemmermann GN, Chyou P, Kato I, Perez-Perez GI, Blaser MJ. *Helicobacter pylori* infection and gastric carcinoma among Japanese Americans in Hawaii. *NEJM,* 1991: 325:1132–1136.

[33] Parsonnet J, Friedman GD, Vandersteen DP, et al. *Helicobacter pylori* infection and the risk of gastric carcinoma. *NEJM,* 1991: 325:1127–1131.

[34] Forman D, Newell DG, Fullerton F, et al. Association between infection with*Helicobacter pylori* and the risk of gastric cancer. *BMJ,* 1991: 302:1302–1305.

[35] Forman D, Webb P, Parsonnet J. *Helicobacter pylori* and gastric cancer. *Lancet,* 1994; 343:243–244.

[36] The Eurogast Study Group. An international association between *Helicobacter pylori* infection and gastric cancer. *Lancet,* 1993; 341: 1359 –1362.

[37] Eck M, Schmausser B, Haas R, Greiner A, Czub S, Muller-Hermelink HK. MALT-type lymphoma of the stomach is associated with *Helicobacter pylori* strains expressing the CagA protein. *Gastroenterology,* 1997; 112:1482–1486.

[38] Wotherspoon AC. Gastric MALT lymphoma and *Helicobacter pylori. Yale J Biol Med,* 1997; 69:61– 68.

[39] Cheli R, Giacosa A. Atrophic gastritis. In: Sherlock P, Morson BC, Barbara L, Veronesi U, eds. *Precancerous Lesions for the Gastrointestinal Tract.* New York: Raven Press, 1983:55.

[40] You WC, Blot WJ, Li JY, et al. Precancerous gastric lesions in a population at high risk of stomach cancer. *Cancer Res,* 1993; 53: 1317–1321.

[41] Walker IR, Strickland RG, Ungar B, Mackay IR. Simple atrophic gastritis and gastric cancer. *Gut,* 1971; 12:906 –911.

[42] Cheli R, Santi L, Ciancamerla G, et al. A clinical and statistical follow-up study of atrophic gastritis. *Am J Dig Dis,* 1973; 18:1061.

[43] Siurala M, Isokoski M, Varis M, et al. Prevalence of gastritis in a rural population: bioptic study of subjects selected at random. *Scand J Gastroenterol,* 1968; 3:211.

[44] Kuipers EJ. *Helicobacter pylori* and the risk and management of associated diseases: gastritis, ulcer disease, atrophic gastritis and gastric cancer. *Aliment Pharmacol Ther,* 1997; 11(suppl 1): 71– 88.

[45] Asaka M, Kimura T, Kudo M, et al. Relationship of *Helicobacter pylori* to serum pepsinogens in an asymptomatic Japanese population. *Gastroenterology,* 1992; 102: 760 –766.

[46] Forman D, Sitas F, Newell DG, et al. Geographic association of *Helicobacter pylori* antibody prevalence and gastric cancer mortality in rural China. *Int J Cancer,* 1990; 46: 608–611.

[47] Correa P, Fox J, Fontham E, et al. *Helicobacter pylori* and gastric carcinoma: serum antibody prevalence in populations with contrasting cancer risks. *Cancer,* 1990; 66: 2569 –2574.

[48] Holcombe C. *Helicobacter pylori*: the African enigma. *Gut,* 1992; 33: 429–431.

[49] Sierra R, Munoz N, Pena AS, et al. Antibodies to *Helicobacter pylori* and pepsinogen levels in children in Costa Rica. *Cancer Epidemiol Biomark Prevent,* 1992; 1: 449 – 1454.

[50] Parsonett J. *Helicobacter pylori* and gastric cancer. *Gastroenterol Clin North Am,* 1993: 22: 89 –104.

[51] Ren, Jian-Song, et al. Pickled Food and Risk of Gastric Cancer—a Systematic Review and Meta-analysis of English and Chinese Literature. *Cancer Epidemiology Biomarkers & Prevention,* 2012; 21(6): 905-915.

[52] Recavarren-Arce S, Leon-Barua R, Cok J, et al. *Helicobacter pylori* and progressive gastric pathology that predisposes to gastric cancer. *Scand J Gastroenterol,* 1991; 181(suppl):51–57.

[53] Borody TJ, Andrews P, Jankiewicz E, Ferch N, Carroll M. Apparent reversal of early gastric mucosal atrophy after triple therapy of *Helicobacter pylori. Am J Gastroenterol,* 1993; 88:1266–1268.

[54] Hack HM, Fennerty MB, Sampliner R, et al. Reversal of intestinal metaplasia after treatment of *H. pylori* infection. *Gastroenterol,* 1994; 106:A87.

[55] Genta RM, Lew GM, Graham DY. Change in the gastric mucosa following eradication of *Helicobacter pylori. Modern Pathol,* 1993; 6: 281–289.

[56] Uemura N, Mukai T, Okamoto S, et al. Effect of *Helicobacter pylori* eradication on subsequent development of cancer after endoscopic resection of early gastric cancer. *Cancer Epidemiol Biomark Prevent.* 1997; 6: 639–642.

[57] Jankiewicz K, Louw JA, Marks IN. Long-term histological consequences of suppression/eradication of *Helicobacter pylori* in antral mucosa. *Eur J Gastroenterol Hepatol,* 1993; 5: 701–705.

[58] Witteman EM, Mravunac M, Becx MJCM, et al. Improvement of gastric inflammation and resolution of epithelial damage one year after eradication of *Helicobacter pylori. J Clin Pathol,* 1995; 48: 250–256.

[59] Borody TJ, Clark IW, Andrews P, Hugh TB, Shortis NP. Eradication of *Helicobacter pylori* may not reverse severe gastric dysplasia. *Am J Gastroenterol,* 1995; 90: 498-499.

[60] Sung JY, Lin SR, Ching JYL, et al. Effects of curing *Helicobacter pylori* infection on precancerous gastric lesions: one-year follow-up of a prospective randomized study in China. *Gastroenterology,* 1998; 114: A296. Abstract.

[61] Figueiredo C, Garcia-Gonzalez MA, Machado JC. Molecular Pathogenesis of Gastric Cancer. *Helicobacter,* 2013; 18.s: 28-33.

[62] Levit L, Balogh E, Nass S, and Ganz PA. *Delivering high-quality cancer care: Charting a new course for a system in crisis.* National Academic Press. Washington, D.C. 2013.

[63] Desch CE et al. American Society of Clinical Oncology/National Comprehensive Cancer Network Quality Measures. *JCO,* 2008; vol 26 (21).

[64] American Society of Clinical Oncology/National Comprehensive Cancer Network Quality Measures. *JCO*, vol 26, num 21, 2008.

[65] Sasako, M. Gastric cancer eastern experience. *Surg Oncol Clin N Am,* 2012; 21(1): 71-7.

[66] Higashi T, Nakamura F, Shimada Y, et al. Quality of gastric cancer care in designated cancer care hospitals in Japan. *International Journal for Quality in Health Care*, 2013; 25(4): 418-28.

[67] Higashi, Takahiro, et al. "Establishing a Quality Measurement System for Cancer Care in Japan." *Japanese journal of clinical oncology*, 2013; 43 (3): 225-232.

[68] Japanese Association for Clinical Cancer Centers. Collaborative Study of Cancer Survivals. http://www.gunma-cc.jp/sarukihan/seizonritu/ (2 September 2010, date last accessed).

[69] Saruki N, Haruo M. Survival statistics publication and web-based calculation publication of survival rates by the Japanese Association of Clinical Cancer Centers. *JACR Monogr,* 2012; 17: 22–7 (in Japanese).

[70] Dikken, Johan L., et al. "Quality of Care Indicators for the Surgical Treatment of Gastric Cancer: A Systematic Review." *Annals of surgical oncology, 2013;* 20 (2): 381-398.

[71] Strong VE, Song KY, Park CH, et al. Comparison of gastric cancer survival following R0 resection in the United States and Korea using an internationally validated nomogram. *Ann Surg,* 2010;251(4):640–6.

[72] Isobe Y, Nashimoto A, Akazawa K, et al. Gastric cancer treatment in Japan: 2008 annual report of the JGCA nationwide registry. *Gastric Cancer,* 2011; 14(4):301–16.

[73] Sant M, Allemani C, Santaquilani M, Knijn A, Marchesi F, Capocaccia R. EUROCARE-4. Survival of cancer patients diagnosed in 1995–1999. Results and commentary. *Eur J Cancer,* 2009;45(6):931–91.

[74] Kouloulias VE, Poortmans PM, Bernier J, et al. The Quality Assurance programme of the Radiotherapy Group of the European Organization for Research and Treatment of Cancer (EORTC): a critical appraisal of 20 years of continuous efforts. *Eur J Cancer,* 2003;39(4):430–7.

[75] Therasse P, De Mulder PH. Quality assurance in medical oncology within the EORTC. European Organisation for Research and Treatment of Cancer. *Eur J Cancer,* 2002;38(Suppl 4):S152–4.

[76] *The Association of Upper Gastrointestinal Surgeons of Great Britain and Ireland.* http://www.augis.org/. Accessed 1 March 2012.

[77] Dutch Upper GI Cancer Audit. http://www.clinicalaudit.nl/duca/. Accessed 1 March 2012.

[78] Jensen LS, Nielsen H, Mortensen PB, Pilegaard HK, Johnsen SP. Enforcing centralization for gastric cancer in Denmark. *Eur J Surg Oncol,* 2010;36 Suppl 1:S50-4.

[79] Viúdez-Berral, Antonio, et al. "Current management of gastric cancer." *Rev Esp Enferm Dig,* 2012; 104(3): 134-141.

[80] Bittoni, Alessandro, et al. "Selecting the Best Treatment for an Individual Patient." *Early Gastrointestinal Cancers.* Springer Berlin Heidelberg, 2012: 307-318.

[81] Waddell T, Verheij M, Allum W, et al. Gastric cancer: ESMO–ESSO–ESTRO Clinical Practice Guidelines for diagnosis, treatment and follow-up. *Annals of Oncology,* 2013; 24.suppl 6: vi57-vi63.

[82] Park JM and Kim YH. Current approaches to gastric cancer in Korea. *Gastrointestinal cancer research,* 2008; 2(3): 137.

[83] Lee JH, Kim KM, Cheong JH, et al. Current management and future strategies of gastric cancer. *Yonsei medical journal,* 2012; 53(2): 248-257.

[84] Siegel R, Naishadham D, Jemal A. Cancer statistics, 2013. *CA Cancer J Cin,* 2013; 63 (1): 11-30.

[85] Qie XD, Chen B, Wang J, et al. Comparison for treatment experience of gastric cancer between China Medical University and University of Tokyo – a report of 2438 cases. *Med J Liaoning.,* 2002; 16:238–240.

[86] 25. Zhu, Xiaodong, and Jin Li. Gastric carcinoma in China: Current status and future perspectives (Review). *Oncology Letters,* 2010; 1(3): 407-412.

[87] Strong VE, Song KY, Park CH, et al. Comparison of Gastric Cancer Survival Following R0 Resection in the United States and Korea Using an Internationally Validated Nomogram. *Annals of Surgery,* 2010; 251(4): 640-646.

[88] Strong VE, Song KY, Park CH, et al. Comparison of disease-specific survival in the United States and Korea after resection for early-stage node-negative gastric carcinoma. *Journal of Surgical Oncology,* 2013; 107(6): 634-640.

[89] Markar SR, Karthikesalingam A, Jackson D, and Hanna GB. Long-Term Survival After Gastrectomy for Cancer in Randomized, Controlled Oncological Trials: Comparison between West and East. *Annals of Surgical Oncology,* 2013; 20: 2328-2338.

[90] Japanese Gastric Cancer Association. Japanese gastric cancer treatment guidelines 2010 (ver. 3). *Gastric Cancer,* 2011; 14: 113-123.

[91] Songun I, Putter H, Kranenbarg EM, et al. Surgical treatment of gastric cancer: 15-year follow-up results of the randomised nationwide Dutch D1D2 trial. *Lancet Oncology,* 2010; 11(5): 439-49.

[92] NCCN Clincal Practice Guidelines in Oncology (NCCN Guidelines). *Gastric Cancer (Including cancer in the proximal 5cm of the stomach). Version* 2.2013. NCCN.org

[93] Waddell T, Verheij M, Allum W, et al. Gastric cancer: ESMO-ESSO-ESTRO Clinical Practice Guidelines for diagnosis, treatment and follow-up. *Annals of Oncology,* 2013; 24(Supplement 6): vi57-vi6.

[94] Cunningham D, Allum WH, Stenning SP, et al. Perioperative chemotherapy versus surgery alone for resectable gastroesophageal cancer. *N Engl J Med,* 2006; 355: 11-20.

[95] Iwasaki Y, Sasako M, Yamamoto S, et al. Phase II study of preoperative chemotherapy with S-1 and cisplatin followed by gastrectomy for clinically resectable type 4 and large type 3 gastric cancers (JCOG0210). *J Surg Oncol,* 2013; 107(7): 741-5.

[96] Fujitani K. Overview of Adjuvant and Neoadjuvant Therapy for Resectable Gastric Cancer in the East. *Dig Surg,* 2013; 30: 119-129.

[97] Yoshikawa T, Nakamura K, Tsuburaya A, et al. Gastric Cancer Surgical Study Group of Japan Clinical Oncology Group: A phase II study of preoperative chemotherapy with S-1 (S) and cisplatin (P) followed by D3 gastrectomy for gastric cancer with extensive lymph node metastasis (ELM): survival results of JCOG 0405. *J Clin Oncol,* 2011; 29(suppl 4): abstract 70.

[98] Smalley SR, Benedetti JK, Haller DG, et al. Updated Analysis of SWOG-Directed Intergroup Study 0116: A Phase III Trial of Adjuvant Radiochemotherapy Versus Observation After Curative Gastric Cancer Resection. *JCO,* 2012; 30(19): 2327-2333.

[99] Huang YY, Yang Q, Zhou SW, et al. Postoperative chemoradiotherapy versus postoperative chemotherapy for completely resected gastric cancer with D2 Lymphadenectomy: a meta-analysis. *PLoS One,* 2013; 8(7): e68939.

[100] Lee J, Lim do H, Kim S, et al. Phase III trial comparing capecitabine plus cisplatin versus capecitabine plus cisplatin with concurrent capecitabine radiotherapy in completely resected gastric cancer with D2 lymph node dissection: the ARTIST trial. *J Clin Oncol,* 2012; 30: 268-273.

[101] Sakuramoto S, Sasako M, Yamaguchi T, et al. Adjuvant chemotherapy for gastric cancer with S-1, an oral fluoropyrimidine. *N Engl J Med,* 2007; 357: 1810-1820.

[102] Bang YJ, Kim YW, Yang HK, et al. Adjuvant capecitabine and oxaliplatin for gastric cancer after D2 gastrectomy (CLASSIC): a phase 3 open-label, randomised controlled trial. *Lancet,* 2012; 379: 315-321.

[103] Bang YJ, Van Cutsem E, Feyereislova A, et al. Trastuzumab in combination with chemotherapy vesus chemotherapy alone for treatment of HER2-positive advanced gastric or gastro-oesophageal junction cancer (ToGA): a phase 3, open-label, randomised controlled trial. *Lancet,* 2010; 376(9742): 687-97.

[104] Sawaki A, Ohashi Y, Omuro Y, et al. Efficacy of trastuzumab in Japanese patients with HER2-positive advanced gastric or gastroesophageal junction cancer: a subgroup analysis of the Trastuzumab for Gastric Cancer (ToGA) study. *Gastric Cancer,* 2012; 15(3): 313-22.

[105] Ohtsu A, Shah MA, Van Cutsem E, et al. Bevacizumab in Combination With Chemotherapy As First-Line Therapy in Advanced Gastric Cancer: A Randomized, Double-Blind, Pacebo-Controlled Phase III Study. *JCO,* 2011; 29(3): 3968-76.

In: Gastric Cancer
Editor: Jasneet Singh Bhullar

ISBN: 978-1-63117-983-9
© 2014 Nova Science Publishers, Inc.

Chapter 2

Gastric Cancer: Focus on Epidemiology, Pathology, Diagnosis and Treatment - A Global Overview

Lan Mo, M.D.[1], Jafar Al-Mondhiry, M.S.[2] and Jennifer Wu, M.D.[3]*
[1] Fellow Physician, Hematology /Oncology Program,
NYU Langone Medical Center,
NYU School of Medicine,
New York, NY, US
[2] Medical Student, NYU School of Medicine,
New York, NY, US
[3] Assistant Professor of Medicine,
Division of Hematology and Medical Oncology,
GI Oncology Section,
NYU School of Medicine, NYU Perlmutter Cancer Center,
New York, NY, US

Abstract

Risk factors for gastric cancer (GC) are highly dependent on dietary habits, *H. pylori* infections and less frequently, genetic syndromes. The pathogenesis of GC from these three risk factors is different and briefly discussed here. Various histology of GC and their potential implications in prognosis are also briefly described. Certain endemic areas with high incidence of GC have instituted effective screening program to detect early stage GC, a strategy worth exploring in the future where GC incidence is amongst the fastest growing cancer in the world.

For local or superficial disease (Stage IA), surgery alone is curative, and the treatment may involve endoscopic mucosal resection, although subtotal or total gastrectomy is still a common choice depending on tumor location. For more advanced disease (Stage IB-III), surgery is the main modality to achieve cure. The various

---

* Corresponding Author: Email: Jennfier.wu@nyumc.org.

techniques of gastrectomies are discussed, especially the differences and controversies of D1 and D2 lymph node dissection.

In addition, adjuvant treatment including either chemoradiation with (5-FU) or chemotherapy alone using capecitabine and oxaliplatin are options of standard care in various parts of the world. A combination of triplet in the perioperative setting, which includes fluoropyramidine, anthracycline and platinum, has also been widely adapted as an effective therapy that improves patient outcome.

For palliation and symptomatic treatment of locally advanced or widely metastatic disease, radiotherapy is especially helpful in relieving stenosis or bleeding in conjunction with stent placement, laser therapy, or occasionally palliative surgery. In the first line metastatic setting, the US standard adopts either a doublet of fluoropyrimidine and platinum or a triplet where a taxane is added, although efficacy improvement from the triplet over the doublet is unsatisfactory. The understanding of HER2 overexpression in a subset of GC patients has led to the success of a novel targeted agent such as trastuzumab in combination of chemotherapy in the first line treatment. In the 2nd line treatment of GC, where no standard treatments dramatically demonstrates efficacy, taxane as a single agent or in combination with platinum, or fluoropyrimidine and irinotecan are all common choices.

Very recent data suggests the survival advantage of anti-angiogenic agent ramucirumab over supportive care, despite discouraging results from another antiangiogenic agent. It thus provides insights into the careful selection of anti-angiogenesis therapy in GC, suggesting that the overexpression of angiogenesis in GC is just the beginning of an exciting journey in our understanding of this disease.The treatment of GC requires the expertise of a multidisciplinary approach. Advances in early detection, surgical techniques and understanding of biology will ultimately help combat this deadly condition.

Keywords: Adjuvant Therapy, Capecitabine, Chemoradiation, Cisplatin, D1, D2, 5-Fluorouracil, Gastrectomy, Gastric Cancer, HER2, *Helicobacter pylori,* Laparoscopic Surgery, Lymphadenectomy, Neoadjuvant Therapy, Perioperative Chemotherapy, Radiation Therapy, Targeted Agents, Trastuzumab, Ramucirumab, VEGFR-2

Abbreviations

CRT: Chemoradiotherapy
CT: Chemotherapy
DCF: Docetaxel, Cisplatin and 5-Fluorouracil
ECF: Epirubicin, Cisplatin and 5-Fluorouracil
EOF: Epirubicin, Oxaliplatin and 5-Fluorouracil
ECX: Epirubicin, Cisplatin and Capecitabine
EOX: Epirubicin, Oxaliplatin and Capecitabine
EOC: Epirubicin, Oxaliplatin, and Capecitabine
EUS: Endoscopic Ultrasound
5-FU: 5-Fluorouracil
FDG-PET: Positron Emission Tomography with Fluorodeoxyglucose
FP: 5-Fluorouracil and Cisplatin
GC: Gastric Cancer
GEJ: Gastroesophageal Junction

H. *Pylori:* Helicobacter *Pylori*
HER2: Human Epidermal Growth Factor Receptor Type 2
LV: Leucovorin
OS: Overall Survival
PFS: Progression-Free Survival
RR: Response Rate
RT: Radiotherapy
S-1: Tegafur, Gimeracil and Oteracil
SP: S-1 and Cisplatin
VEGFR-2: Vascular Endothelial Growth Factor Receptor Type 2
XP: Capecitabine and Cisplatin.

Introduction

This chapter focuses on the epidemiology, risk factors, pathology, pathogenesis, diagnosis and treatment of GC adenocarcinoma. It involves adenocarcinoma of gastroesophageal junction and stomach. Each section is discussed separately, with an emphasis on treatment of GC.

1. Prevalence

The World Health Organization (WHO) ranks GC 4th globally in incidence and 2nd highest in mortality [1]. In 2013, an estimated 21,600 people will be diagnosed and 10, 990 people will eventually die of this disease in the United States [2]. The epidemiology of GC has significantly changed over the past several decades especially in developed countries. There is a recognized decrease in incidence and mortality of distal or non-cardia (the lower body and antrum of stomach) GC and an increase in incidence and mortality of proximal gastroesophageal junction (GEJ) cancer.

Specifically, the incidence of GC originating from the cardia (the top portion of the stomach near the junction of the esophagus) follows the distribution of esophageal cancer. In the United States, an estimated 17,990 cases of esophageal cancer will be diagnosed in 2013, and 15,210 deaths are expected from this disease [2]. GC mortality rate closely follows its incidence; however, incidence varies widely by geographical region (Figure 1).

Non-cardia gastric adenocarcinoma shows marked geographic variation in countries such as Japan, Korea, China, Costa Rica and the former Soviet Union [3] (Figure 1). In the next three decades, GC is ranked the fastest growing cancer in both Europe and the United States [4], determining the reason for the considerable rise in the incidence of adenocarcinoma of proximal stomach and distal esophagus remains a challenge, making GC one of the most important diseases to understand in the 21st century.

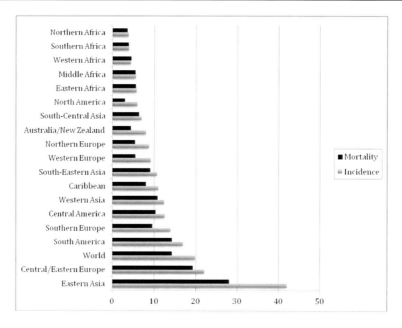

Figure 1. Geographic Distribution of Gastric Cancer Incidence and Mortality (Age-Standardized Rates per 100,000).

2. Histology and Molecular Profile

A. All Subtypes of GC

WHO categorizes GC into five histological subtypes which includes adenocarcinoma, papillary, mucinous, tubular, and signet ring cell [5, 6] (Figure 2A). Most of GEJ cancers are adenocarcinoma, which are further divided into two distinct types, intestinal (well-differentiated) and diffuse (undifferentiated); each has distinct morphologic appearance, epidemiology, pathogenesis, and genetic profile [7] (Table 1).

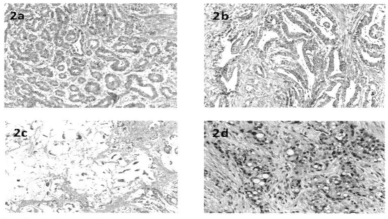

Figure 2A. Historical subtypes of gastric cancer. The WHO classification of gastric adenocarcinomas: papillary (2a), tubular (2b), mucious (2c), and signet ring cell (2d).

Gastric Cancer

Table 1. Clinical types of gastric cancer

Subtypes	Non-Cardia Gastric Cancer	Cardia (GEJ) Gastric Cancer	Diffuse Gastric Cancer
Environmental	Tobacco(OR 1.5) High dietary salt	*H. Pylori* infection (OR 3.0) Use of NSAIDs/Aspirin	None specifically identified
Clinical	Tobacco Use Alcohol Use	Obesity/High BMI, GERD	Family history Inherited syndromes
Genetic	Immune regulatory SNPs	None specifically identified	E-cadherin gene (CDH1)mutation
Gender	Male : Female(2:1)	Male: female (5:1)	Women increase the risk of breast cancer
Age	Incidence increases with age (peak age 50-70)	Wide age range	Median age at diagnosis is 38 years old
Race	White: Black (1:4)	White: Black (2:1) Industrialized nations	

OR: odds ratio; SNP: single nucleotide polymorphism, CDH1: Cadherin-1

Table 2. Risk Factors for Gastric Cancer

Dietary	High salt and nitrate intake Smoked and cured foods A diet low in Vitamins A and C Poor-quality drinking water
Toxins	Occupational exposure: rubber, coal Radiation exposure Smoking
Infections	*Helicobactor pylori*
Family History of gastric cancer	Remnant Stomach (2-3%)
Genetic predisposition syndromes	Hereditary Diffuse Gastric Cancer (3-5%) HNPCC (Lynch Syndrome, 1-2%) FAP (Familial Adenomatous Polyposis, 1%) Li-Fraumeni syndrome(<1%) Peutz-Jeghers syndrome(<1%)
Unbalance of stomach acid	Pernicious anemia Atrophic gastritis
Blood group	Type A
Obesity	High BMI
Gender	Male
Age	Elderly

B. Subtypes of Gastric Adenocarcinoma

Lauren first categorized adenocarcinoma of GC into intestinal and diffuse subtypes in 1965 based on microscopic appearance and growth patterns (Figure 2B). The intestinal type resembles normal intestinal mucosa, and usually originates from pre-existing chronic atrophic gastritis. In contrast, the diffuse type consists of discohesive poorly differentiated cells without recognizable gland formation and infiltrates insidiously [8]. Tumors containing both diffuse and intestinal histology are classified as mixed type. Signet ring cells are often a component of poorly differentiated diffuse GC [9] (Figure 2B). Linitis plastica ("leather bottle stomach") refers to the diffuse infiltration of poorly differentiated gastric adenocarcinoma in the submucosa and muscularis propria throughout the entire stomach. Diffuse subtype cancers have a poor prognosis and a high propensity to develop metastasis with rapid progression.

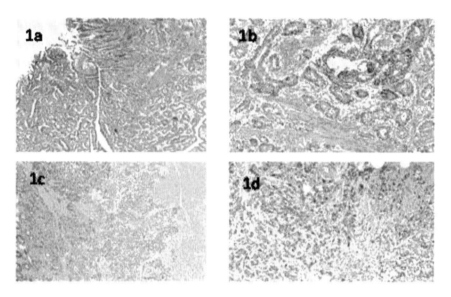

Figures 2A and 2B were courtesy by Dr. Fang-Ming Deng, MD, Ph. D, Pathologist at NYU Langone Medical Center.

Figure 2B. Historical subtypes of gastric cancer. The Lauren classification of gastric adenocarcinomas of intestinal (1a-1b) and diffuse subtype (1c-1d). Note the well formed gland structures in intestinal type, while individual or poorly formed nest of cells growing an infiltrated growth pattern in diffuse type.1a and 1c, low power;1b and 1d, high power.

C. Genetic Profile

Most recent study in Singapore [10] identified the genetic expression of 248 gastric-tumor cell lines using microarray data. The gene-expression profiles suggested three subtypes of gastric tumors — proliferative, metabolic, and mesenchymal; each with distinct genomic and epigenomic properties. The subtypes were validated in profiles of 70 tumors from Australian patients. Drug sensitivities of each type were based on clinical survival data and high-throughput screening of cell lines.

The proliferative tumors had high genetic instability, *TP53* mutations, and DNA hypomethylation. Metabolic tumors were more sensitive to 5-fluorouracil. Mesenchymal tumor cells had features of stem cells and were more sensitive to phosphatidylinositol-3-kinase–AKT–mTOR inhibitors in vitro. The conclusion suggested that gene-expression patterns can be used to classify GC into the three subtypes, which have differences in molecular and genetic features. These differences may correlate with response to specific treatments. If these findings can be verified in a broader spectrum of GC, they could have a major impact on treatment approaches and potential of a more-effective personalized therapy.

D. HER2

Up to 15% of GEJ cancer overexpress HER2 protein, more frequently encountered in intestinal type rather than diffuse type of tumor; its therapeutic implication will be discussed under the treatment section. Biology and immunohistochemistry (IHC) characteristics are different in GEJ cancer compared to breast cancer. In contrast to breast cancer, HER2 staining in GEJ tumors is heterogeneous, with incomplete membrane staining. The HER2 IHC scoring system for GEJ adenocarcinomas differs from that of breast carcinoma.

Automated image analysis, validated for scoring of HER2 IHC in breast cancer, has a low correlation between HER2 IHC 2+ and IHC 3+ cases scored by conventional light microscopy and cannot be reliably used in the interpretation of HER2 IHC expression in GEJ adenocarcinomas [11]. Therefore, IHC staining of HER2 in GC is still most reliably done by pathologists' experienced manual interpretation.

3. Risk Factors and Pathogenesis

A. Infection

There is general consensus that *H. pylori* causes distal GC and does not increase the risk of proximal GEJ cancer [12]. Much of the incidence variation in geographic areas can be explained by differences in diet and the prevalence of *H. Pylori* infection in the developing world.

Several studies have demonstrated an increased likelihood of *H. pylori* infection in patients with GC, particularly cancer of the distal stomach (non-cardia) [13]. *H. pylori* has the ability to colonize gastric mucosa and incite a series of inflammatory and immune reactions, which in turn lead to mucosal damage, intestinal metaplasia, and dysplasia [14] (Figure 3). This is thought to be secondary to *H. pylori* strain-specific virulence factors, most notably cytotoxin associated gene A (cagA) and vacuolating cytotoxin gene (vacA). In Western countries, about 60% of *H. pylori* isolated are cagA positive, where in Japan; nearly 100% of this strain possesses cagA.

A large Chinese study showed no benefit in the prevention of GC with the eradication of *H. pylori*. In a prospective, randomized, placebo-controlled, population-based primary prevention study, 1630 patients with *H. pylori* infection, were randomly assigned to receive *H pylori* eradication treatment or placebo from 1994-2002. Among the 18 new cases of GC that developed, no overall reduction was observed in participants who received *H. pylori* eradication treatment (n = 7) compared with those who did not (n = 11) (P =.33) [15].In contrast, a recent meta-analysis suggested that eradication could indeed reduce the risk of GC. In this study, overall 37 of 3388 (1.1%) treated patients developed GC compared with 56 of 3307 (1.7%) untreated (control) participants. In a pooled analysis of 6 studies with a total of 6695 participants followed from 4 to 10 years, the relative risk for GC was 0.65 (95% CI,

0.43 to 0.98) [16]. A multicenter, prospective cohort study conducted in Japan from 2000-2007, 4133 patients with *H. pylori* positive peptic ulcer elected to undergo *H. pylori* eradication or standard antacid therapy, 56 GC cases developed with mean follow-up of 5.6 years, overall there was no significant difference in incidence between the two groups(incidence ratio:0.58, 95% CI: 0.28-1.19) [17]. At the present time, treatment of patients with this infection should be reserved for patients with demonstrated symptomatic ulcer disease rather than *H.* pylori carriers. Chemoprevention strategy to achieve eradication of *H. pylori* is still controversial.

Dietary-Related Gastric Cancer	H. pylori-Related Gastric Cancer	Genetic related Gastric Cancer
	Colonization of Gastric Mucosa	Gene Mutation
	↓	↓
Chronic Superficial Gastritis		Genetic Instability
↓	Expression of Bacterial NO2 / NO Mutagens	↓
Parietal Cell Loss		Uncontrolled cell proliferation
↓	↓	↓
Hypochlorhydria	Inflammatory Immune Reaction	Abnormal cell architecture
↓		↓
Serum Gastrin Increase	↓	Mucosal Damage
↓	Mucosal Damage	↓
Gastric Epithelial Cell Proliferation	↓	Dysplasia
↓	Intestinal Metaplasia	↓
Genetic Instability / Uncontrolled Proliferation	↓	Carcinoma
↓	Colonic Metaplasia	
Dysplasia	↓	
↓	Dysplasia	
Carcinoma	↓	
	Carcinoma	

Figure 3.Pathogenesis of Gastric Cancer.

B. Diet

GC has been correlated with diets high in salted or smoked foods, as well as dried meats and fish, along with poor-quality drinking water [18]. Such foods are believed to cause GC through a combination of chronic superficial gastritis, parietal cell loss and resulting hypochlorhydria, compensatory serum gastrin increase, and gastric epithelial cell proliferation [19] (Figure 3). Conversely, diets high in fruit and vegetable intake were inversely correlated to rates of GC (Table 2).

C. Other Factors

Not surprisingly, gastric ulcer disease, atrophic gastritis, and pernicious anemia which all follow pathogenesis similar to poor dietary habit, are associated with increased risk of GC development [20]. Gastroesophageal reflux disease (GERD) is a principle risk factor for Barrett's esophagus, only 1%-3% of patients will develop GC [21]. Obesity predisposes patients at risk for GERD; the rising incidence of GEJ cancer can at least be partially attributed to the increase in obesity across the globe.

Certain toxics such as radiation exposure can cause an increased risk of many cancers, including GC [22]. In the U.S., GC is seen far more in non-white race, male gender, and advanced age, its incidence increases with age starting in the fifth decades [23]. This male predominance is seen universally, with men carrying twice the risk for this cancer, independent of geography. The lowest incidences for GC are in Western countries and in people of higher socioeconomic status.

D. Genetic Syndromes

A lack of adhesion molecules in diffuse carcinomas allows the individual tumor cells to grow and invade adjacent structures without forming tubules or glands. Genetic predisposition syndromes consist of 10-15% of all GC.

Hereditary diffuse GC (HDGC) syndrome presents as early onset diffuse GC, as well as lobular breast cancer [24]. With germline mutation in E-cadherin gene (*CDH1*), it has 60-80% penetrance with an autosomal dominant inheritance [25]. E-cadherin is a cell-adhesion protein, critical to cell development, differentiation and architecture. *CDH1* can also present as somatic mutations in GC (in up to 40% of cases) and is associated with poor prognosis [26]. Criteria for testing for E-cadherin gene mutation is developed by the International GC linkage consortium (Table 3). Prophylactic gastrectomy reportedly eliminates the risk of GC [27].

Table 3. Criteria for E-cadherin gene mutation testing

Two or more documented cases of gastric cancer in first degree relatives, with at least one documented case of diffuse gastric cancer diagnosed before the age of 50 years.
Three or more cases of documented diffuse gastric cancer in first –or second-degree relatives, independent of age if onset
Diffuse gastric cancer before the age of 40 years without a family history
Families with diagnoses of both diffuse gastric cancer and lobular breast cancer, with one case before the age of 50 years
In addition, in cases where expert pathologists detect carcinoma in situ adjacent to diffuse-type gastric cancer, genetic testing should be considered since this is rarely, if ever, seen in sporadic cases.

Other infrequently described inherited syndromes that may manifest as GC include Lynch syndrome with microsatellite instability (MSI) [deficiencies in MutL homolog 1 or 2 (*MLH1, MSH2*)], familial adenopolyposis coli (FAP) (Adenomatous polyposis coli, *APC*), Cowden's syndrome (loss of phosphatase and tensin homolog, *PTEN*), Peutz-Jager syndrome (*PJS1*), Li-Fraumeni syndrome (*TP53*) [28]. Similar to *CDH1*, many of the inherited genes are more commonly presented as somatic mutations in GC, particularly *TP53*, which is reported in as high as 77% of the cases [29].

E. Remnant Stomach

Remnant gastric carcinoma has been reported in 2–3 % of patients who have undergone gastrectomy for carcinoma or benign disease and account for 1.8 % of all GC in a large series [30].

F. Summary

The risk of GC development is strongly influenced by nutritional, environmental, socioeconomic factors and genetic predisposition. GC's variation in global incidence is closely related to differences in such as diet, which is in turn associated with environmental toxin exposure and *H.pylori* infection. The steady decline in incidence of distal cancer could be attributed to better dietary habits and water quality, however, the rise in proximal GC could be related to the obesity epidemic. Gene expression profile may be used to classify GC into the three subtypes. We need better understanding of the risk factors to accurately determine population at risk for GC and to create effective tools for early detection.

4. Screening

A. Background

The value of screening asymptomatic individuals for GC remains controversial [31].GC has a clinically silent course making timely diagnosis and treatment a continuous challenge. Clinically, patients may complain of weight loss, fatigue, abdominal pain, or postprandial fullness. Such symptoms may warrant a double-contrast barium upper GI series, but these are relatively non-specific signs, and often only accompany advanced disease (Table 4).

Table 4. Symptoms of Advanced Gastric Cancer

Weight loss
Abdominal Pain
Abdominal Mass
Postprandial Fullness
Anorexia
Nausea or Vomiting
Bleeding or Hematemesis

B. International Consensus

Annual mass screening for GC has been provided in some countries with high incidence of GC such as Japan, Venezuela, and Chile, with the aim of detecting GC in its earliest stage when the prognosis is better [32]. International consensus on the appropriate screening intervals or even methods does not exist, and there is considerable variability even within graphical regions with similar prevalence.

C. Korea and Japan

In South Korea, upper gastrointestinal series or upper endoscopy is offered every two years to all individuals, beginning at age 40 [33]. In Japan, the use of barium studies precedes the use of endoscopy as the main population-based screening, including conventional double contrast barium x-ray with photofluorography or the new double contrast barium x-ray with digital radiography; endoscopy is then performed if any abnormality is detected. This standard was developed through efficacy studies in Japan comparing barium studies to upper endoscopy, *H. pylori* testing, and serum pepsinogen testing, with the greatest balance of sensitivity, specificity, cost-effectiveness, and five-year survival coming from the barium cohort [34]. While this regimen is offered annually to all individuals over 40 years old in Japan, recent studies are exploring the use of esophago-gastro-duodenoscopy for younger patients, interval vary according to cancer risk [35]. In Japan and Korea, where screening is performed widely, early detection of GC is often possible.

D. US and Europe

In the U.S. and Western Europe, where GC rates remain relatively low, the use of such screening is reserved with those with particular risk factors, including family history, genetic syndromes, atrophic gastritis, pernicious anemia, recent immigration from high-incidence regions, and those with a history of partial gastrectomy [36].

5. Diagnosis

A. Pathology

Definitive diagnosis always demands biopsy of the suspected lesion. Multiple biopsies (6-8 biopsies), using standard size endoscopy forces are recommended to provide sufficient material for histologic interpretation, especially in the setting of an ulcerated lesion [37].

B. Staging

(a). Methodology in Staging

(i). Current Staging System
Oncological staging is established primarily through the TNM system developed by the American Joint Committee on Cancer (AJCC). The current 7th edition AJCC TNM staging system was recently updated in 2010 [38]. It accounts for depth of tumor invasion (T) and lymph node involvement (N); in addition, for patients with GEJ adenocarcinoma, tumor grade (G1 well, G2 moderately, G3 poorly, G4 undifferentiated) was included as well.

(ii). Validation of Current Staging System

Several studies using patient cohorts have found that the application of the 7th International Union for Cancer Control (UICC)-AJCC staging system resulted in a better prognostic stratification of overall survival compared to the 6th edition [39]. In contrast, others have reported that the increased complexity of the 7th edition staging system is accompanied by improvements in the predictive value of nodal staging as compared to the 6th edition, but not better in overall stage-specific predictive accuracy. These authors suggested that future refinements of the TNM staging system should consider whether increased complexity is balanced by improved prognostic accuracy [40]. It is controversial whether to include stage II/III GEJ cancer within the TNM-gastric adenocarcinoma (TNM-GC) or TNM-esophageal adenocarcinoma (TNM-EC) system; it has been reported that 163 II/III GEJ GC patients were better classified by the TNM-GC compared to the TNM-esophageal cancer staging system, potentially impacting the next TNM revision for GEJ tumors [41].

(iii). Techniques for Staging

In order to assess the depth of invasion, several different technologies are employed, including computed tomography (CT), positron emission tomography with fluorodeoxyglucose uptake (FDG-PET), and most importantly endoscopic ultrasound (EUS). PET scans are not yet recommended as standard diagnostic procedure in view of limited sensitivity but can be helpful to determine resectability of GC in select cases [42]. EUS has been shown to offer the most accurate prediction of tumor invasion, with that of surgical and endoscopic resection, with particularly good utility in assessing small T1 lesions and regional lymph node involvement [43]. In addition, many new technologies such as magnifying endoscopy with narrow band imaging have emerged as important new tools in diagnosing early stage GC by allowing observation of microvascular architecture and greater assessment of tumor depth and invasion [44,45].

(b). Staging and Prognosis

GC is an aggressive disease, very often patients present with early lymph node (LN) involvement. The five-year survival rates are 90%, 60%, and 15% for stages I, II, and III diseases, respectively. The five-year survival drops from 65% to 15% if there is LN involvement. About 75% of patients will have positive LNs (LN+) at the time of presentation in Western countries where routine screening has not been implemented [39]. Reflected in the TNM staging, poor prognostic factors include the number of involved LNs, and differentiation grade for GEJ. Other poorly prognostic factors not included in the TNM system include extracapsular LN spread, differentiation grade, lymphovascular and perineural invasion.

6. Treatment

Therapies are divided into four main components: surgical resection, chemotherapy, targeted agents and radiotherapy. While their uses as individual modality or combination will depend on the particular stage of cancer and patient's clinical factors, for the purposes of this chapter, we will discuss each separately.

A. Surgical Resection

The potentially curative treatment approach for patients with GC is surgical resection. Total or subtotal gastrectomy remains a key element of treatment in most stages. The primary goal of surgery is to accomplish a complete resection with negative margins (R0 resection); R1 indicates microscopic residual disease (positive margin) and R2 indicates gross (macroscopic) residual disease in the absence of distant metastasis [46].

(a). Endoscopic Mucosal Resection (EMR)

For intraepithelial tumors or tumors limited to the muscularis mucosa or lamina propria (T1a or earlier stage), EMR is a less invasive option that provides curative relief. Japanese treatment guidelines recommend EMR as a standard treatment for well differentiated mucosal gastric tumors less than 2cm in size without signs of ulceration [47]. Such techniques have matured to allow en bloc resections possible through endoscopic procedures fitted with flex-knife, patients benefit from less surgical complications and preserved quality of life compared to gastrectomy [48]. While far less common in the United States, EMR has become the standard of treatment for early GC in countries like Japan that have extensive experience with this technique.

(b). Laparoscopic Gastrectomy

Advances in laparoscopic techniques have expanded its use in the treatment of GC. Lymphadenectomy, local resection, total and subtotal gastrectomy (proximal or distal), and even multiple forms of reconstruction (including esophagojejunostomy and esophagus-remnant anastomosis) are all now possible intra-abdominally. A retrospective analysis of 1,294 patients in Japan has shown the safety and non-inferiority of this laparoscopic gastrectomy, with cure rates exceeding those of laparotomy with lower surgery-related mortality and complications [49]. Likewise, a concomitant rise in the use of robotic-assisted surgery is changing the surgical management of GC, as expertise and technology mature with this technique that promises greater scale of hand movement, multi-articulated motion, and a reduction in hand tremor.

Most recent study using laparoscopic total gastrectomy (LTG) compared with open total gastrectomy (OTG) for gastric remnant gastric cancer (GRC), of 1,247 consecutive patients who underwent gastrectomy for GC from January 1996 to May 2012, the overall 3-year survival rate was comparable between the LTG and OTG groups (77.8 % vs. 100 %;p = 0.9406) [50].

(c) Lymphadenectomy

(i). D1 vs. D2 Lymphadenectomy

While lymphadenectomy remains an essential component in GC management across the world, the extent of lymphadenectomy differs by region. The type of surgery performed differs between Asia and the United States. D2 resection, the standard surgery in Japan, involves the meticulous resection of all lymph nodes surrounding the left gastric artery, common hepatic artery, celiac axis, splenic artery, and proper hepatic artery (Figure 4) [47]. In the United States, D1 resection (removal of only perigastric lymph nodes) has long been the standard approach. Retrospective data suggest that the outcome for D2 resection is better than the outcome for D1 resection; however, the disparity might be caused by a fundamental difference in the disease biology itself, rather than the surgical techniques.

(ii). Randomized Studies with No Difference between D1 and D2 Lymphadenectomy

Randomized trials initially did not clearly demonstrate a survival benefit for patients undergoing a D2 compared with a D1 dissection [51]. In Europe, two major phase III clinical studies failed to prove the efficacy of D2 over D1 lymphadenectomy, and thus D1 lymphadenectomy has become the standard of treatment both in Europe and the United States when curative resection is possible [52, 53]. However, certain issues in these two studies limited its widespread acceptance in the world; these two studies showed that the relatively high morbidity and mortality in the patients who underwent D2 lymphadenectomy, and frequent use of splenectomy and distal pancreatectomy (unnecessary under current standards), all indicated inadequate surgical technique [54] that may have compromised the efficacy of D2 dissection.

(iii). Randomized Study with Advantage of D2 Lymphadenectomy

After a 15-year follow-up of a randomized Dutch trial with 1078 patients, D2 lymphadenectomy was associated with lower locoregional recurrence (12% vs. 22%) and GC-related death rates (37% vs. 48%) than D1 surgery [55]. Although D2 dissection was associated with higher operative morbidity, these data suggest that D2 lymphadenectomy could be considered the surgical standard of care.

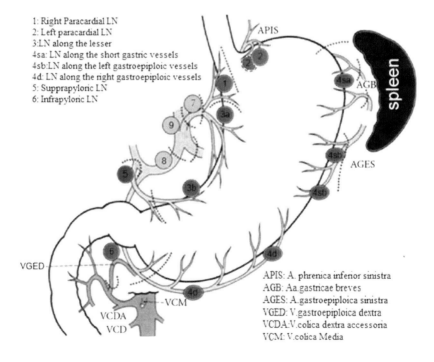

Figure 4. (Continued).

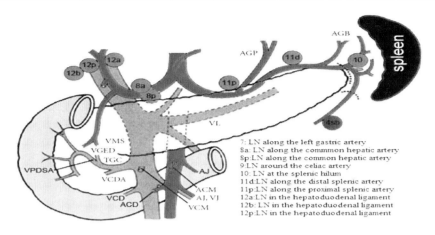

Figure 4. D1 (1-6) vs. D2 (1-12) Lymphadenectomy.

(iv). Japan and Eastern Asian Perspective

In Japan and East Asian countries where the incidence of GC is considerably higher than the rest of the world, D2 lymphadenectomy remains the gold standard for surgery, although no recent studies in the region support the safety or effectiveness over D1 dissection [56]. In Japan, the JCOG 9501 study investigated the use of D2 plus paraaortic lymphadenectomy (D3) over D2 lymphadenectomy, but failed to demonstrate any significant differences in 5-year survival, although safety was comparable between these two techniques [57].

B. Chemotherapy and Radiation Therapy for Curative Intent

Curative Therapies

(a). **Chemoradiotherapy**

(i). MacDonald Regimen

In the U.S., the Macdonald phase III trial explored the utility of adjuvant chemoradiation therapy (CRT). Patients with stage I to IV (M0) GEJ cancer or GC were randomized assigned to receive either surgery alone or surgery followed by bolus 5-FU/LV based chemotherapy (Mayo clinic regimen), with sandwiched radiation therapy (45 GY) with bolus 5-FU/LV as radiosensitizer. This study showed an approximate 20% improvement in survival for the group receiving the combined-modality therapy. The median OS was 36 months vs. 27 months and relapse-free survival of 30 months vs. 19 months in the adjuvant CRT group as compared to those receiving surgery alone. The hazard ration (HR) for death and relapse in the surgery-only arm and CRT arm were 1.35(95% CI [1.09, 1.66]; p=0.005) and 1.52(95%CI (1.23, 1.86); p<0.001), respectively [58]. The Macdonald regimen has become one of the standards of treatment in the U.S. for adjuvant therapy following curative resection. It should be noted, however, that the level of lymph node dissection performed on this cohort patients was far short of what most patients receive today. Most patients (54 percent) had undergone a D0 dissection, only 10 percent of patients in this trial received full D2 lymphadenectomy. Thus, it is very possible that the benefits of adjuvant radiation in addition to surgery and chemotherapy were overestimated due to the amount of residual disease in the group; patients had post-surgery, favoring benefits of radiation in this group. While varying standards exist throughout the world for the role of lymph node dissection in GC treatment (see 'SURGERY' above), it is generally recognized that the results of the MacDonald study suffer from this limitation. Nevertheless, Macdonald study provided the long lasting OS benefit using combined modality in the adjuvant setting. The most updated 10 years following up of the Macdonald study demonstrated the benefit of the CRT despite a slightly increased in secondary malignancy in the combined modality group [59].

(ii) ARTIST Trial

Following the MacDonald study, the ARTIST trial compared the utility of radiotherapy (RT) added to the chemotherapy regimen of capecitabine and cisplatin (XP) as adjuvant treatment after curative resection with D2 lymphadenectomy. Stratified analysis of 3-year disease-free survival of patients with lymph node metastasis showed a statistically significant difference, with 77.5% vs. 72.3% disease-free survival in the XP plus RT group over XP therapy alone [60]. However, the primary endpoint of 3-year disease-free survival did not show statistical significant effectiveness of RT (78.2% vs. 74.2%, respectively). The study showed high tolerability and low hematological and non-hematological toxicities in those receiving RT, encouraging further exploration of the use of RT in adjuvant settings in the proper patient population.

(iii) C80101 Study and CRITICS Trial

More recently, a large CALGB-led intergroup trial (C80101) trial tried to improve upon the results obtained with bolus 5-FU/LV plus radiation therapy by randomly assigning patients with resected GC to the standard MacDonald regimen, radiation with epirubicin, cisplatin and 5-FU (ECF) (61). The study did not demonstrate any difference in outcome between the two arms.

The CRITICS trial, currently being conducted by a group in the Netherlands examining perioperative ECF therapy against the Macdonald regimen embraced in the U.S., may offer guidance on future recommendations [62].

(b). **Neoadjuvant and Adjuvant Therapy**

Several years after the publication of the MacDonald study, perioperative chemotherapy with ECF regimen administrated before and after surgery for resectable GC also has shown a significant overall survival benefit compared with surgery alone. In the MAGIC trial, a group of European patients with GC, GEJ cancer, and lower esophageal cancer were randomized to surgery alone vs. surgery with 3 cycles of ECF before and 3 cycles of ECF after surgery. The 5-year survival rate for the surgery plus perioperative ECF group was 36%, significantly higher than the 23% in surgery alone group. In addition, the combined modality also prolonged progression-free survival with increased down-staging rate [63]. It is of note that only approximately 55% of patients in the perioperative chemotherapy group actually received postoperative therapy, which suggests that the main component responsible for the improved outcome was the preoperative treatment phase. Despite these successes, the completion rate for postoperative ECF therapy suffered (only 42% in this trial), prompting further investigation before ECF therapy can become the standard of therapy. The Magic study, however, provided a RT free option for resectable GC patients.

(c). Neoadjuvant Chemotherapy

Neoadjuvant chemotherapy has been shown to shrink primary tumors and regional lymph nodes in phase II clinical trials with intriguing results [64]. These small studies, however, have not established any definitive role for preoperative neoadjuvant chemotherapy in facilitating resection of initially unresectable tumors.

(d). Adjuvant Chemotherapy

(i) ECF intensified

The results of trials investigating the role of adjuvant chemotherapy without additional radiation therapy are mixed. An Italian study using an intensified, ECF-based treatment regimen as adjuvant therapy after GC resection did not demonstrate a benefit in outcome [65].

(ii) S-1

On the other hand, a Japanese phase III trial of S-1(an oral fluoropyrimidine), as adjuvant therapy after D2 lymphadenectomy of stage II or III GC demonstrated an OS benefit, with a 3-year OS rate of 80.1% in the S1 group and 70.1% in the surgery-only group (HR 0.68, 95% CI [0.52, 0.87]; p=0.003) [66]. The improvement in overall survival was confirmed after 5-year follow-up [67].

(iii) CLASSIC

At the 2011 ASCO annual meeting, a South Korean phase III trial in 1035 patients with D2-resected stage II/III GC identified adjuvant therapy with capecitabine plus oxaliplatin as superior to surgery alone, with significant improvement in 3-year disease-free survival(74% vs. 60%, respectively; HR 0.56; p<0.0001). This is the so called CLASSIC study [68], which has now become one of the standard adjuvant chemotherapy treatments (Table 5).

Table 5. Chemotherapy in Resectable Gastric Cancer EAST meets WEST

Study	Regimens	Primary Endpoint	Primary Endpoint results	P Value	% Benefit
CLASSIC (Korea)	Surgery vs surgery+ adjuvant Capecitabine/Oxaliplatin	3-yr DFS	59% vs 74%	0.0001	15
MAGIC (Europe)	Surgery vs surgery+ Periop ECF	5-yr OS	23% vs 36%	0.009	13
Sakuramoto (Japan)	Surgery vs surgery+ Adjuvant S-1	3-yr OS	70% vs 80%	0.003	10
CALGB 80101(US)	Postop 5-FU/LV CRT vs ECF CRT	OS	37 vs. 38 months	0.80	1
ARTIST (Korea)	Postop CT vs. CRT (capecitabine/cisplatin)	3-yr DFS	74% vs 78%	0.086	2

(iv) Meta-analysis

A recent meta-analysis of 17 trials with 3,838 patients confirmed that adjuvant chemotherapy without radiation after GC resection was associated with a significant overall survival benefit of 20%, with an HR of 0.82(95% CI[0.79, 0.9]; p<0.001) [69], again suggesting that adjuvant chemotherapy alone could benefit patients in the post surgery setting.

(v) Intraperitoneal Therapy with Immunological Agent

Recently, intraperitoneal injection of a rat-mouse hybrid monoclonal antibody, catumaxomab, was investigated after curative intent resection of GC in a small 54-patient trial, achieving a promising 2-year survival of 75%. Catumaxomab binds to epithelial cell adhesion molecule (EpCAM) antigens via one arm and to CD3 on T lymphocytes via the other arm, and also to an antigen-presenting cell (macrophage, a natural killer cell, or a dendritic cell) via the heavy chains, facilitating an immunological reaction towards the tumor cells. This approach merits further testing, as it may enhance clearance of microscopic GC disseminated to the peritoneum (whether detected by peritoneal washings or not), with potential of improving long term outcomes of perioperative approaches [70].

Patients with advanced disease, a retrospective study from Taiwan, were divided into two groups, one group that underwent surgery alone and another group that underwent surgery with a hyperthermic intraperitoneal chemotherapy (HIPEC) as an adjuvant treatment. These were patients with locally advanced GC and serosal invasion. A total of 29 patients underwent gastrectomy with HIPEC and 83 patients who underwent gastrectomy alone. The 5-year survival rates were 43.9% and 10.7% for the combined group vs. surgery alone respectively. The 5-year median survival were 22.66 (17.55-25.78) and 34.81 (24.97-44.66) months (p = 0.029), respectively. The carcinomatosis recurrence time was longer in patients who underwent gastrectomy with HIPEC and received R0 resection [71].

(e) Summary

Based on the previously mentioned trials and meta-analysis, either postoperative chemoradiation (FU/RT) in the United States, perioperative(pre- and postoperative) chemotherapy ECF(or similar) in US and Europe(United Kingdom), or adjuvant chemotherapy either with capecitabine/oxaliplatin or S-1 alone after D2 resection in Asia can be regarded as standards of care for the management of resectable GC.

C. Primary Systemic Therapy for Unresectable Gastric Cancer

About 40-50% of patients will present with unresectable disease. Amongst the most widely used treatment regimens for unresectable GC, multiple agents are active, including:

(i) Anti-metabolites: fluoropyrimidine (5-FU), capecitabine, S-1 and methotrexate.
(ii) DNA damaging agents: platinum agents, mitomycin-C, Topoisomerase I/II inhibitors such as epirubicin/doxorubicin, etoposide, irinotecan
(iii) Anti-microtubule agents: taxanes (paclitaxel and docetaxel)
(iv) Anti-angiogenic agents: ramucirumab

(v) Anti-HER2 agent: trastuzumab for HER2-overexpressing GC.

(a). First –Line Chemotherapy

(1). Doublets
(i) FP

Combination regimens are associated with higher response rate (RR) and longer OS when compared with single-agent therapies [72]. A combination of fluoropyrimidines such as 5-FU in combination with platinum such as cisplatin remains the standard of chemotherapy, and is often used as the reference arm in current clinical trials [73, 74].

(ii) XP

Oral derivatives of 5-FU, including capecitabine (a 5-FU prodrug) and a novel compound labeled S-1 (a synthetic combination of tegafur, gimeracil, and oteracil), have been developed and used exclusively. The ML-17032 trial compared a combination of 5-FU and cisplatin (FP) compared with capecitabine and cisplatin (XP). Outcomes demonstrated the non-inferiority of XP therapy to FP therapy, with an overall survival (OS) of 10.5 months and 9.3 months respectively [73].

(iii) SP

With regards to S-1 therapy, the SPIRITS trial demonstrated significantly longer OS for S-1 used in combination with cisplatin over S-1 monotherapy (13.0 vs. 11.0 months, respectively) [74]. Likewise, the FLAGS trial in the U.S. compared FP therapy to a combination of S-1 and cisplatin (SP), and showed that the median OS was 8.6 months in the cisplatin/S-1 arm and 7.9 months in the cisplatin/infusion fluorouracil arm (HR, 0.92; 95% CI, 0.80 to 1.05; P = .20) demonstrating the superiority of SP therapy (75). It is important to note that SP has already become the first choice of primary treatment for unresectable GC in Japan. In a subset analysis, SP produced statistically superior OS for patients with diffuse type histology. Additional studies are needed to confirm the activity of S-1 in the US and the rest of western hemisphere.

(2). Triplets
(i) DCF

The V-325 trial, studied the benefit of triple-drug regimen in US patients. It was a phase III trial involving 445 patients with GC that demonstrated superiority with the addition of docetaxel to cisplatin and 5-FU (DCF) compared with cisplatin and 5-FU (FP) alone, in terms of response rate (37% VS. 25%; P=0.01), time-to-progression (5.6 vs. 3.7 months; P<0.001)) and OS (9.2 vs. 8.6 months; P=0.02)) [76]. However, the DCF group suffered considerable toxicities, including neutropenia and diarrhea, a high rate of febrile neutropenia (30%), which cautions against its widespread acceptance as a first-choice. This study established the feasibility of triplet therapy in the first line in GC and the REAL study followed the same path of triplet therapy, a potential effective regimen for a highly selective group of patients with excellent performance status who can be monitored very closely.

(ii) ECF and EOX

The REAL-2 trial also studied various combinations of triple-therapy, including the use of capecitabine instead of 5-FU and oxaliplatin in place of cisplatin. In a 2x2 factorial design, the conventional combination of ECF was studied against regimens replacing 5-FU with capecitabine (ECX), oxaliplatin replacing cisplatin (EOF), and one arm of treatment containing both experimental treatments (EOX). The combination of EOX was found to be less toxic and at least as active as the ECF combination, with all efficacy parameters trending toward superiority. Median OS in the ECF (control arm), ECX, EOF and EOX group were 9.9 months, 9.9 months, 9.3 months, and 11.2 months respectively; survival rate at 1 year were 37.7%, 40.8%, 40.4%, 46.8%, respectively. In a secondary analysis, OS was longer with EOX than that of ECF, achieved HR of 0.8 when EOX group was compared to ECF group (95% CI [0.66, 0.97]; p=0.02). PFS and RR did not differ significantly between the regimens. Looking at OS as a primary endpoint, both capecitabine and oxaliplatin were shown to be non-inferior to 5-FU and cisplatin-based regimens (hazard ratio 0.86 and 0.92, respectively) [77]. The toxicity profile for the experimental EOX group was favorable, with higher incidence of diarrhea and peripheral neuropathy but lower incidence of alopecia and neutropenia.

(iii) Summary

While trials are still ongoing to determine the best combination of therapy recommendable, EOX therapy is emerging as a viable forerunner. Given the limited number of options available (principally involving either taxanes or platinum-based agents), development of new anti-cancer agents will be a key element moving forward.

(b). Second-Line Chemotherapy

Many patients with advanced GC are refractory to first-line chemotherapy or experience disease progression after a short response to treatment. About 70-80% of patients with refractory GC receive second or later lines chemotherapy in Asia, but less than 30% of patients receive second line therapy in US/Europe. Irinotecan or docetaxel is commonly considered as second line chemotherapy option.

(i) Clinical Trial data

A phase III trial compared XP with irinotecan plus 5-FU in 333 patients with advanced GC who progressed on 1st line chemotherapy [78]. No difference in outcome measures (RR, PFS, OS) could be found. The non-cisplatin, irinotecan-based regimen was less toxic and, thus could be an alternative for patients who are not candidates for a platinum-based treatment. Two recent randomized trials of chemotherapy versus best supportive care clearly demonstrated improvement in OS with use of second –line chemotherapy with either irinotecan or taxane after failure of first-line fluoropyrimidine/platinum therapy [79, 80]. Etoposide also demonstrated some benefit as an alternative second-line option in selected patients [81]. Another phase III trial compared palliative chemotherapy using docetaxel or irinotecan plus best care support (n=133) with best care support alone (n=69), OS was 5.3 vs 3.8 months respectively (HR 0.66, 95%CI: 0.48-0.89, p=0.007) [82].

(ii) Meta-analysis

A recent meta-analysis analyzed 578 studies, two of which were randomized phase III trials that compared chemotherapy with supportive care. A total of 410 patients were eligible for analysis, of whom 150 received docetaxel chemotherapy, and 81 received irinotecan chemotherapy. A significant reduction in the risk of death [HR = 0.64, 95% CI 0.52–0.79, P < 0.0001] was observed with salvage chemotherapy. When the analysis was restricted to irinotecan or docetaxel, there was still significant reduction in the risk of death with each chemotherapeutic agent separately. The HR was 0.55(95% CI 0.40–0.77, P = 0.0004) for irinotecan and 0.71 (95% CI 0.56–0.90, P = 0.004) for docetaxel [83].

(iii) Summary

Based on these trial data, a combination regimen with three drugs including a platinum agent (cisplatin or oxaliplatin) plus fluoropyrimidine as a backbone with the addition of epirubicin or docetaxel can be considered first-line standard of care in the palliative treatment of advanced GC. Second-line chemotherapy is a standard of care for medically-fit patients with advanced GC pretreated with fluoropyrimidines and platinum. Adding second-line chemotherapy to best care support achieves a significant OS improvement. OS benefit was seen across all prognostic subgroups, including those with two prior chemotherapies or with Eastern Cooperative Oncology Group (ECOG) performance status of 1. Chemotherapy (e.g., docetaxel) is superior to BSC (best supportive care) in the second-line setting in patients who are fit enough to receive treatment. Irinotecan has clearly demonstrated activity and could be integrated in a sequential approach (Figure 5).

(c) Molecularly Targeted Agents

Advances in novel targeted anti-cancer agents have revolutionized the treatment of breast, colorectal, and lung cancer, and have slowly been introduced to the field of GC. The role of targeted agents, in particular drugs targeting the vascular endothelial growth factor (VEGF) and EGFR/HER2 system (Figure 6), has been investigated in several recent trials.

(1). First-Line Targeted Therapy

(i) HER2 overexpression

Recent studies from 2012 showed that as many as 13-20% of GC and approximately 30% of GEJ adenocarcinoma over-express HER2. This has prompted interest in the use of trastuzumab, a human monoclonal antibody against HER2 that has well-documented use in the treatment of breast cancer [84, 85].

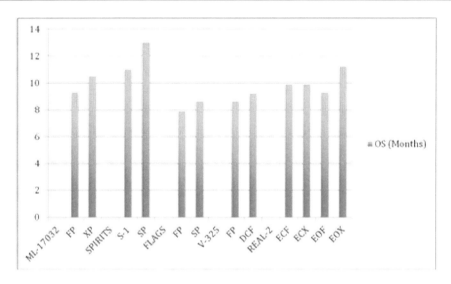

Figure 5. Median Survival Time of Phase III trials of Chemotherapy for Unresectable Gastric Cancer.

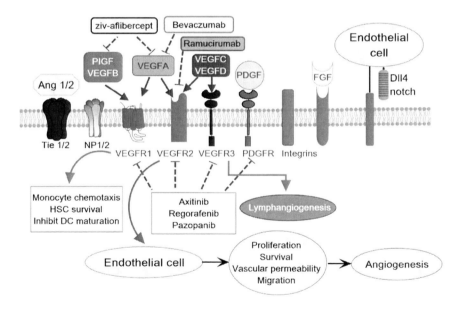

Figure 6. Proangiogenic signals and VEGFR activity.

(ii) ToGA Study

The global ToGA trial explored the effectiveness of adding trastuzumab to chemotherapy (either FP or XP) for HER2 positive GC patients. Of 3,807 tumors from patients with GC who were tested, 810(22.1%) were positive for HER2 overexpression using IHC and fluorescence in situ hybridization (FISH) analysis. Eventually, 584 patients were randomly assigned to receive a fluoropyrimidine plus cisplatin with or without trastuzumab (8mg/kg loading dose followed by 6mg/kg. Cycles were repeated every 3 weeks for 6 cycles, and trastuzumab was subsequently continued every 3 weeks until disease progression. For those who received trastuzumab along with chemotherapy, OS was significantly longer than those receiving chemotherapy alone (13.8 months vs. 11.1 months, respectively, HR 0.74, 95%CI [0.6, 0.91]; p=0.0046) and overall RR were also improved in the trastuzumab arm (47.3% vs. 34.5%, p=0.0017). There were no significant differences in the toxicity between the two treatment arms, with even longer survival for those patients strongly positive for HER2 (16 months) [86]. The ToGA trial was the first phase III trial to demonstrate a survival advantage with the addition of a biologic agent, trastuzumab, to standard chemotherapy in advanced GC.

(iii) Additional Studies Using Targeted Therapies

Combination therapies of trastuzumab added to standard chemotherapy have emerged as the standard of care in patients with metastatic, HER2 –overexpressing gastric and gastroesophageal cancer. Stratification of patients by immunochemistry and FISH analysis for HER2 positivity has become an important tool, as trastuzumab plus chemotherapy has become the new standard of treatment for this subset of patients in the United States. Several phase III trials are investigating the role of other EGFR/HER2 inhibitors such as lapatinib, cetuximab, and panitumumab in GC.

(iv) REAL3 Study

In the European REAL3 trial, panitumumab was added to epirubicin, oxaliplatin, and capecitabine (EOC) therapy, with an OS of 8.8 months in the panitumumab plus EOC group vs. 11.3 months in those receiving just EOC therapy, which was statistically significant [87]. It should be noted, however, the chemotherapy doses in the panitumumab group were significantly lower than those used in the control EOC group.

(v) EXPAND Trial

The EXPAND trial looked at the effectiveness of adding cetuximab to chemotherapy, but found no significant differences in OS, PFS or response rate [88].

(vi) AVAGAST Study

In contrast to these positive results from trastuzumab in HER2 overexpressing GC, bevacizumab failed to demonstrate an OS advantage when added to cisplatin/fluoropyrimidine (mainly capecitabine) in patients with GEJ and gastric adenocarcinoma. However, the AVAGAST trial demonstrated higher RR and longer PFS for the bevecizumab-containing arm, overall RR (46% vs. 37%; p=0.0315) and PFS (6.7 vs. 5.3 months; p=0.0037) compared to chemotherapy alone. However, while OS was longer in the bevacizumab group (12.1 months vs. 10.1 months), the difference was not statistically significant [89].

(2). Second-Line Targeted Therapy

Even though the OS difference between chemo alone versus bevacizumab plus chemotherapy was not statistically significant in the AVAGAST study, there was a trend toward OS advantage with the bevacizumab, therefore hinting that angiogenesis may still have value in the treatment of GC.

(i) REGARD Study

Table 6. Trials of Molecularly Targeted Agents

ToGA	Trastuzumab + CT: 13.8 months CT: 11.1 months
AVAGAST	Bevacizumab + CT: 12.1 months CT: 10.1 months * Not statistically significant
REAL-3	Panitumumab + EOC: 8.8 months EOC: 11.3 months
EXPAND	Cetuximab + CT vs. CT: No difference
REGARD	Ramucirumab + Supportive Care: 5.2 months Supportive Care: 3.8 months * Second-line therapy and patients who progressed within 6 months of adjuvant chemotherapy

This phase III trial showed promising results using of ramucirumab in patients in whom GC or GEJ cancers progressed on first line therapy within 6 months. In conjunction with supportive care, ramucirumab, a vascular endothelial growth factor receptor type 2 (VEGFR-2) antagonist – has been shown to extend OS in an international group of patients from 3.8 months to 5.2 months compared to supportive care alone [90]. Ramucirumab offered a preferable alternative to other cytotoxic chemotherapy regimens for use in second-line therapy, and is generally well tolerated. Thus, while ramucirumab has become an important addition to the armament against GC, to date trastuzumab is the only molecularly targeted agent that has shown to be effective in combination with chemotherapy (Table 6).

(ii) Future Direction

The expansion of this field will likely continue to play an important role in the future of GC, and many phase III clinical trials are ongoing to look at the role of agents such as the therapy using everolimus, a mammalian target of rapamycin (mTOR) inhibitor. The utility of combination to ramucirumab with chemotherapy are also actively under investigation.

D. Radiation Therapy

(a) Resectable Disease

Radiation therapy was assessed in randomized trials in both the preoperative and postoperative setting in patients with resectable GC. Two randomized trials have compared surgery alone to surgery plus RT in patients with GC. In the first trial conducted by the British Stomach Cancer Group, 423 patients were randomized to undergo surgery alone, followed surgery by RT or chemotherapy. At 5-year follow –up, no survival benefit was seen for patients receiving postoperative RT or chemotherapy compared with those who underwent surgery alone. But there was a significant reduction in locoregional recurrence with the addition of RT to surgery (27% with surgery vs. 10% for surgery plus RT and 19% for surgery plus chemotherapy). In the second trial, were randomized 370 patients to preoperative RT or surgery alone. There was a significant improvement in survival with preoperative RT (30% vs. 20%; p=0.0094) [91]. Resection rates were also higher in the preoperative RT arm (89.5%) compared to surgery alone (79%), suggested that preoperative RT improves local control and survival.

(b) Unresectable Disease

Several historical studies demonstrated the efficacy of concurrent chemoradiotherapy in GC treatment over the use of radiotherapy or chemotherapy alone. A 1968 study in the US demonstrated a significantly longer survival time with the use of concurrent chemoradiotherapy over radiotherapy (11.6 months vs. 5.7 months, respectively) [92]. One year later, Falkson published a comparison of concurrent chemoradiotherapy, radiotherapy alone and chemotherapy alone, and found that RR with concurrent chemoradiotherapy (55% of patients) far exceeded that of chemotherapy alone (17%) or radiotherapy alone (0%) [93]. For unresectable GC, radiotherapy - has shown in several Japanese studies to play an important palliative role in shrinking larger tumors and addressing problems such as pain, stenosis, and bleeding [94,95]. However, an important study by the Eastern Cooperative Oncology Group (ECOG) failed to show any direct survival benefit from the use of RT plus 5-FU vs. 5-FU monotherapy in patients with unresectable gastric and pancreatic cancer (8.2 months vs. 9.3 months, respectively) [96]. While radiotherapy is generally well tolerated, the rapidly changing chemotherapy regimens and the introduction of novel, molecularly targeted agents may prompt a re-evaluation of the role radiotherapy in both resectable and unresectable GC.

Conclusion

The treatment of GC varies considerably based on geographical region, incidence, local expertise and resources, and the current state of research. For local or superficial disease (Stage IA), the treatment may include endoscopic mucosal resection, although subtotal or total gastrectomy is still a common choice depending on tumor location, with some level of lymph node dissection. For more advanced disease (Stage IB-III), treatment includes both surgical resection and the use of perioperative or adjuvant chemoradiotherapy. Addition of pre and post-surgery chemotherapy consistently demonstrates benefit vs. surgery alone. Novel molecularly targeted anticancer agents are also being tested with this group of patients, with promising evidence for the addition of trastuzumab in patients expressing HER2.

For palliation and symptomatic treatment of widely metastatic disease (Stage IV), radiotherapy is especially helpful, along with certain chemotherapy regimens, stent placement, laser therapy, or surgical treatment of blockage or bleeding.

Very recent studies suggest the utility of using single agent ramucirumab in those failing chemotherapy in advanced disease or in patients who progressing quickly on adjuvant chemotherapy. Treatment advances will likely hinge on the continued expansion of molecularly targeted therapy, as well as continued research in biomarkers domestically and internationally in setting optimum standards for the adjuvant and perioperative use of chemoradiotherapy for each patient population.

Disclosure of Conflict of Interests

There are no conflicts of interests from three authors.

Author Responsibility:

Lan Mo expanded the manuscript on pathology, pathogenesis, and provided all final figures and tables.

Jafar Al-Mondhiry assembled the literature and drafted the manuscript, provided drafted the tables and figures of the manuscript

Jennifer Wu developed the outline of the manuscript, created the flow of each section and provided references, wrote the abstract and the chemotherapy section of the manuscript and edited the final manuscript for approval

Acknowledgments

We are grateful to Dr. Fang-Ming Deng at the Department of Pathology at NYU Langone Medical Center who provides all the pathology figures for this chapter.

We are indebted to Dr. Lawrence Peter Leichman, Professor of Medicine, Director of GI Oncology of NYU Perlmutter Cancer Center, for his expert review of this chapter to allow final approval of its publication.

References

[1] Ferlay J, Shin HR, Bray F, Forman D, Mathers C, Parkin DM. GLOBOCAN 2008, Cancer Incidence and Mortality Worldwide: IARC Cancer Base No. 10 [GLOBOCAN. database]. Lyon, France: International Agency for Research on Cancer, 2010.

[2] Siegel R, Naishadham D, Jemal A. Cancer Statistics, 2013. *CA Cancer J.Clin.* 2013 Jan;63(1):11-30.

[3] Corley DA, Buffler PA. Esophageal and gastric cardia adenocarcinomas: analysis of regional variation using the Cancer Incidence in Five Continents database. *Int. J. Epidemiol.* 2001 Dec;30(6):1415-1425.

[4] Kubo A, Corley DA. Body mass index and adenocarcinoma of esophagus or gastric cardia: a systemic review and meta-analysis. *Cancer Epidemiol. Biomarkers prev.* 2006; 15:872-888.

[5] Dicken BJ, Bigam DL, Cass C, Mackey JR, Joy AA, Hamilton SM. Gastric adenocarcinoma: review and considerations for future directions. *Ann. Surg.* 2005; 241(1):27-39.

[6] Werner M, Becker KF, Keller G, Hofler H. Gastric adenocarcinoma: Pathomorphology and molecular pathology. *J. Cancer Res. Clin. Oncol.* 2001;127(4):207-216.

[7] Shah MA, Khanin R, Tang L, Janjigian YY, Klimstra DS, Gerdes H, Kelsen DP. Molecular classification of gastric cancer: a new paradigm. *Clin. Cancer Res.* 2011;17(9):2693-2701.

[8] Volk J, Parsonnet J. Epidemiology of Gastric Cancer and Helicobacter pylori. Springer Science + Business Media LLC, New York, New York, USA, 2009.

[9]   Taghavi S, Jayarajan SN, Davey A, Willis AI. Prognostic significance of signet ring gastric cancer. *J. Clin.Oncol*. 2012;30 (28):3493-3498.

[10] Lei Z, Tan IB, Das K, Deng N, Zouridis H, Pattison S, Chua C, Feng Z, Guan YK, Ooi CH, Ivanova T, Zhang S, Lee M, Wu J, Ngo A, Manesh S, Tan E, Teh BT, So JB, Goh LK, Boussioutas A, Lim TK, Flotow H, Tan P, Rozen SG. Identification of molecular subtypes of gastric cancer with different responses to PI3-kinase inhibitors and 5-fluorouracil. *Gastroenterology*. 2013;145:554–565.

[11] Jeung J, Patel R, Vila L, Wakefield D, Liu C. Quantitation of HER2/neu expression in primary gastroesophageal adenocarcinomas using conventional light microscopy and quantitative image analysis. *Arch Pathol. Lab. Med*. 2012;136:610-617.

[12] Brenner H, Rothenbacher D, Arndt V. Epidemiology of stomach cancer. *Methods Mol. Biol*. 2009;472:467-477.

[13] Eslick GD, Lim LL, Byles JE, Xia HH, Talley NJ. Association of helicobacter pylori infection with gastric carcinoma: a meta-analysis,. *Am. J.Gastroenterol*1999;94(9): 2373-2379.

[14] Compare D, Rocco A, Nardone G. Risk factors in gastric cancer. Eur *Rev. Med.Pharmacol. Sci*. 2010 Apr;14(4):302-308.

[15] Wong BC, Lam SK, Wong WM, Chen JS, Zheng TT, Feng RE, Lai KC, Hu WH, Yuen ST, Leung SY, Fong DY, Ho J, Ching CK, Chen JS . Helicobacter *pylori* eradication to prevent gastric cancer in a high-risk region of China: a randomized controlled trial. *JAMA* 2004; 291: 187-194.

[16] Fuccio L, Zagari RM, Eusebi LH, Laterza L, Cennamo V, Ceroni L, Grilli D, Bazzoli F.Meta-analysis: can Helicobacter pylori eradication treatment reduce the risk of gastric cancer? *Ann. Intern. Med*. 2009; 151(2): 121-128.

[17] Mabe K, Takahashi M, Oizumi H, Tsukuma H, Shibata A, Fukase K, Matsuda T, Takeda H, Kawata S. Does Helicobacter pylori eradication therapy for peptic ulcer prevent gastric cancer? *World J. Gastrioeterol*. 2009; 15(34):4290-4297.

[18] Liu C, Russell RM. Nutrition and gastric cancer risk: an update. *Nutr. Rev*. 2008; 66: 237-249.

[19] Correa P. A human model of gastric carcinogenesis. *Cancer Res*.1988; 48(13):3554-3560.

[20] Devita VT, Lawrence TS, Rosenberg SA, DePinho RA, Weinberg A. Principles and practice of oncology, Ninth, North American Edition, Lippincott Williams & Wilkins, Philadelphia, Pennsylvania, USA 2011.

[21] Jemal A, Bray F, Center MM, Ferlay J, Ward E, Forman D. Global cancer statistics. *CA Cancer J. Clin*. 2011;61(2):69-90.

[22] Kelley JR, Duggan JM. Gastric cancer epidemiology and risk factors. *J. Clin.Epidemiol*.2003: 56(1); 1-9.

[23] Howlader N, Noone AM, Krapcho M, Garshell J, Neyman N, Altekruse SF, Kosary CL, Yu M, Ruhl J, Tatalovich Z, Cho H, Mariotto A, Lewis DR, Chen HS, Feuer EJ, Cronin KA (eds). SEER Cancer Statistics Review, 1975-2010, National Cancer Institute. Bethesda, MD, http://seer.cancer.gov/csr/1975_2010/, based on November 2012 SEER data submission, posted to the SEER web site, 2013.

[24] Kangelaris KN, Gruber SB. Clinical implications of founder and recurrent CDH1 mutations in hereditary diffuse gastric cancer. *JAMA* 2007; 297:2410-2411.

[25] Richards FM, Mckee SA, Rajpar MH, Cole TR, Evans DG, Jankowski JA, Mckeown C, Sanders DS, Maher ER. Germline E-cadherin gene (CDH1) mutations predispose to familial gastric cancer and colorectal cancer. *Hum. Mol. Genet.*1999;8(4):607-610.

[26] Corso G, Carvalho J, Marrelli D, Vindigni C, Carvalho B, Seruca R, Roviello F, Oliveira C. Somatic mutations and deletions of the e-cadherin gene predict poor survival of patients with gastric cancer. *J. Clin.Oncol.*2013;31(7):868-875.

[27] Fitzgerald RC, Hardwick R, Huntsman D, Carneiro F, Guilford P, Blair V, Chung DC, Norton J, Ragunath K, Van Krieken JH, Dwerryhouse S, Caldas C. Hereditary diffuse gastric cancer: updated consensus guidelines for clinical management and directions for future research. *J. Med. Genet.*2010;47(7):436-444.

[28] Kaurah P, Huntsman DG. Hereditary diffuse gastric cancer. In: Gene Reviews. RA Pagon, TD Bird, CR Dolan, K Stephens, MP Adam (Eds.). University of Washington Press, Seattle, Washington, USA, 1993.

[29] Fenoglio-Preiser CM, Wang J, Stemmermann GN, Noffsinger A. TP53 and gastric carcinoma: a review. *Hum. Mutat.*2003;21(3):258-270.

[30] Nozaki I, Nasu J, Kubo Y, Tanada M, Nishimura R, Kurita A.Risk factors for metachronous gastric cancer in the remnant stomach after early cancer surgery. *World J. Surg.*2010;34(7):1548–1554.

[31] Leung WK, Wu MS, Kakugawa Y, Kim JJ, Yeoh KG, Goh KL, Wu KC, Wu DC, Sollano J, Kachintorn U, Gotoda T, Lin JT, You WC, Ng EK, Sung JJ; Asia Pacific Working Group on Gastric Cancer. Screening for gastric cancer in Asia: current evidence and practice. *Lancet Oncol.* 2008;9(3):279-287.

[32] Pisani P, Oliver WE, Parkin DM, Alvarez N, Vivas J. Case-control study of gastric cancer screening in Venezuela. *Br. J. Cancer.* 1994;69(6):1102-1105.

[33] Yoo KY. Cancer control activities in the Republic of Korea. *Jpn J. Clin.Oncol.*2008; 38(5):327-333.

[34] Hamashima C, Shibuya D, Yamazaki H, Inoue K, Fukao A, Saito H, Sobue T. The Japanese guidelines for gastric cancer screening. *Jpn J. Clin.Oncol.*2008; 38(4):259-267.

[35] Kobayashi D, Takahashi O, Arioka H, Fukui T. The optimal screening interval for gastric cancer using esophago-gastro-duodenoscopy in Japan. *BMC Gastroenterol.* 2012; 12(10):144-150.

[36] Hirota WK, Zuckerman MJ, Adler DG, Davila RE, Egan J, Leighton JA, Qureshi WA, Rajan E, Fanelli R, Wheeler-Harbaugh J, Baron TH, Faigel DO. ASGE guideline: the role of endoscopy in the surveillance of premalignant conditions of the upper GI tract. *Gastrointest Endosc.* 2006; 63(4):570-580.

[37] Hatfield AR, Slavin G, Segal AW, Levi AJ. Importance of the site of endoscopic gastric biopsy in ulcerating lesions of the stomach. *Gut.* 1975 Nov;16(11):884-886.

[38] Edge SBB, Compton CC, Fritz AG, Greene FL, Trotti A. (Eds.). AJCC Cancer Staging Handbook, Springer, New York, New York, USA, 2009.

[39] Talsma K, Van Hagen P, Grotenhuis BA, Steyerberg EW, Tilanus HW, Van Lanschot JJ, Wijnhoven BP. Comparison of the 6th and 7th Editions of the UICC-AJCC TNM Classification for Esophageal Cancer. *Ann. Surg.Oncol* 2012;19 (7):2142-2148.

[40] Dikken JL, Van De Velde CJ, Gonen M, Verheij M, Brennan MF, Coit DG. The new American Joint Committee on Cancer/International Union against cancer staging

system for adenocarcinoma of the stomach: increased complexity without clear improvement in predictive accuracy. *Ann. Surg.Oncol.* 19(8):2443-2451, 2012.

[41] Hasegawa S, Yoshikawa T, Aoyama T, Hayashi T, Yamada T, Tsuchida K, Cho H, Oshima T, Yukawa N, Rino Y, Masuda M, Tsuburaya A. Esophagus or stomach? The seventh TNM classification for Siewert type II/III junction adenocarcinoma. *Ann. Surg. Oncol.* 2013;20(3):773-779.

[42] Herrmann K, Ott K, Buck AK, Lordick F, Wilhelm D, Souvatzoglou M, Becker K, Schuster T, Wester HJ, Siewert JR, Schwaiger M, Krause BJ. Imaging gastric cancer with PET and the radiotracers 18F-FLT and 18F-FDG: a comparative analysis. *J.Nucl. Med.* 2007;48(12):1945-1950.

[43] Choi J, Kim SG, Im JP, Kim JS, Jung HC, Song IS. Comparison of endoscopic ultrasonography and conventional endoscopy for prediction of depth of tumor invasion in early gastric cancer. *Endoscopy* 2010; 42(9):705-713.

[44] Ezoe Y. Muto M. Uedo N. Doyama H. Yao K. Oda I. Kaneko K. Kawahara Y. Yokoi C. Sugiura Y. Magnifying narrowband imaging is more accurate than conventional white-lite imaging in diagnosis of gastric mucosal cancer. *Gastroenterology* 2011; 141:2017- 2025.

[45] Nagahama T. Yao K. Maki S. Yasaka M. Takaki Y. Matsui T. Tanabe H. Iwashita A. Ota A. Usefulness of magnifying endoscopy with narrow-band imaging for determining the horizontal extent of early gastric cancer when there is an unclear margin by chromoendoscopy (with video) *Gastrointest. Endosc.* 2011; 74:1259- 1267.

[46] Hermanek P, Wittekind C. Residual tumor (R) classification and prognosis. Semin Surg Oncol. 1994;10(1):12-20.

[47] Japanese Gastric Cancer Association (JGCA). Japanese gastric cancer treatment guidelines 2010 (ver. 3) *Gastric. Cancer* 2011; 14: 113 -123.

[48] Ono H, Kondo H, Gotoda T, Shirao K, Yamaguchi H, Saito D, Hosokawa K, Shimoda T, and Yoshida S. Endoscopic mucosal resection for treatment of early gastric cancer. *Gut.* 2001; 48(2): 225–229.

[49] Kitano S. Shiraishi N. Uyama I. Sugihara K. Tanigawa N. Japanese Laparoscopic Surgery Study Group A multicenter study on oncologic outcome of laparoscopic gastrectomy for early cancer in Japan *Ann. Surg.* 2007; 245: 68- 72.

[50] Nagai E, Nakata K, Ohuchida K, Miyasaka Y, Shimizu S, Tanaka M. Laparoscopic total gastrectomy for remnant gastric cancer: feasibility study. *Surg Endosc.* 2014;28 (1): 289-296.

[51] Bonenkamp JJ, Hermans J, Sasako M, van de Velde CJ, Welvaart K, Songun I, Meyer S, Plukker JT, Van Elk P, Obertop H, Gouma DJ, van Lanschot JJ, Taat CW, de Graaf PW, von Meyenfeldt MF, Tilanus H; Dutch Gastric Cancer Group. Extended lymph-node dissection for gastric cancer. *N. Engl. J. Med.* 1999;340(12):908-914.

[52] Cuschieri A, Weeden S, Fielding J, Bancewicz J, Craven J, Joypaul V, Sydes M, Fayers P. Patient survival after D1 and D2 resection for gastric cancer: Long-term results of the MRC randomized surgical trial. Surgical Co-operative Group *Br. J. Cancer.* 1999; 79: 1522- 1530.

[53] Hartgrink HH, van de Velde CJ, Putter H, Bonenkamp JJ, Klein Kranenbarg E, Songun I, Welvaart K, van Krieken JH, Meijer S, Plukker JT. Extended lymph node dissection for gastric cancer: Who may benefit? Final results of the randomized Dutch Gastric Cancer Group Trial. *J. Clin. Oncol.* 2004; 22: 2069- 2077.

[54] Biffi R, Chiappa A, Luca F. Extended lymph node dissection without routine spleno-pancreatectomy for treatment of gastric cancer: low morbidity and mortality rates in a single center series of 250 patients. *J. Surg.Oncol.* 2006;93(5): 394–400.

[55] Songun I, Putter H, Kranenbarg EM, Sasako M, van de Velde CJ. Surgical treatment of gastric cancer: 15-year follow-up results of the randomized nationwide Dutch D1D2 trial. *Lancet Oncol.* 2010; 11(5):439-449.

[56] Takahashi T, Saikawa Y, Kitagawa Y. Gastric cancer: Current status of diagnosis and treatment. *Cancers.* 2013; 5: 48-63.

[57] Sasako M, Sano T, Yamamoto S, Kurokawa Y, Nashimoto A, Kurita A, Hiratsuka M, Tsujinaka T, Kinoshita T, Arai K. D2 lymphadenectomy alone or with para-aortic nodal dissection for gastric cancer. *N. Engl. J. Med.* 2008; 359: 453- 462.

[58] Macdonald JS, Smalley SR, Benedetti J, Hundahl SA, Estes NC, Stemmermann GN, Haller DG, Ajani JA, Gunderson LL, Jessup JM. Chemoradiotherapy after surgery compared with surgery alone for adenocarcinoma of the stomach or gastroesophageal junction. *N. Engl. J. Med.* 2001; 345: 725- 730.

[59] Smalley SR, Benedetti JK, Haller DG, Hundahl SA, Estes NC, Ajani JA, Gunderson LL, Goldman B, Martenson JA, Jessup JM, Stemmermann GN, Blanke CD, Macdonald JS. Updated analysis of SWOG-directed intergroup study 0116: a phase III trial of adjuvant radiochemotherapy versus observation after curative gastric cancer resection. *J. Clin. Oncol.* 2012 ;30(19):2327-33.

[60] Lee J, Lim DH, Kim S, Park SH, Park JO, Park YS, Lim HY, Choi MG, Sohn TS, Noh JH. Phase III trial comparing capecitabine plus cisplatin vesus capecitabine plus cisplatin with concurrent capecitabine radiotherapy in completely resected gastric cancer with D2 lymph node dissection: The ARTIST trial. *J. Clin. Oncol.* 2012;30(3): 268 -273.

[61] Fuches CS, Tepper JE, Niedzwiecki D, Hollis D, Mamon HJ, Swanson R, Haller DG, Dragovich T, Alberts SR, Bjarnason GA, Willett CG, Enzinger PC, Goldberg RM, Venook AP, Mayer RJ. Postoperative adjuvant chemoradiation for gastric or gastroesophageal junction (GEJ) adenocarcinoma using epirubicin, cisplatin and infusion (CI) 5-FU (ECF) before and after CI 5-FU and radiotherapy(CRT) compared with bolus 5-FU/LV before and after CRT: intergroup trial CALGB 80101. *J. Clin.Oncol.* 2011 ASCO annual meeting Abstracts. Vol 29, No.15_suppl, 2011:4003.

[62] Dikken J.L. van Sandick J.W. Mauritis Swellengrebel H.A. Lind P.A. Putter H. Jansen E.P. Boot H. van Grieken N.C. van de Velde C.J. Verheij M. Neo-adjuvant chemotherapy followed by surgery and chemotherapy or by surgery and chemoradiotherapy for patients with resectable gastric cancer (CRITICS). *BMC Cancer* 2011; 11: 329-334.

[63] Cunningham D, Allum WH, Stenning SP, Thompson JN, Van de Velde CJ, Nicolson M, Scarffe JH, Lofts FJ, Falk SJ, Iveson TJ, Smith DB, Langley RE, Verma M, Weeden S, Chua YJ, MAGIC Trial Participants. Perioperative chemotherapy versus surgery alone for resectable gastroesophageal cancer. *N. Engl. J. Med.* 2006; 355(1): 11- 20.

[64] Cascinu S, Scartozzi M, Labianca R, Catalano V, Silva RR, Barni S, Zaniboni A, D'Angelo A, Salvagni S, Martignoni G, Beretta GD, Graziano F, Berardi R, Franciosi V; Italian Group for the Study of Digestive Tract Cancer (GISCAD). High curative resection rate with weekly cisplatin, 5-fluorouracil, epidoxorubicin, 6S-leucovorin, glutathione and filgastrim in patients with locally advanced, unresectable gastric cancer:

a report from the Italian Group for the Study of Digestive Tract Cancer(GISCAD). *Br. J. Cancer* 2004; 90(8): 1521-1525.

[65] Cascinu S, Labianca R, Barone C, Santoro A, Carnaghi C, Cassano A, Beretta GD, Catalano V, Bertetto O, Barni S, Frontini L, Aitini E, Rota S, Torri V, Floriani I; Italian Group for the Study of Digestive Tract Cancer, Pozzo C, Rimassa L, Mosconi S, Giordani P, Ardizzoia A, Foa P, Rabbi C, Chiara S, Gasparini G, Nardi M, Mansutti M, Arnoldi E, Piazza E, Cortesi E, Pucci F, Silva RR, Sobrero A, Ravaioli A. Adjuvant treatment of high –risk, radically resected gastric cancer patients with 5- fluorouracil, leucovorin, cisplatin, and epidoxorubicin in a randomized controlled trial. *J. Natl. Cancer Inst.*2007; 99(8):601-607.

[66] Sakuramoto S, Sasako M, Yamaguchi T, Kinoshita T, Fujii M, Nashimoto A, Furukawa H, Nakajima T, Ohashi Y, Imamura H, Higashino M, Yamamura Y, Kurita A, Arai K; ACTS-GC Group. Adjuvant chemotherapy for gastric cancer with S-1, an oral fluoropyrimidine. *N. Engl. Med.* 2007; 357(18); 1810-1820.

[67] Sasako M, Sakuramoto S, Katai H, Kinoshita T, Furukawa H, Yamaguchi T, Nashimoto A, Fujii M, Nakajima T, Ohashi Y. Five-year outcome of a randomized phase III trial comparing adjuvant chemotherapy with S-1 verus surgery alone in stage II or III gastric cancer: *J. Clin.Oncol*2011; 29(33): 4387-4393.

[68] Bang YJ, Kim YW, Yang HK, Chung HC, Park YK, Lee KH, Lee KW, Kim YH, Noh SI, Cho JY, Mok YJ, Kim YH, Ji J, Yeh TS, Button P, Sirzén F, Noh SH. Adjuvant capecitabine and oxaliplatin for gastric cancer after D2 gastrectomy (CLIASSIC): a phase 3, open-label, randomized controlled trial. *Lancet* 2012:379(9813); 315-321.

[69] Paoletti X, Oba K, Burzykowski T, Michiels S, Ohashi Y, Pignon JP, Rougier P, Sakamoto J, Sargent D, Sasako M, Van Cutsem E, Buyse M. Benefit of adjuvant chemotherapy for resectable gastric cancer: a meta-analysis. *JAMA.* 2010; 303(17): 1729-1737.

[70] Bokemeyer CRK, Atanackovic D, Arnold D, Woell E, Büchler MW. Two-year follow-up of a phase II study on catumaxomab as part of a multimodal approach in primarily resectable gastric cancer. *J. Clin.Oncol.* 2012; 30: abstr #4095.

[71] Kang LY, Mok KT, Liu SI, Tsai CC, Wang BW, Chen IS, Chen YC, Chang BM, Chou NH. Intraoperative hyperthermic intraperitoneal chemotherapy as adjuvant chemotherapy for advanced gastric cancer patients with serosal invasion. *J. Chin. Med. Assoc.* 2013;76(8):425-431.

[72] Wagner AD, Grote W, Hearting J, Kleberg G, Grote A, Fleeing WE. Chemotherapy in advanced gastric cancer: a systemic review and meta-analysis based on aggregate data. *J. Clin.Oncol.* 2006; 24(18):2903-2909.

[73] Kang YK, Kang WK, Shin DB, Chen J, Xiong J, Wang J, Lichinitser M, Guan Z, Khasanov R, Zheng L, Philco-Salas M, Suarez T, Santamaria J, Forster G, McCloud PI. Capecitabine/cisplatin versus 5-fluorouracil/cisplatin as first-line therapy in patients with advanced gastric cancer: A randomised phase III noninferiority trial. *Ann. Oncol.* 2009; 20(4): 666- 673.

[74] Koizumi W, Narahara H, Hara T, Takagane A, Akiya T, Takagi M, Miyashita K, Nishizaki T, Kobayashi O, Takiyama W, Toh Y, Nagaie T, Takagi S, Yamamura Y, Yanaoka K, Orita H, Takeuchi M. S-1 plus cisplatin versus S-1 alone for first-line treatment of advanced gastric cancer (SPIRITS trial): A phase III trial. *Lancet Oncol.* 2008; 9(3) :215 -221.

[75] Ajani JA, Rodriguez W, Bodoky G, Moiseyenko V, Lichinitser M, Gorbunova V, Vynnychenko I, Garin A, Lang I, Falcon S. Multicenter phase III comparison of cisplatin/S-1 with cisplatin/infusional fluorouracil in advanced gastric or gastroesophageal adenocarcinoma study: The FLAGS trial. *J. Clin. Oncol*. 2010; 28: 1547- 1553.

[76] Van Cutsem E, Moiseyenko VM, Tjulandin S, Majlis A, Constenla M, Boni C, Rodrigues A, Fodor M, Chao Y, Voznyi E, Risse ML, Ajani JA. Phase III study of docetaxel and cisplatin plus fluorouracil compared with cisplatin and fluorouracil as first-line therapy for advanced gastric cancer: a report of the V325 Study Group. *J. Clin.Oncol.* 2006;24(31):4991-4997.

[77] Cunningham D, Starling N, Rao S, Iveson T, Nicolson M, Coxon F, Middleton G, Daniel F, Oates J, Norman AR. Capecitabine and oxaliplatin for advanced esophagogastric cancer. *N. Engl. J. Med*. 2008; 358(1): 36 -46.

[78] Dank M, Zaluski J, Barone C, Valvere V, Yalcin S, Peschel C, Wenczl M, Goker E, Cisar L, Wang K, Bugat R. Randomized phase III study comparing irinotecan combined 5-fluororacil and folinic acid to cisplatin combined with 5-fluororacil in chemotherapy naïve patients with advanced adenocarcinoma of the stomach or esophagogastric junction. *Ann.Oncol.*2008; 19(8): 1450-1457.

[79] Park SH, Lim DH, Park K. A multicenter, randomized phase III trial comparing second-line chemotherapy(SLC) plus best supportive care(BSC) with BCS alone for pretreated advanced gastric cancer(AGC). *J. Clin.Oncol. ASCO Annual Meeting*, 2011; Vol 29, Abstract# 4004.

[80] Thuss-Patience PC, Kretzschmar A, Bichev D, Deist T, Hinke A, Breithaupt K, Dogan Y, Gebauer B, Schumacher G, Reichardt P. Survival advantage for irinotecan versus best supportive care as second-line chemotherapy in gastric cancer-A randomized phase III study of the Arbeitsgemeinschaft Internistische Onkologie (AIO) . *Eur. J. Cancer.* 2011; 47(15): 2306-2314.

[81] Taal BG, Teller FG, ten Bokkel Huinink WW, Boot H, Beijnen JH, Dubbelman R. Etoposide, leucovorin, 5-fluororacil (ELF) combination chemotherapy for advanced gastric cancer: experience with two treatment schedules incorpotating intravenous or oral etoposide. *Ann.Oncol.*1994; 5(1):90-92.

[82] Kang JH, Lee SI, Lim do H, Park KW, Oh SY, Kwon HC, Hwang IG, Lee SC, Nam E, Shin DB, Lee J, Park JO, Park YS, Lim HY, Kang WK, Park SH. Salvage chemotherapy for pretreated gastric cancer: a randomized phase III trial comparing chemotherapy plus best supportive care with best supportive care alone. *J. Clin.Oncol.* 2012;30(13):1513-1518.

[83] Kim HS, Kim HJ, Kim SY, Kim TY, Lee KW, Baek SK, Kim TY, Ryu MH, Nam BH, Zang DY. Second-line chemotherapy versus supportive cancer treatment in advanced gastric cancer: a meta-analysis. *Ann.Oncol.* 2013;24(11):2850-2854.

[84] Terashima M, Kitada K, Ochiai A, Ichikawa W, Kurahashi I, Sakuramoto S, Katai H, Sano T, Imamura H, Sasako M. Impact of expression of human epidermal growth factor receptors EGFR and ERBB2 on survival in Stage II/III gastric cancer. *Clin. Cancer Res.* 2012;18: 5992- 6000.

[85] Janjigian YY, Werner D, Pauligk C, Steinmetz K, Kelsen DP, Jäger E, Altmannsberger HM, Robinson E, Tafe LJ, Tang LH, Shah MA, Al-Batran SE. Prognosis of metastatic

gastric and gastroesophageal junction cancer by HER2 status: A European and USA international collaborative analysis. *Ann. Oncol.* 2012; 23(10): 2656 -2662.

[86] Bang YJ, Van Cutsem E, Feyereislova A, Chung HC, Shen L, Sawaki A, Lordick F, Ohtsu A, Omuro Y, Satoh T, Aprile G, Kulikov E, Hill J, Lehle M, Rüschoff J, Kang YK; ToGATrial Investigators. Trastuzumab in combination with chemotherapy versus chemotherapy alone for treatment of HER2-positive advanced gastric or gastro-oesophageal junction cancer (ToGA): A phase 3, open label, randomised controlled trial. *Lancet.* 2010; 376(9742): 687- 697.

[87] Chau I, Okines AF, Castro DG, Saffery Y, Barbachano A, Wotherspoon L, Puckey S, Hulkki Wilson FY, Coxon GW, Middleton DR. REAL3: A multicenter randomized phase II/III trial of epirubicin, oxaliplatin, and capecitabine (EOC) versus modified (m) EOC plus panitumumab (P) in advanced oesophagogastric (OG) cancer—Response rate (RR), toxicity, and molecular analysis from phase II. *J. Clin. Oncol. ASCO Annual Meeting*, 2011, Vol 29.

[88] Lordick F, Kang YK, Chung HC, Salman P, Oh SC, Bodoky G, Kurteva G, Volovat C, Moiseyenko VM, Gorbunova V, Park JO, Sawaki A, Celik I, Götte H, Melezínková H, Moehler M. Capecitabine and cisplatin with or without cetuximab for patients with previously untreated advanced gastric cancer (EXPAND): a randomised, open-label phase 3 trial. *Lancet Oncol.* 2013;14(6):490-9.

[89] Ohtsu A, Shah MA, van Cutsem E, Rha SY, Sawaki A, Park SR, Lim HY, Yamada Y, Wu J, Langer B. Bevacizumab in combination with chemotherapy as first-line therapy in advanced gastric cancer: A randomized, double-blind, placebo-controlled phase III study. *J. Clin.Oncol.* 2011; 29(30): 3968- 3976.

[90] Fuchs CS, Tomasek J, Cho JY, Dumitru F, Passalacqua R, Goswami C, Safran H, Vieira dos Santos L, Aprile G, Ferry DR, Melichar B, TehfeM, Topuzov E, Tabernero J, Zalcberg JR, Chau I, Koshiji M, Hsu Y, Schwartz JD, Ajani JA. Ramucirumab monotherapy for previously treated advanced gastric or gastro-oesophageal junction adenocarcinoma (REGARD): an international, randomized, multicenter, placebo-controlled, phase 3 trial. *Lancet.* 2014; 383 (9911):31-39.

[91] Zhang ZX, Gu XZ, Yin WB, Huang GJ, Zhang DW, Zhang RG. Randomized clinical trial on the combination of preoperative irradiation and surgery in the treatment of adenocarcinoma of gastric cardia (AGC)--report on 370 patients. *Int. J.Radiat.Oncol. Biol. Phys.* 1998;42(5):929-934.

[92] Childs DS Jr, Moertel CG, Holbrook MA, Reitemeier RJ, Colby M Jr. Treatment of unresectable adenocarcinomas of the stomach with a combination of 5-fluorouracil and radiation. *Am. J.Roentgenol. Radium Ther.Nucl. Med.* 1968; 102(3) :541- 544.

[93] Falkson G. Falkson H.C. Fluorouracil and radiotherapy in gastrointestinal cancer *Lancet.* 1969;2: 1252- 125.

[94] Yoshikawa T, Tsuburaya A, Hirabayashi N, Yoshida K, Nagata N, Kodera Y, Takahashi N, Oba K, Kimura M, Ishikura S. A phase I study of palliative chemoradiation therapy with paclitaxel and cisplatin for local symptoms due to an unresectable primary advanced or locally recurrent gastric adenocarcinoma. *Cancer Chemother. Pharmacol.* 2009; 64:1071-1077.

[95] Hashimoto K, Mayahara H, Takashima A, Nakajima TE, Kato K, Hamaguchi T, Ito Y, Yamada Y, Kagami Y, Itami J. Palliative radiation therapy for hemorrhage of

unresectable gastric cancer: A single institute experience. *J. Cancer Res.Clin.Oncol.* 2009; 135:1117-1123.

[96] Klaassen DJ, MacIntyre JM, Catton GE, Engstrom PF, Moertel CG. Treatment of locally unresectable cancer of the stomach and pancreas: A randomized comparison of 5-fluorouracil alone with radiation plus concurrent and maintenance 5-fluorouracil—An Eastern Cooperative Oncology Group Study. *J. Clin.Oncol.* 1985; 3:373- 378.

In: Gastric Cancer
Editor: Jasneet Singh Bhullar

ISBN: 978-1-63117-983-9
© 2014 Nova Science Publishers, Inc.

Chapter 3

Gastric Cancer Staging

Matthew Dixon[1,] Abraham El-Sedfy[2] and Natalie Coburn[3]
[1]Department of Surgery, Maimonides Medical Center, Brooklyn, NY, US
[2]Department of Surgery, Saint Barnabas Medical Center, Livingston, NJ, US
[3]Department of Surgery, University of Toronto, Toronto, Ontario, Canada

Abstract

Worldwide, gastric adenocarcinoma is one of the most commonly found malignancies, and one of the most common causes of cancer-related death. Although adjuvant therapies have improved survival, resection remains the fundamental curative option for gastric cancer patients. Accurate staging forms the basis for which treatments are selected. An understanding of the staging systems commonly used is important for physicians involved in the treatment of gastric cancer. In addition, several staging modalities are routinely prescribed in an attempt to accurately stage the patient with gastric cancer. Each of these staging modalities has their own benefits and drawbacks with varying degrees of accuracy, sensitivity and specificity. The following staging modalities will be reviewed in detail: computed tomography, magnetic resonance imaging, abdominal ultrasound, [18]Fluorodeoxyglucose-positron emission tomography, esophagogastroduodenoscopy, endoscopic ultrasound, staging laparoscopy, peritoneal cytology and sentinel lymph node biopsy. The ultimate goal is correlation between staging modalities and pathology findings such that accurate staging is performed with delivery of the most appropriate stage-specific treatment.

Introduction

Curative treatment of gastric adenocarcinoma requires surgical or endoscopic resection. In recent years, the addition of adjuvant therapies has demonstrated an improvement in overall survival [1-4], but this has increased the complexity of clinical decision-making. Management decisions for the treatment of gastric cancer by a multidisciplinary team are stage-specific and thus rely heavily on accurate staging.

Inappropriate pre-operative evaluation and planning could potentially lead to under-staging, resulting in positive resection margins, or an unnecessary laparotomy for patients with incurable disease. It is also possible for patients to be over-staged, leading to the unfortunate circumstance of a potentially curative patient being incorrectly recommended for palliation, rather than surgical resection.

Staging Systems

Two staging systems for gastric cancer have been proposed: the Tumor-Node-Metastasis (TNM) staging system outlined by the Union Internationale Contre le Cancer (UICC) / American Joint Committee on Cancer (AJCC) [5] and the Japanese classification of gastric cancer as defined by the Japanese Gastric Cancer Association (JGCA) [6]. The two systems are similar, as they both describe the depth of the primary tumor invasion, the extent of lymph node (LN) involvement, and the presence or absence of distant metastasis.

UICC/AJCC T Stage

The T component of the TNM staging system corresponds to the depth of tumor invasion within the corresponding organ. The deeper the tumor invades into the wall of the organ, the higher the T stage assigned.

In the updated 7th edition of the AJCC staging manual, the T categories for gastric cancer have been modified to be consistent with those corresponding to cancers of the esophagus, small intestine and large intestine.

A stage of T0 is assigned when there is no evidence of a primary tumor. Carcinoma in situ, which is denoted by Tis, represents pathology demonstrating malignant cells which have not yet violated the basement membrane of the mucosa. Any tumor greater than Tis has violated the basement membrane and is considered to be a malignant lesion. T1a lesions are confined to the mucosa, while T1b lesions have invaded through the mucosa into the submucosa. It can be important to differentiate between T1a and T1b lesions, as some T1a lesions may be amenable to endoscopic resection. From a series of 1549 cases of surgically resected patients, the median 5-year survival of patients with T1a and T1b lesions are 90.2% and 86.7%, respectively [7]. (Figure 1) When a cancer invades through the submucosa and into the muscularis propria, it is classified as a T2 lesion. The median 5-year survival of patients with these lesions is 75.2% [7]. T3 lesions invade the subserosa, but do not invade the serosa or any of the structures adjacent to the stomach. The median 5-year survival of these patients is 54.9% [7]. T4 lesions, the highest classification assigned, are split into two subcategories. T4a lesions invade through the serosa and are exposed to the peritoneal cavity. T4b lesions are cancers that not only invade through the serosa, but invade adjacent structures as well. The 5-year survival of patients with T4a and T4b lesions are 31.1% and 17.5%, respectively [7]. (Figure 1).

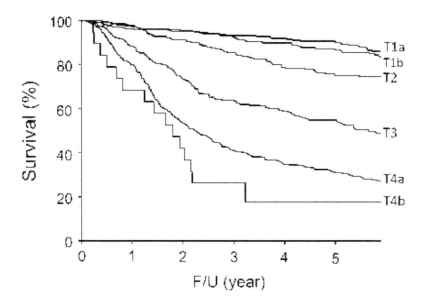

Figure 1. Kaplan-Meier curve of 5-year survival of patients with gastric cancer by T-stage. (From Fang WL, Huang KH, et al., *World J. Surg.* 2011; 35(12):2723-9).

Table 1. T staging of gastric cancer

T Stage	Description
TX	The primary tumor is not feasible
T0	No evidence of a primary tumor
Tis	Carcinoma in situ
T1	Tumor invasion of the lamina propria, muscularis mucosa, or submucosa
	T1a: Tumor invasion of the lamina propria or muscularis mucosa
	T1b: Tumor invasion of the submucosa
T2	Tumor invasion of the muscularis propria
T3	Tumor penetration of the subserosal connective tissue without evidence of visceral peritoneum or adjacent structures
T4	Tumor invasion of serosa or adjacent structures
	T4a: Tumor invasion of serosa
	T4b: Tumor invasion of adjacent structures

Knowledge of a tumor being classified as T4b can be crucial in pre-operative planning, as these lesions may require a multivisceral resection. For example, if a tumor is found to be invading the pancreas or colon, then en-bloc resection will be necessary for curative intent [8]. Survival in these advanced cases is also influenced by burden of LN involvement, thus in these cases of advanced disease, a neoadjuvant approach may be considered by the multidisciplinary team.

UICC/AJCC N Stage

The N component of the TNM staging system corresponds to the degree to which LN harbor gastric cancer. Nodal status is one of the most important prognostic indicators in many cancers, including gastric cancer.

Over the years, the UICC/AJCC have evolved their classification system for N staging in gastric cancer. Prior to 1997, nodal staging was based upon the distance from involved LN to the primary cancer. In their fifth edition, in order to improve the ability to reliably compare nodal stage between series/institutions, to align the staging of gastric cancer to that of other gastrointestinal malignancies, and to minimize the impact of surgical dissection on staging accuracy, the AJCC/UICC recommended that N stage be based upon the number of LNs involved. They recommended a minimum assessment of 15 LN with N1 = 1–6 positive LN; N2 = 7–15 positive LN; and N3 = more than 15 positive LN. The cut-points were derived from retrospective databases [9]. Subsequent examinations [10, 11] have demonstrated the superior predictive ability of LN staging based on number of nodes involved rather than location of nodal involvement [12]. Part of the superior predictive ability has been attributed to the category N3 (>15 LN positive), a group with extremely poor prognosis. In the 7th edition, the UICC/AJCC revised the nodal classification system such that N1 = 1–2 positive LNs; N2 = 3-6 positive LN; N3a = 7-15 positive LN; and N3b = 16 or more positive LN [13]. 5-year survival rates based on N-stage have also been defined. N0 disease has a 5-year survival of 83.5%; 57.8% for N1; 27.4% for N2, and 11.4% for N3 disease [7]. (Figure 2).

As such, the UICC/AJCC now recommends that a minimum of 16 LN be assessed for accurate nodal staging [14]. Unfortunately, if an inadequate number of LN are assessed, significant stage migration can occur [13, 15]. An appropriately performed resection should yield enough LN for adequate staging, as an average of 15 LN can be harvested from a D1 lymphadenectomy, 27 nodes from a D2 lymphadenectomy, and 43 nodes from a D3 lymphadenectomy [15]. A D0 lymphadenectomy, an incomplete dissection of N1 level LN, is inadequate for staging.

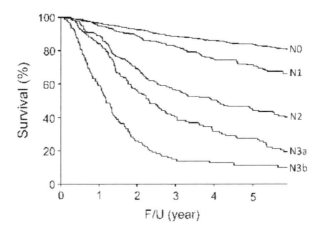

Figure 2. Kaplan-Meier curve of 5-year survival of patients with gastric cancer by N-stage. (From Fang WL, Huang KH, et al., *World J. Surg.* 2011; 35(12):2723-9).

There is a strong correlation between T and N stages. In patients with disease that is limited to the mucosa (i.e., T1a lesions), there is an approximate 3-5% risk of LN involvement. This risk increases to 11-25% in cases where disease is limited to the submucosa (i.e., T1b lesions). More advanced cancers have a substantial increase in risk of LN involvement, with T2 tumors having a risk of 50%, while T3 tumors have an 83% risk of involvement [16-18]. This can be attributed, in part, to the complex lymphatic system of the stomach, which freely communicates with other equally complex intermuscular and subserosal lymphatic networks [19, 20].

UICC/AJCC M Stage

The M component of the TNM staging system corresponds to the presence of any distant metastases, and is denoted by M1. M stage is highly predictive of patient survival. While the 5-year survival of patients with metastatic disease is 7%, those without evidence of metastatic disease have an estimated 5-year survival of up to 78% [21]. Unfortunately, over 30% of patients will have evidence of metastatic disease at presentation [22]. Common manifestations of distant metastases include the presence of liver metastases, ascites, carcinomatosis (diffuse peritoneal metastases), Blummer shelf (palpable mass on rectal examination secondary to drop metastases into the pelvis), Virchow node (palpable supraclavicular LN), or Sister Mary Joseph node (palpable periumbilical mass) [23, 24].

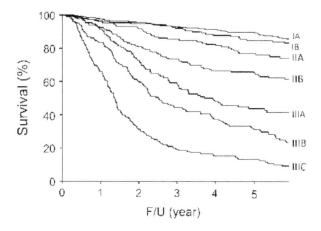

Figure 3. Kaplan-Meier curve of 5-year survival of patients with gastric cancer by Stage. (From Fang WL, Huang KH, et al., *World J. Surg.* 2011; 35(12):2723-9).

All of the possible combinations of T, N, and M status have been organized into different stages of disease; stage I disease represents the earliest malignant disease, while stage IV represents metastatic spread. Updates to the 7th edition of the UICC/AJCC staging system include the splitting of stage II disease into stage IIA and stage IIB, and the addition of stage IIIC. Additionally, all TNM stages now considered to be stage IIB were previously classified as stage IIIA, with the exception of T1N3M0, which was previously considered to be stage IV disease.

In the previous edition of the UICC/AJCC staging manual, N3 disease was considered to represent stage IV disease, regardless of T or M stage. This is no longer the case, as now only patients with distant nodal or visceral metastases are considered to have stage IV disease [5]. Figure 3 shows the 5-year survival of patients by each stage with the exception of stage IV [7].

Japanese Gastric Cancer Association Staging Classification

The Japanese Gastric Cancer Association (JGCA) updated their staging classification system in 2011 with the release of the 3rd edition [6], which is very similar to the 7th edition of the UICC/AJCC.

However, the JGCA classification system offers more detailed descriptions of the cancer than the TNM staging system. The primary tumor is described in the JGCA by six characteristics: (1) size and number of lesions, (2) tumor location, (3) macroscopic types, (4) histological classification, (5) depth of tumor invasion, and (6) cancer stromal volume, infiltrative pattern, and capillary invasion.

For the size and number of lesions, the tumor is described in its two greatest dimensions. If there are multiple lesions, then the largest of the lesions is classified.

In describing the tumor's location, the stomach is anatomically divided into three areas: the upper (U), middle (M) and lower (L) portions. Gastric cancers are then described by the area of the stomach involved by tumor. In cases where the tumor involves more than one portion of the stomach, those portions are described in descending order of the degree of involvement, with the portion containing most of the tumor described first.

For example, if tumor on the lesser curvature involves the upper and middle portions of the stomach, and most of the tumor is in the middle portion of the stomach, then it is described as MU. The macroscopic type describes the tumor by its appearance, and whether it has an infiltrative or an ulcerative pattern of growth, or a combination of both (Table 5).

Table 2. N staging of gastric cancer

N stage	Description
NX	Regional lymph nodes cannot be assessed
N0	No evidence of lymph node metastases
N1	Metastases in ≤ 2 regional lymph nodes
N2	Metastases in 3-6 regional lymph nodes
N3	Metastases in ≥ 7 regional lymph nodes
	N3a : Metastases in 7-15 regional lymph nodes
	N3b : Metastases in 16 or more regional lymph nodes

Table 3. M staging of gastric cancer

M stage	Description
M0	No evidence of metastases
M1	Evidence of distant metastases

Table 4. TNM staging system of gastric cancer

Stage	T stage	N stage	M stage
Stage 0	Tis	N0	M0
Stage IA	T1	N0	M0
Stage IB	T2	N0	M0
	T1	N1	M0
Stage IIA	T3	N0	M0
	T2	N1	M0
	T1	N2	M0
Stage IIB	T4a	N0	M0
	T3	N1	M0
	T2	N2	M0
	T1	N3	M0
Stage IIIA	T4a	N1	M0
	T3	N2	M0
	T2	N3	M0
Stage IIIB	T4b	N0	M0
	T4b	N1	M0
	T4a	N2	M0
	T3	N3	M0
Stage IIIC	T4b	N2	M0
	T4b	N3	M0
	T4a	N3	M0
Stage IV	Any T	Any N	M1

Table 5. Macroscopic types of gastric cancer

Type	Description
Type 0 (superficial)	Typical of T1 tumor
Type 1 (mass)	Polypoid tumor with sharp demarcation from surrounding mucosa
Type 2 (ulcerative)	Ulcerated tumor with raised margins; surrounded by thickened gastric wall; clear margins
Type 3 (infiltrative ulcerative)	Ulcerated tumor with raised margins; surrounded by thickened gastric wall; unclear margins
Type 4 (diffuse infiltrative)	Marked ulceration or raised margins; gastric wall is thickened and indurated; unclear margin
Type 5 (unclassifiable)	Tumor cannot be classified

For the histological classification system, if there is more than one subtype, the different components are recorded in descending order of the amount of surface area occupied. Additionally, tumors are described by stromal volume, infiltrative pattern and capillary invasion. Stromal volume must be recorded for tumors whose depth of invasion is deeper than T1b and is classified by being medullary (containing scanty stroma), scirrhous (containing abundant stroma) or intermediate type.

Table 6. Tumor infiltrative (INF) pattern into surrounding tissues

Type	Description
INFa	Expanding growth with distinct border from surrounding tissue
INFb	Intermediate pattern between INFa and INFc
INFc	Infiltrative growth with no distinct border with surrounding tissue

Table 7. Lymphatic invasion pattern by gastric tumors

Type	Description
ly0	No lymphatic invasion
ly1	Minimal lymphatic invasion
ly2	Moderate lymphatic invasion
ly3	Marked lymphatic invasion

Table 8. Venous invasion pattern by gastric tumors

Type	Description
v0	No venous invasion
v1	Minimal venous invasion
v2	Moderate venous invasion
v3	Marked venous invasion

Tables 6, 7 and 8 summarize the classification schemes for infiltrative pattern, lymphatic invasion and venous invasion, respectively.

With recent changes, the depth of tumor invasion follows the T staging from the 7th edition of the UICC/AJCC, as outlined in Table 1. The 2nd edition of JGCA described tumor depth of invasion from T1 to T4 without any sub-classification [9]. Thus, differences between the 2nd and 3rd JGCA classifications system include expansion of T1 lesions into T1a and T1b lesions, as well as expansion of T4 lesions into T4a and T4b.

The evolution of the JGCA classification system from the 2nd to the 3rd edition has seen an abandonment of the classification of LN metastases based on anatomic location, and adoption of classification of LN metastases based on the number of involved nodes [6, 9]. The 2nd edition of the JCGA system classified LN involvement with respect to anatomic location of the primary tumor. N1 disease was metastases to group 1 nodes, which refer to perigastric nodes. N2 disease was classified as metastases to group 2 nodes, which refer to the nodes along the celiac axis and its branches. Finally, N3 disease was classified as involvement of group 3 nodes, which refer to retropancreatic or para-aortic nodes. Description of N stage by the JGCA currently follows the 7th edition of the UICC/AJCC staging manual (Table 2). Description of M stage by the JGCA classification system also follows the 7th edition of the UICC/AJCC staging manual, as outlined in Table 3. They further sub-classify metastases based on three locations: peritoneal metastases, positive peritoneal cytology, and hepatic metastases. Finally, definition of disease stage is the same as the 7th edition of the UICC/AJCC staging manual (Table 4).

Summary of Staging Systems

Pre-operative staging allows clinicians to stratify patients as early gastric cancer (EGC) or advanced gastric cancer (AGC) and influences the type of resection planned. For EGC staging, the JGCA classification system's increased granularity is very important in Asia, as endoscopic and limited resections are more often employed. In addition, pre-operative confirmation of M stage in gastric cancer is a necessary and important component of staging.

The presence of distant metastases has important implications on treatment. While patients without evidence of metastatic disease should undergo curative-intent resection and possibly adjuvant therapy, patients with M1 disease should be referred for systemic chemotherapy, clinical trial enrollment, best supportive care or palliative treatments if symptomatic [25].

Radiology and Pre-Operative Staging

The management and treatment of gastric cancer is complex and resource intensive [26]. Once the diagnosis of gastric cancer is confirmed on esophagogastroduodenoscopy (EGD), accurate staging of tumor depth (T), regional lymph node (LN) involvement (N) and distant metastases (M) form the basis of treatment planning. This clinical baseline stage provides clinicians with information required to establish treatment strategies. Clinical staging accuracy has greatly improved, secondary to the refinement of several diagnostic technologies for pre-operative evaluation, including computed tomography (CT), magnetic resonance imaging (MRI), positron emission tomography (PET), abdominal ultrasound (AUS), endoscopic ultrasound (EUS) and staging laparoscopy [27-29]. Several published guidelines represent careful and systematic investigation of the latest literature resulting in rational, evidence based recommendations [30-33].

It is believed that standardization of staging and pre-operative workup may lead to improved outcomes by improving accuracy in pre-operative staging, resulting in a decrease of margin-positive resection rates, a decrease in unnecessary laparotomies and a decrease in peri-operative mortality [26, 34].

Computed Tomography

The computed tomography (CT) scan (Figure 4) is the standard non-invasive imaging modality used in the pre-operative staging of the gastric cancer patient. Although limited in accuracy of determination of T stage [35], it is a powerful tool for examining LN involvement, ascites, pelvic involvement, liver metastases and peritoneal dissemination.

Drawbacks of CT include exposure to ionizing radiation and iodine-based intravenous contrast agents, which can potentially result in contrast-induced nephropathy or anaphylaxis [36].

Importantly, there are considerable differences among CT scanners. Traditional single detection CT scanners are limited by large section thickness, low image resolution, and slow scanning, which lead to respiratory motion artifacts. Additionally, traditional CT scanners are unable to provide multi-planar reformations [37, 38], which can be especially useful when planning an operative approach.

MDCT has improved the speed at which images are acquired (which minimizes or eliminates respiratory motion artifact) [38], and allows for more accurate timing of contrast boluses during arterial, venous or parenchymal phases [28]. MDCT also has improved the spatial resolution and quality of the multi-planar reformation images, allowing the radiologist to choose the optimal imaging plane in which to accurately evaluate tumor depth of invasion of the gastric wall and perigastric fat plane infiltration [37]. Distention of the gastric wall with water or other low attenuation agents and intravenous contrast injection are required for optimal imaging [28]. MDCT has an overall accuracy of T stage determination of 80% [35]. With multi-planar reformation images, this increases to 82% [35].

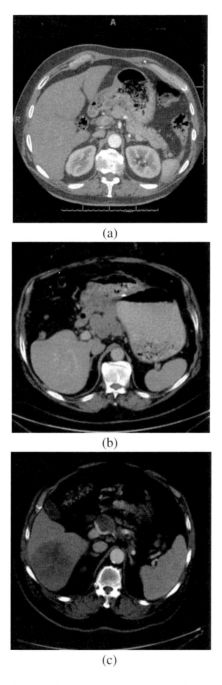

Figure 4. (a) CT Abdomen showing gastric cancer (Stage IIA) involving the antrum. (Figure courtesy of Dr. John Hagen, University of Toronto); (b) CT Abdomen demonstrating invasion of the neck of the pancreas. (Figure courtesy of Dr. Caitlin McGregor, University of Toronto); (c) CT Abdomen demonstrating liver metastases (Figure courtesy of Dr. Caitlin McGregor, University of Toronto).

Determination of N stage with CT, while important, also suffers from low accuracy. The ability of many imaging modalities to detect potentially metastatic nodes is determined primarily by the size of the nodes [39]. It should be noted that not all tumor positive LN are enlarged [40]. Similarly, not all enlarged LN contain metastases [41], making accuracy of N staging suboptimal with any modality that evaluates primarily based upon size or shape criteria, including CT, ultrasound, or MRI. Most studies examining the utility of CT scan in diagnosing nodal involvement define it as enlarged LN, with heterogeneity of the definition, ranging from >6mm to >1cm [37]. Correlation of LN metastases with LN shape has also been examined. Irregularly shaped LN have been suggested to have a higher risk of malignancy than consistently shaped nodes. However, most benign and malignant appearing LN were round in shape, thus the shape of the LN does not often allow for correct differentiation between benign and malignant nodes [42, 43]. The reported sensitivities and specificities for determining nodal involvement range from 50 to 95% and 40 to 99%, respectively. Typically, specificity is higher than sensitivity for nodal involvement, but this is not consistent between studies [44, 45]. A recent meta-analysis by our group found MDCT with multi-planar reformation images has the highest overall accuracy in predicting LN status (71%) [35]. Inaccuracies in true nodal status make pre-operative determination of disease spread difficult and must be taken into account in reports of pre-operative staging for neoadjuvant and peri-operative therapies and treatment decision-making.

CT scan is perhaps most useful in the determination of M stage, allowing examination of the entire abdomen and evaluation for the presence of metastases to the liver, viscera, distant LN and malignant ascites. The addition of CT scan of the pelvis allows for the evaluation of drop metastases into the pelvis, as well as the presence of Krukenberg tumors in the ovaries. The accuracy of demonstrating metastases on a CT scan is 81.2%, with sensitivity of 71.8% to 88.9% and specificity of 82.6% to 100% [35]. CT evaluation of the chest may also play a role in the staging of some patients. For gastroesophageal junction cancers, a CT chest is important for full evaluation of local disease, and surgical planning of esophagogastrectomy. CT chest is also useful for examining mediastinal lymphadenopathy and pulmonary metastases. The incidence of lung metastases is infrequent, ranging from 0.5 to 16% in reported series [46]. Therefore, routine use of CT chest in the staging of gastric cancer is not specifically advocated by all guidelines [31-33].

Several published practice guidelines advocate for the use of CT scans in the preoperative evaluation of patients with gastric cancer. Guidelines from the Association of Upper Gastrointestinal Surgeons of Great Britain and Ireland (AUGIS)/British Gastroenterology Society (BGS) [32] recommend that initial staging should be performed with a CT including multi-planar reformation images of the thorax, abdomen and pelvis to determine the presence of metastatic disease.

The European Society Medical Oncology/World Congress Gastrointestinal Cancer (ESMO/WCGIC) 2010 meeting [33] concluded that CT scan is the method of choice for evaluation of local extension and distant metastases. Guidelines from the Scottish Intercollegiate Guidelines Network (SIGN) [47] recommend that CT chest and abdomen with IV contrast and gastric distention with oral contrast or water be performed routinely, and that the liver should be evaluated in the portal venous phase for any metastases. Finally, the National Comprehensive Cancer Network (NCCN) [31] has recommended CT chest and abdomen be a part of the work-up for the patient suspected of harboring gastric cancer, and CT pelvis in those where it is clinically indicated.

Although imperfect in terms of accuracy, CT scans are crucial in pre-operative staging. CT scans of the abdomen should be obtained in order to evaluate local disease, while CT scans of the chest and pelvis can give important information about distant metastases.

Positron Emission Tomography

[18]Fluorodeoxyglucose-positron-emission tomography (FDG-PET) scans have found a role in the staging of many cancers and have evolved as a promising metabolic imaging modality for demonstrating tumor morphology and pathological metabolic activity. This imaging modality takes advantage of the fact that tumor cells, which have uncontrolled growth and division, are generally a metabolically active tissue, with their primary energy source being glucose. FDG, a radioactive detector molecule, is injected, phosphorylated by hexokinase, and then metabolized through normal aerobic respiration. In general, highly metabolically active cancer cells concentrate more FDG than normal tissues.

The PET scanner detects pairs of gamma rays emitted by the [18]Fluoride isotope, and uses a semi-quantitative method, the standardized uptake value (SUV), to assess the uptake of FDG and localize the tumor [48]. When these tumor cells are located in tissues whose cells have a lower metabolic activity, FDG-PET (Figure 5) allows imaging based on the altered glucose metabolism in these tumor cells, and distinguishes the tumor from normal tissue. In tissues such as the brain and heart, which are highly metabolically active, it is difficult to adequately distinguish the tumor from the surrounding normal tissue. FDG-PET scans appear to have decreased diagnostic accuracy for gastric cancer compared to CT imaging. Unfortunately, the number of studies examining the use of FDG-PET in preoperative staging is small with low patient accrual. Dassen and colleagues (2009) review of the role of FDG-PET revealed that tumor location, tumor size and gastric cancer histological type are determinants that influenced sensitivity and specificity [41].

The overall accuracy with which FDG-PET can detect a primary GC ranges between 58.1% and 95.9% [45, 49-53] with a pooled overall primary tumor detection rate of 80% [35]. FDG-PET has a poorer accuracy for detecting earlier stage gastric cancers (26-63%) in comparison to advanced gastric cancers (83-100%) [45, 51, 53]. Detection of early gastric carcinomas by FDG-PET can be complicated by background signaling secondary to high physiological uptake of FDG by the normal gastric wall [41].

There is also variability in the ability of FDG-PET to detect the various histological subtypes. Overall accuracy for detecting intestinal type ranges from 65.5-83%, non-intestinal type 41-79% [50-52], poorly differentiated adenocarcinomas 61.5%-79% and signet ring cell carcinoma 0-78% [50, 51]. This reflects the variable metabolic utilization of the subtypes and appears to be directly related to over-expression of the glucose transporter-1 (GLUT-1) transmembrane transporter protein [41]. FDG-PET cannot differentiate depth of invasion, and thus cannot assign T stages [48]. As with N-staging for CT scan, FDG-PET leaves much to be desired with an overall accuracy of 60%, and a sensitivity of 40% for detecting N+ disease. In patients with large or advanced cancers, enhancement of local LN may be obscured by a stronger signal from the primary [54]. However, the specificity of FDG-PET scans for N-staging is 98% [35], the highest of any imaging modality, suggesting that FDG-PET may find a role in clarifying true nodal positivity in pre-operative planning. M staging by FDG-PET boasts an overall accuracy of 75.5% to 100% [45, 55, 56], which is comparable to CT scan. Some authors suggest that, for the detection and confirmation of solid organ and distant metastases, FDG-PET may be a superior modality. One study found that FDG-PET had a higher sensitivity (90% (95% CI: 80-97%)) than U/S, CT or MRI for detecting hepatic metastases in a series of mixed gastrointestinal malignancies, including gastric cancer [57]. However, another study of only gastric cancer patients reported that the sensitivity and specificity of FDG-PET were 85% and 74%, respectively for liver metastases, and 67% and 88% for lung metastasis [58].

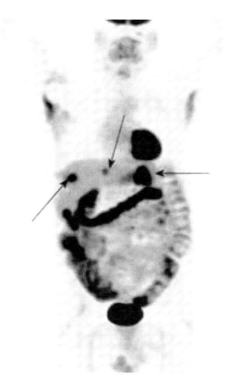

Figure 5. FDG-PET scan demonstrating proximal gastric cancer with liver metastasis. (From Smyth EC and Shah MA. *World J Gastroenterol* 2011; 17(46): 5059-5074).

The pre-operative use of FDG-PET scans proved to be controversial amongst guidelines. It is interesting to note that SIGN guidelines, published earliest amongst the mentioned guidelines, do not advocate the routine use of PET scans in the staging of gastric cancer [47]. The ESMO/WCGIC guidelines state that FDG-PET may offer additional information for gastroesophageal junction tumors, but not gastric tumors [33]. NCCN guidelines state that FDG-PET alone is not an adequate diagnostic procedure in the detection and pre-operative staging of GC, but that it could be helpful when used in conjunction with CT scan [31]. NCCN guidelines recommend a PET-CT if there is no evidence of M1 disease on CT evaluation and state that it is not appropriate for T1 patients [31]. AUGIS/BSG guidelines state that FDG-PET scans can be used in combination with endoscopic ultrasound and CT for esophageal and gastroesophageal junction cancers, but not necessarily for gastric cancer [32, 59]. More recently, an international expert panel from a RAND/UCLA Appropriateness Method study defining processes of care in the optimal management of gastric cancer concluded that, PET scans are *not* routinely indicated in staging because their utility in changing management has not yet been defined [60].

Due to the high costs associated with this modality and its poorer overall accuracy when compared to CT scans, it is not used routinely as a primary radiologic staging modality. However, it may be useful as an adjunct staging modality in selected cases, especially if a finding of M1 disease will change management.

Magnetic Resonance Imaging

Magnetic resonance imaging (MRI) is a powerful imaging tool and features high soft-tissue contrast, multi-planar imaging capability, provision of biochemical and anatomic information, versatility of sequence selection and modification, as well as an absence of ionizing radiation [54]. However, CT scan has traditionally been favored over MRI for the staging of gastric cancer because of associated higher costs. (Figure 6) Furthermore, historically, the lack of a suitable oral contrast medium for MRI had made it more difficult to obtain clear images secondary to variable distensibility and artifacts caused by active peristalsis, cardiovascular pulsation and respiration [54, 61-69].

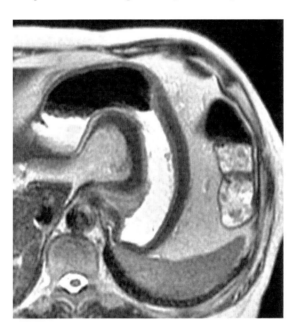

Figure 6. MRI demonstrating gastric cancer of the greater curvature. (Figure courtesy of Dr. John Hagen, University of Toronto).

Recent technological advancements in MRI have improved gastric cancer imaging. First, faster MRI processing allows for images to be obtained during a single breath-hold minimizing motion artifact and improving image quality [54, 65, 68]. The rapid administration of intravenous contrast medium using an automatic power injector has improved the enhancement of the gastric wall and gastric tumors [68]. Administration of anti-peristaltic agents has also allowed for improved image quality by reducing active peristalsis [54]. Subtraction imaging can decrease signal intensities of perigastric fatty tissue, facilitating demonstration of the different layers of the gastric wall [68]. Additionally, the use of phased array coils has increased the signal-to-noise ratio and has improved the spatial resolution of MR images [54]. These advancements have allowed MRI to become a more promising imaging modality for gastric cancer.

The ability of MRI to detect gastric cancers is strongly influenced by tumor size and morphology. The spatial resolution of MR images prohibits it from detecting early gastric cancers [68], limiting the applicability of MRI. Advanced gastric cancers, on the other hand, are easily detectable on MRI because the infiltrated wall is visualized as a thickened area, which is distinguished from the normal wall [65].

Arterial-dominant phase scanning is useful in detecting the tumor and evaluating tumor extent along the gastric wall [68]. Differing degrees of enhancement of the gastric wall can allow for layer differentiation. The inner mucosal layer shows rapid and marked enhancement, while the outer low-signal intensity submucosal and muscular layers have delayed enhancement [65]. Advanced gastric cancers show gradual enhancement from the inner mucosal side to the outer serosal side [68]. Therefore, depiction of the entire tumor is most clearly seen on the delayed images [68].

T staging has been possible with MR images. One study demonstrated that up to five layers of the gastric wall can be differentiated with MRI, comparable to endoscopic ultrasound [61]; however this was an ex vivo study, and no in vivo studies have recorded such visualization of the gastric wall [54]. Clinical studies have demonstrated that two [65] to three [68] layers of the normal gastric wall can be identified on dynamic MRI of the stomach. When two layers are identifiable, the first layer corresponds to the mucosa while the second layer corresponds to the submucosa and muscularis together. These layers are differentiated by degrees of enhancement [65]. When a third layer is visible, this allows differentiation of the submucosa and muscularis [68].

Identification of T4 lesions is important for surgical decision-making and planning for whether there is a need for a multi-visceral resection or a neoadjuvant approach. Identification of pancreatic invasion is possible by observation of obscuring fat signals between the stomach and the pancreas [65]. Invasion of the transverse colon is suggested by arresting peristalsis with the administration of intravenous hyocine butylbromide [65], and observation of an obscuring fat plane. Invasion of the left lobe of the liver can also be suggested by observing interruption of the low signal intensity between the liver and the stomach [65]. T staging performance of MRI has been examined by three studies [54, 61, 65, 66, 68] and was found to have an overall accuracy of 83% [35], which is comparable to MDCT scan. However, this data is based on only 3 studies examining a total of 109 patients [35], potentially representing a publication bias towards good results.

As with CT scans, determination of LN involvement by MRI is primarily based on size criteria. Accurate assessment of metastatic lymph nodes can be difficult when they are grouped together, or are in close proximity to the gastric mass [54]. Overall accuracy of N stage for MRI has been reported in only two studies, and is reported to be 52.2% to 55.2% [54, 65]. Only one study reported sensitivity and specificity of 85% and 75%, respectively [65]. While this reported sensitivity is the highest of the available imaging modalities, this is only reported in a single study. Therefore, MRI alone cannot reliably confirm or exclude the presence of LN metastases [35, 43].

The use of intravenous contrast may improve detection of LN by MRI. Tatsumi et al., examined the identification of LN on MRI using ferumoxtran-10, a lymphotropic contrast agent for MRI with efficacy in detecting metastatic LN in a variety of other cancers [70]. MRI findings were correlated with histopathologic findings in surgical specimens. The overall accuracy using ferumoxtran-10 was 94.8%, with sensitivity and specificity of 100% and 92.6%, respectively [70]. The positive predictive value and negative predictive value were 85.5% and 100%, respectively. This suggests that use of newer contrast agents for MRI may improve identification of LN metastases in the future [70]. M staging for MRI has not been closely examined. Reports of accuracy, sensitivity and specificity are lacking. MRI is of limited utility for determination of an M stage as the entire abdomen is not routinely imaged. Additionally, some authors have found that peritoneal carcinomatosis without ascites is difficult to detect on staging MR images [54]. However, MRI may serve an important purpose for clarification of possible metastatic lesions found on CT or ultrasound in the liver or ovaries [54].

MRI may be a useful alternative to CT due to its high resolution of soft tissue, its multi-planar imaging capability and its lack of ionizing radiation [54]. While practice guidelines do not recommend the routine use of MRI in the staging of gastric cancer [32, 33], it may be a useful staging modality, reserved for patients who cannot undergo CT [47] because of renal impairment, pregnancy, or hypersensitivity to CT contrast materials [54].

Abdominal Ultrasound

Abdominal ultrasound (AUS) (Figure 7) has become a very versatile imaging technique. Cost effective and portable, AUS has found applicability in a wide variety of clinical settings. Specific to gastric cancer, AUS has difficulty accurately evaluating the fundus, greater curvature, lymph node basins [71, 72], the diaphragm and the splenic hilum [73]. Moreover, the presence of bowel gas can disrupt adequate examination and it is operator dependent.

The overall accuracy for T staging with AUS is 67.8% [35], which does not compare favorably to CT or MRI. Only two studies, based on 168 patients, have evaluated the accuracies of each T stage [42, 73]. Accuracy of identifying T1 disease is 37.5% to 55.6%, 75.0% to 90.0% for T2, 56.2% to 87.3% for T3 and 0% to 71.1% for T4. Although identification of T1 lesions was least accurate, Liao et al., described identification of T1 lesions in only 9 patients, 4 of which were over-staged [42]. Three of these patients had ulcerative carcinoma, and Liao et al., found that in these cases, the normally hyper-echoic submucosal layer becomes hypo-echoic secondary to inflammation or edema around the tumor, giving it similar echogenicity to that of muscularis propria [42].

Accuracy for identifying T2 and T3 lesions is better. The normal serosal layer is seen as a thin, smooth hyper-echoic band. When the tumor remains below this hyper-echoic band, it is diagnosed as T2. When the tumor histologically invades the serosa, interruption of this smooth hyper-echoic band is visualized sonographically [42], and T3 status is assigned. AUS cannot reliably diagnose T4 lesions due to difficulty in visualizing perigastric organs [42]. However, a diagnosis of a T4 lesion may be made when there is interruption of the serosal layer of the gastric wall and it is indistinguishable from adjacent organs, the tumor and organs move synchronously, or there is no tumor movement with the patient's breathing. In their study, Liao et al., correctly identified invasion of the transverse colon with AUS in 1 out of 3 patients [42]. In a patient with identified invasion of the transverse colon, there was circumferential involvement. When the tumor only invaded one luminal side of the transverse colon, luminal gas interfered with the diagnosis, suggesting that AUS will have difficulty in identifying this relationship.

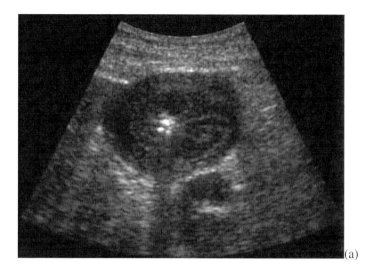

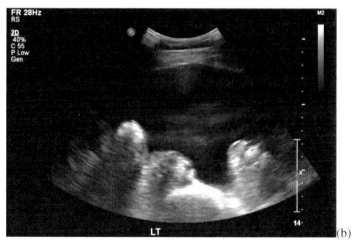

Figure 7. (a) Abdominal ultrasound showing a 5 cm diameter stomach with its wall being abnormally thickened due to cancer. The bright area is gas in the stomach (Figure courtesy of Dr. John Hagen, University of Toronto); (b) Abdominal ultrasound demonstrating ascites from gastric cancer. (Figure courtesy of Dr. Caitlin McGregor, University of Toronto).

N staging with AUS suffers from the same drawbacks as CT and MRI in that it is based primarily on size of the LN. Overall accuracy for N staging by AUS is found to be 68.1% [35]. Again, this analysis is based on only two studies [42, 73] of 168 patients, suffering from low power. Overall sensitivity and specificity is 63.0% and 78.8%, respectively. While the specificity compares to that of CT and MRI, given the low number of cases evaluated, more studies are needed. Furthermore, MDCT, especially with multi-planar reformatted images has a higher specificity.

Irregularly shaped LN seen on AUS have been suggested to have a higher risk of malignancy than consistently shaped nodes. However, most benign and malignant appearing lymph nodes were round in shape. Therefore, the shape of the lymph node does not often allow for correct differentiation between benign and malignant nodes [42]. AUS can also evaluate echogenicity of LN. Some authors report that most malignant lymph nodes were hypo-echoic, while most benign lymph nodes were iso-echoic to slightly hyper-echoic [74, 75]. On the other hand, Heinz et al., state that echogenicity of nodes seen on endoscopic ultrasound does not allow for correct differentiation between benign and malignant lymph nodes [76]. Therefore, differentiation of benign and malignant nodes based on echogenicity remains unclear.

The overall accuracy for M staging by AUS is only 64.7% [35]. Kayaalp et al., found that the sensitivity for detecting metastatic disease is unacceptably low [77]. The sensitivity for detection of liver metastases, peritoneal metastases and ascites was 50%, 9% and 64%, respectively. Although AUS is associated with low sensitivities, its reported specificities for detecting liver metastases, peritoneal metastases, and ascites are 98%, 98% and 93%, respectively [77].

None of the published practice guidelines mention the use of AUS as a staging modality for gastric cancer given the inherit limitations of this technique.

Endoscopy

Upper endoscopy, or esophagogastroduodenoscopy (EGD) was first introduced in the 1970s and is one of the most commonly performed and important modalities in the diagnosis of gastric cancer (Figure 8). Upper endoscopy is frequently used in the screening of asymptomatic patients, as well as the diagnosis and work-up of patients with pathological processes of the upper GI tract [78]. The sensitivity and specificity of endoscopy for detection of gastric cancers is reported to be 93% and 100%, respectively [79]. Despite the importance of endoscopy in the diagnosis of gastric cancer, the information obtained at endoscopy offers little in terms of oncologic staging.

An advantage of endoscopy in evaluation of the gastric cancer patient is its ability to directly visualize the luminal surface of the stomach, facilitating examination of the tumor appearance and allowing for biopsy of the lesion. Endoscopy is important in surgical planning, as assessment of proximal and distant disease extent can facilitate anticipated need for resection of the duodenum or esophagus in order to obtain negative margins.

As such, reporting for upper endoscopy should be performed in a standard, systematic manner. A complete upper endoscopy is recommended to include a thorough visualization from the upper esophageal sphincter to the second portion of the duodenum, including retroflexion [78]. Adequate documentation of the tumor size and appearance, description of the tumor location within the stomach relative to the gastroesophageal (GE) junction and/or duodenum, and description of any involvement of the esophagus, GE junction or duodenum constitutes a complete EGD report, which is necessary for appropriate pre-operative planning. If the above information is not clearly documented, it may be necessary to repeat the EGD prior to resection.

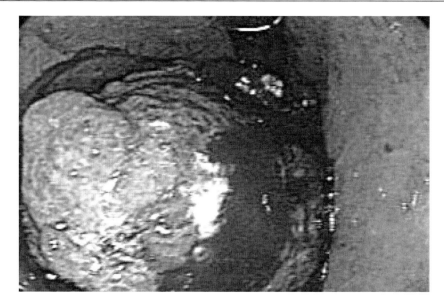

Figure 8. Esophagogastroduodenoscopy demonstrating a gastric mass on the greater curvature. (Figure courtesy of Dr. John Hagen, University of Toronto).

Endoscopic Ultrasound

Endoscopic ultrasound (EUS) was first introduced in the 1980s, providing a method for examining local tumor infiltration by allowing evaluation of the individual layers of the gastric wall [80, 81] without any interference from interposed fat, or bowel gas [82]. EUS is able to evaluate regional LN that may be enlarged, identify liver metastases, and detect ascites [83]. EUS, however, is not without its drawbacks. Like endoscopy, it is operator dependent, and is a very demanding endoscopic procedure. As such, advanced training and extensive experience is required in order to obtain usable images with the echoendoscope [84]. Echoendoscopes provide frequencies at 5-12 MHz, while miniature probes are capable of ultra-high frequencies of 12-30 MHz. Higher frequencies yield higher resolution of the tumor at the expense of depth of penetration, thus limiting nodal examination [80]. The echoendoscope must be well positioned in order to obtain high quality images and permit full visualization of the tumor, which can be difficult, especially if the tumor causes strictures [28].

An important goal of performing EUS in gastric cancer is determining an accurate T stage for treatment decisions, such as whether the patient is a candidate for an endoscopic resection. The diagnostic accuracy for overall T staging by EUS and for each individual T stage is summarized in Table 9. For overall T stage, the diagnostic accuracy ranges from 56.9% to 87.7%, with a pooled accuracy of 75%. The diagnostic accuracy for T1 cancer by EUS ranges from 14% to100%, with a pooled accuracy of 77%. For T2 lesions, the diagnostic accuracy ranges from 24% to 90%, with a pooled accuracy of 65% [84].

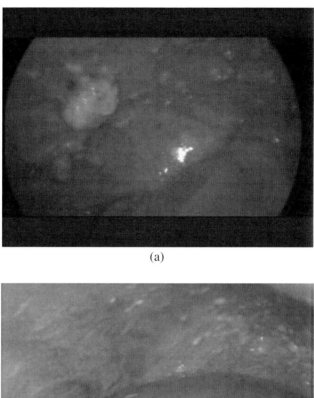

Figure 9. (a) Peritoneal carcinomatosis of the underlying anterior abdominal wall found during staging laparoscopy for gastric cancer. A large lesion with multiple smaller lesions surrounding the larger lesion is identifiable. (Figure courtesy of Dr. John Hagen, University of Toronto); (b) Liver metastases discovered during staging laparoscopy. Carcinomatosis is also seen on the inferior surface of the diaphragm. (Figure courtesy of Dr. Peter Stotland, University of Toronto).

This low to moderate diagnostic accuracy for T staging in early gastric cancer raises concerns as to whether or not this is, in fact, the ideal modality for T staging, especially for the identification of candidates for endoscopic resection. Kim et al., found that early gastric cancer with undifferentiated histopathologic features was more frequently associated with an incorrect assessment of true tumor invasion depth by EUS [85].

Although of more limited clinical value, the pooled diagnostic accuracies for advanced gastric cancers (i.e., T3-4) is 79% to 85% [83]. Patients with such lesions, assuming they are candidates, would proceed to gastrectomy with or without peri-operative chemotherapy. Detection of invasion of adjacent organs could be important for clinical decision-making, as a multi-visceral resection, or neo-adjuvant approach could be planned.

N staging, to a certain degree, is also possible with EUS, as enlarged LN in the peri-gastric nodal basin (i.e., Group 1 nodes) can be visualized. More distant nodal basins (i.e., Group 2 or 3 nodes) are not within the range of tissue penetration for the EUS, and therefore may not be visualized. The range of accuracies for N staging in published studies was found to be 30% to 90% with a pooled accuracy of only 64% [83]. Therefore, while EUS can identify and biopsy enlarged regional LN in the peri-tumoral area, N-staging by EUS is of limited value in the pre-operative assessment [86]. Similarly, although the left lobe of the liver can be assessed by EUS, the entire liver cannot be visualized, allowing only for a partial metastatic hepatic assessment. Furthermore, EUS is of limited use in the overall assessment of more distant metastatic spread [28].

Some practice guidelines have supported the optional use of EUS with or without fine needle aspiration of suspicious lymph nodes for further staging of esophageal and GEJ tumors prior to the administration of curative therapy, but this recommendation does not necessarily apply to more distally located gastric cancer. Although EUS allows for the evaluation of individual layers of the gastric wall [80], the lack of unanimous support by experts may be secondary to the fact that it often does not change management strategies for resectable tumors, unless there is anticipation for an endoscopic resection [26]. The SIGN guidelines recommend an EUS for patients with GEJ tumors who are candidates for curative resection [47]. ESMO guidelines have not provided a complete consensus on the application of EUS, however maintain that there may be a role to guide pre-operative treatment for certain patients with superficial disease or with *linitis plastic* [33]. AUGIS/BSG guidelines recommend an EUS for patients with GEJ tumors [32]. NCCN guidelines recommend that an EUS is indicated for assessing the depth of tumor invasion and if there is no evidence of M1 disease [31].

Table 9. Summary of range of diagnostic accuracies and pooled accuracies for all T staging by EUS, and for each individual T stage as reported by Cardoso et al. [83]

T stage	Range of Accuracy	Pooled Accuracy
Overall	56.9% to 87.7%	75%
T1	14% to 100%	77%
T2	24% to 90%	65%
T3	50% to 100%	85%
T4	25% to 100%	79%

Staging Laparoscopy

Since the inception of laparoscopic surgery, staging laparoscopy has evolved into a highly accurate modality for identification of metastatic spread before the undertaking of a formal resection [34, 87-89]. Staging laparoscopy can identify metastatic disease too small to be detected on available pre-operative radiographic staging modalities, hence avoiding an unnecessary laparotomy (Figure 9). A complete staging laparoscopy should include the inspection of the stomach, diaphragm, liver and ovaries [26, 90]. With thorough laparoscopic inspection, the accuracy for detecting intra-abdominal M1 disease is 94% to 100% [87, 88].

However, with improvement of image resolution of MDCT scans, the question of whether or not performing a staging laparoscopy is still relevant has been raised. Despite improvements in imaging accuracy, a recent study found that almost one third of patients who were identified by other staging modalities as M0, had radiologically occult intra-abdominal metastases, which were discovered by staging laparoscopy [89]. Sarela et al., evaluated 657 patients with potentially resectable gastric cancer over a 10 year period and discovered that 31% had M1 disease [89]. Another study found staging laparoscopy changed management in 25% to 54% of patients with advanced gastric cancer [88].

Therefore, even with the combined accuracy of performing multiple staging modalities in the work-up process, suboptimal identification of incurable disease by radiologic staging alone, results in high rates of unnecessary laparotomies in gastric cancer patients, with resultant morbidity and mortality. In a large population based series that did not account for indication, the median hospital length of stay is shorter with staging laparoscopy compared to a negative laparotomy (2 days vs. 10 days, p <0.001) [91]. Furthermore, the in-hospital mortality of patients undergoing a staging laparoscopy is only 5.3%, compared to 13.1% for patients who underwent a futile laparotomy (p<0.001) [91].

Laparoscopy, however, should not be routinely performed on all patients. The diagnostic yield of performing a staging laparoscopy on a patient with early gastric cancer (i.e., T1-2) is low. The SIGN guidelines indicate that laparoscopy should be considered in patients with suspected full thickness gastric wall tumor involvement [47]. ESMO recommends performing a staging laparoscopy pre-operatively [33]. AUGIS/BSG recommend performing a laparoscopy in all patients with gastric cancer, and NCCN guidelines recommend that laparoscopy was deemed a necessary pre-operative maneuver for patients considered for chemoradiotherapy or surgical resection and in patients with suspected T3 or T4 tumors [31]. In summary, practice guidelines have recommended that staging laparoscopy be reserved for advanced gastric cancer (i.e., T3-4), where there is a higher likelihood of metastases [47, 92]. Given its diagnostic accuracy, its ability to change management in appropriately selected patients, and the benefits to the patient in terms of reduction in hospital length of stay and mortality, staging laparoscopy should be utilized in the staging of all patients with advanced gastric cancer.

Peritoneal Washings

Peritoneal washings for cytological analysis have been advocated for the identification of free intraperitoneal cancer cells, despite the absence of any evidence of gross peritoneal disease. The etiology of these free intraperitoneal cancer cells is not fully understood, however, they are thought to arise from where the primary tumor invades the serosa [93]. Positive cytology is associated with advanced T stage, but not with N positivity [94].

Positive cytology of peritoneal washings is a poor prognostic indicator [94, 95] and a strong independent predictor of recurrence even after an R0 resection [96]. In gastric cancer, peritoneal dissemination is one of the most common patterns of metastasis and recurrence [97]. Reported recurrence rates for patients with positive cytology range from 11% to 100% [98], but appear to be dependent upon the method used to detect cancer cells in peritoneal washings and the length of time that the patients are observed for recurrence.

Although the UICC/AJCC have defined positive peritoneal cytology as M1 disease [5], the treatment implications of this microscopic disease are debated. While some authors state that positive cytology is a contra-indication to resection [31, 99], others feel that positive peritoneal cytology is useful for identifying patients who are unlikely to benefit from resection alone, and would require additional treatment in order to improve survival [100]. Some authors have suggested that the early detection and eradication of intraperitoneal cancer cells may improve patient survival [101, 102]. Lorenzen et al., reported that 37% of gastric cancer patients with positive peritoneal cytology were subsequently converted to negative after a minimum of 6 weeks of neoadjuvant chemotherapy [103]. These patients had improved median survival (36.1 vs. 9.2 months; $p = 0.002$) and 2-year survival (71.4 vs. 25%; $p = 0.002$) compared to patients who had persistently positive cytology [103]. However, the 5-year survival of patients in whom peritoneal lavage was converted from positive to negative was only 14.3% [103].

Some groups have also suggested that the prognosis of patients with positive peritoneal cytology may be improved with intraperitoneal chemotherapy. The use of extensive peritoneal lavage followed by intraperitoneal chemotherapy has been shown to improve 5-year survival of patients with positive peritoneal cytology over those with intraperitoneal therapy alone (43.8% vs. 4.6%, $p < 0.0001$) [104]. Intraperitoneal chemotherapy has been demonstrated to be prophylactic against peritoneal recurrence and results in improved survival [105, 106]. Therefore, identification of intraperitoneal cancer cells may have an impact on management decisions with regards to peri-operative therapy.

Current guidelines are inconsistent in their recommendations for peritoneal washings. Obtaining peritoneal washings at the time of diagnostic laparoscopy is recommended by SAGES [89]. ESMO, on the other hand, does not consider obtaining peritoneal washings a necessary practice [33]. The NCCN guidelines do not explicitly incorporate peritoneal washings into the gastric cancer treatment algorithm, despite later considering positive peritoneal cytology a criterion of unresectable disease [31].

An argument can be made for performing peritoneal washings at the time of staging laparoscopy because the length of time added to the procedure in order to obtain the washings is not significant. However, as there is no reliable mechanism for intra-operative assessment of cytology, performance of peritoneal washings must be planned several days prior to scheduled resection, necessitating two separate operations if resection is performed.

Sentinel Lymph Node

Accurate assessment of lymph node status is an integral part to determination of clinical outcomes and for therapeutic planning in gastric cancer. EGC is associated with 5-year OS rates of greater than 90% and pathological data have suggested that the majority of lymph nodes resected do not contain metastases [107-110]. Further, extensive lymphadenectomies are associated with increased risk of complications [111]. Sentinel lymph node (SLN) biopsy is well-established in the treatment of breast cancer and melanoma, and allows for lymph node assessment with limited dissection and reduced complications [112]. SLN biopsy has been investigated as an alternative to extensive lymphadenectomy in the treatment of EGC. Mapping for SLN biopsy has been completed with dye, radio-colloid, as well as combinations of dye and radio-colloid. Potential anatomical limitations to SLN mapping exist in gastric cancer, due to the complex and unpredictable lymphatic drainage of the stomach, increasing the likelihood of skip metastases.

A systematic review on the accuracy of SLN biopsy in gastric cancer was performed by Cardoso et al., which revealed an overall calculated false negative rate (FNR) of 34.7% with dye alone, 18.5% with radio-colloid alone, and 13.1% for the combination of dye and radio-colloid [113]. A recent systematic review performed by Faith-Can et al., reveals accuracy rates ranged from 78% to 100% [114]. Worldwide, evaluation of metastasis to the SLN is mainly accomplished by hematoxylin and eosin (H&E) staining, however recent studies have shown potential for routine use of immunohistochemical staining (IHC) and reverse transcription-polymerase chain reaction (RT-PCR) [114]. Hirayama et al., performed a comparison study to assess diagnosis of LN metastasis using H&E, IHC staining for cytokeratin and RT-PCR of carcinoembryonic antigen mRNA [115]. RT-PCR, using lymph node washings, is a rapid diagnostic tool and allows for conservation of lymph nodes as permanent specimens [115]. RT-PCR had an slightly inferior specificity to that of H&E (94.5% vs. 100%) but had superior sensitivity (91.9% vs. 78.4%) [115]. In regards to this intraoperative test for detecting metastasis, significance is placed on the superior sensitivity [115].

More recently, there has been the publication of the results of a multicenter trial (JCOG 0302), which evaluated the feasibility and accuracy of diagnosis using SLN biopsy in T1 gastric cancer [116]. Final results revealed a high FNR and accrual was suspended early. Primary analysis revealed a FNR of 46 % (13/28) and 7 of 13 patients had nodal metastases outside the lymphatic basin [116]. However, a recent prospective multicenter trial in Japan performed by Kitagawa et al., revealed a higher accuracy of nodal evaluation for metastasis (93%) and lower FNR (7%) compared to JCOG 0302 results [117]. This drastic difference in results may be explained by the difference in the procedural learning phase in both studies [117]. In JCOG 0302, only five cases were required as the minimum for the initial leaning phase, while a minimum of 30 cases were required for the learning phase in the multicenter trial performed by Kitagawa et al., [117]. Thus at present, SLN biopsy remains an experimental treatment modality in gastric cancer [116].

Conclusion

The importance of accurate staging of patients with gastric cancer cannot be overstated, and is the foundation for providing the most appropriate stage-specific treatment. Establishment of uniformity and identification of appropriate and necessary practices in the pre-operative management of gastric cancer is vital to ensuring accurate staging and adequate treatment. Importantly, accurate pre-operative staging radiographically and laparoscopically allows us to stratify patients into optimal stage-specific treatments and therefore improve survival outcomes. Under-staging can lead to under-treating patients who are falsely diagnosed with highly aggressive local disease, while over-staging can lead to futile attempts at treatment with curative intent where palliation is the more appropriate.

Several investigative techniques for the staging of gastric cancer are available. Unfortunately, none of these techniques are perfect, and simply performing one of these techniques for the purposes of staging may be inadequate. However, the combination of several techniques will increase the chances of diagnosing the correct stage and allowing patients to be correctly allocated to appropriate treatment algorithms.

References

[1] Cunningham D, Allum WH, Stenning SP, et al., Perioperative chemotherapy versus surgery alone for resectable gastroesophageal cancer. *N. Engl. J. Med.* 2006 Jul 6;355(1):11-20.

[2] Macdonald JS, Smalley SR, Benedetti J, et al., Chemoradiotherapy after surgery compared with surgery alone for adenocarcinoma of the stomach or gastroesophageal junction. *N. Engl. J. Med.* 2001 Sep 6;345(10):725-30.

[3] Paoletti X, Oba K, Burzykowski T, et al., Benefit of adjuvant chemotherapy for resectable gastric cancer: a meta-analysis. *JAMA.* 2010 May 5;303(17):1729-37.

[4] Sakuramoto S, Sasako M, Yamaguchi T, et al., Adjuvant chemotherapy for gastric cancer with S-1, an oral fluoropyrimidine. *N. Engl. J. Med.* 2007 Nov 1;357(18):1810-20.

[5] American Joint Committee on Cancer. Chapter 11: Stomach. In: Edge S, Byrd D, Compton C, et al., eds. AJCC Cancer Staging Manual 7th ed. New York: Springer.

[6] Japanese Gastric Cancer Association. Japanese classification of gastric carcinoma: 3rd English edition. *Gastric Cancer.* 2011;14:101-12.

[7] Fang WL, Huang KH, Chen JH, et al., Comparison of the survival difference between AJCC 6th and 7th editions for gastric cancer patients. *World J. Surg.* 2011 Dec;35(12):2723-9.

[8] Brar SS, Seevaratnam R, Cardoso R, et al., Multivisceral resection for gastric cancer: a systematic review. *Gastric Cancer.* 2011 Sep;15 Suppl 1:S100-7.

[9] Japanese Gastric Cancer Association. Japanese classification of gastric carcinoma- 2nd English edition. *Gastric Cancer.* 1998;1:10-24.

[10] Bland JM, Altman DG. Multiple significance tests: the Bonferroni method. *BMJ.* 1995 Jan 21;310(6973):170.

[11] Viera AJ, Garrett JM. Understanding interobserver agreement: the kappa statistic. *Fam. Med.* 2005 May;37(5):360-3.

[12] Smith DD, Schwarz RR, Schwarz RE. Impact of total lymph node count on staging and survival after gastrectomy for gastric cancer: data from a large US-population database. *J. Clin. Oncol.* 2005 Oct 1;23(28):7114-24.

[13] Bouvier AM, Haas O, Piard F, Roignot P, Bonithon-Kopp C, Faivre J. How many nodes must be examined to accurately stage gastric carcinomas? Results from a population based study. *Cancer.* 2002 Jun 1;94(11):2862-6.

[14] UICC/AJCC. American Joint Committee on Cancer, Cancer Staging Manual. 1988-2002. http://cancerstaging.org/references-tools/ deskreferences/Pages/default.aspx. Available at.

[15] Wagner PK, Ramaswamy A, Ruschoff J, Schmitz-Moormann P, Rothmund M. Lymph node counts in the upper abdomen: anatomical basis for lymphadenectomy in gastric cancer. *Br. J. Surg.* 1991 Jul;78(7):825-7.

[16] Coburn NG. Lymph nodes and gastric cancer. *J. Surg. Oncol.* 2009 Mar 15;99(4):199-206.

[17] de Gara CJ, Hanson J, Hamilton S. A population-based study of tumor-node relationship, resection margins, and surgeon volume on gastric cancer survival. *Am J. Surg.* 2003 Jul;186(1):23-7.

[18] Onate-Ocana LF, Aiello-Crocifoglio V, Mondragon-Sanchez R, Ruiz-Molina JM. Survival benefit of D2 lympadenectomy in patients with gastric adenocarcinoma. *Ann. Surg. Oncol.* 2000 Apr;7(3):210-7.

[19] Jamieson JK, Dobson JF. Lectures on the lymphatic system of the stomach. *The Lancet.* 1907;169(4364):1061-6.

[20] Kay EB. Regional lymphatic metastases of carcinoma of the stomach. *Ann. Surg.* 1941 Jun;113(6):1059-61.

[21] Hundahl SA, Phillips JL, Menck HR. The National Cancer Data Base Report on poor survival of U.S. gastric carcinoma patients treated with gastrectomy: Fifth Edition American Joint Committee on Cancer staging, proximal disease, and the "different disease" hypothesis. *Cancer.* 2000 Feb 15;88(4):921-32.

[22] Wanebo HJ, Kennedy BJ, Chmiel J, Steele G, Jr., Winchester D, Osteen R. Cancer of the stomach. A patient care study by the American College of Surgeons. *Ann. Surg.* 1993 Nov;218(5):583-92.

[23] Baumgart DC, Fischer A. Virchow's node. *Lancet.* 2007 Nov 3;370(9598):1568.

[24] Powell FC, Cooper AJ, Massa MC, Goellner JR, Su WP. Sister Mary Joseph's nodule: a clinical and histologic study. *J. Am. Acad. Dermatol.* 1984 Apr;10(4):610-5.

[25] Mahar AL, Coburn NG, Singh S, Law C, Helyer LK. A systematic review of surgery for non-curative gastric cancer. *Gastric Cancer.* 2012 Sep;15 Suppl 1:S125-37.

[26] Dixon M, Cardoso R, Tinmouth J, et al., What studies are appropriate and necessary for staging gastric adenocarcinoma? Results of an international RAND/UCLA expert panel. *Gastric Cancer.* 2013 Apr 30.

[27] Abdalla EK, Pisters PW. Staging and preoperative evaluation of upper gastrointestinal malignancies. *Semin. Oncol.* 2004 Aug;31(4):513-29.

[28] Kwee RM, Kwee TC. Imaging in local staging of gastric cancer: a systematic review. *J. Clin. Oncol.* 2007 May 20;25(15):2107-16.

[29] Weber WA, Ott K. Imaging of esophageal and gastric cancer. *Semin Oncol.* 2004 Aug;31(4):530-41.

[30] Roberts P, Seevaratnam R, Cardoso R, Law C, Helyer L, Coburn N. Systematic review of pancreaticoduodenectomy for locally advanced gastric cancer. *Gastric Cancer.* 2011 Sep;15 Suppl 1:S108-15.

[31] Ajani JA, Bentrem DJ, Besh S, et al., Gastric cancer, version 2.2013: featured updates to the NCCN Guidelines. *J. Natl. Compr Canc. Netw.* 2013 May 1;11(5):531-46.

[32] Allum WH, Blazeby JM, Griffin SM, Cunningham D, Jankowski JA, Wong R. Guidelines for the management of oesophageal and gastric cancer. *Gut.* 2011 Nov;60(11):1449-72.

[33] Van Cutsem E, Dicato M, Geva R, et al., The diagnosis and management of gastric cancer: expert discussion and recommendations from the 12th ESMO/World Congress on Gastrointestinal Cancer, Barcelona, 2010. *Ann. Oncol.* 2011 Jun;22 Suppl 5:v1-9.

[34] Smith BR, Stabile BE. Gastric adenocarcinoma: reduction of perioperative mortality by avoidance of nontherapeutic laparotomy. *J. Gastrointest Surg.* 2007 Feb;11(2):127-32.

[35] Seevaratnam R, Cardoso R, McGregor C, et al., How useful is preoperative imaging for tumor, node, metastasis (TNM) staging of gastric cancer? A meta-analysis. *Gastric Cancer.* 2011 Sep;15 Suppl 1:S3-18.

[36] Halvorsen RA. Which study when? Iodinated contrast-enhanced CT versus gadolinium-enhanced MR imaging. *Radiology.* 2008 Oct;249(1):9-15.

[37] Chen CY, Wu DC, Kang WY, Hsu JS. Staging of gastric cancer with 16-channel MDCT. *Abdom Imaging.* 2006 Sep-Oct;31(5):514-20.

[38] Kim AY, Kim HJ, Ha HK. Gastric cancer by multidetector row CT: preoperative staging. *Abdom Imaging.* 2005 Jul-Aug;30(4):465-72.

[39] Lim JS, Yun MJ, Kim MJ, et al., CT and PET in stomach cancer: preoperative staging and monitoring of response to therapy. *Radiographics.* 2006 Jan-Feb;26(1):143-56.

[40] Kwee RM, Kwee TC. Imaging in assessing lymph node status in gastric cancer. *Gastric Cancer.* 2009;12(1):6-22.

[41] Dassen AE, Lips DJ, Hoekstra CJ, Pruijt JF, Bosscha K. FDG-PET has no definite role in preoperative imaging in gastric cancer. *Eur. J. Surg. Oncol.* 2009 May;35(5):449-55.

[42] Liao SR, Dai Y, Huo L, et al., Transabdominal ultrasonography in preoperative staging of gastric cancer. *World J. Gastroenterol.* 2004 Dec 1;10(23):3399-404.

[43] Takao S, Tadano S, Taguchi H, et al., Accurate analysis of the change in volume, location, and shape of metastatic cervical lymph nodes during radiotherapy. *Int. J. Radiat. Oncol. Biol. Phys.* 2011 Nov 1;81(3):871-9.

[44] Bhandari S, Shim CS, Kim JH, et al., Usefulness of three-dimensional, multidetector row CT (virtual gastroscopy and multiplanar reconstruction) in the evaluation of gastric cancer: a comparison with conventional endoscopy, EUS, and histopathology. *Gastrointest Endosc.* 2004 May;59(6):619-26.

[45] Chen J, Cheong JH, Yun MJ, et al., Improvement in preoperative staging of gastric adenocarcinoma with positron emission tomography. *Cancer.* 2005 Jun 1;103(11):2383-90.

[46] Kemp CD, Kitano M, Kerkar S, et al., Pulmonary resection for metastatic gastric cancer. *J. Thorac. Oncol.* 2010 Nov;5(11):1796-805.

[47] Alderson D. Scottish Intercollegiate Guidelines Network (SIGN) 87--the management of oesophageal and gastric cancer. *Clin. Oncol.* (R Coll Radiol). 2008 Sep;20(7):530-1.

[48] Ozkan E, Soydal C, Araz M, Kir KM, Ibis E. The role of 18F-FDG PET/CT in detecting colorectal cancer recurrence in patients with elevated CEA levels. *Nucl. Med. Commun.* 2012 Apr;33(4):395-402.

[49] Kim SK, Kang KW, Lee JS, et al., Assessment of lymph node metastases using 18F-FDG PET in patients with advanced gastric cancer. *Eur. J. Nucl. Med. Mol. Imaging.* 2006 Feb;33(2):148-55.

[50] Mochiki E, Kuwano H, Katoh H, Asao T, Oriuchi N, Endo K. Evaluation of 18F-2-deoxy-2-fluoro-D-glucose positron emission tomography for gastric cancer. *World J. Surg.* 2004 Mar;28(3):247-53.

[51] Mukai K, Ishida Y, Okajima K, Isozaki H, Morimoto T, Nishiyama S. Usefulness of preoperative FDG-PET for detection of gastric cancer. *Gastric Cancer.* 2006;9(3):192-6.

[52] Stahl A, Ott K, Weber WA, et al., FDG PET imaging of locally advanced gastric carcinomas: correlation with endoscopic and histopathological findings. *Eur. J. Nucl. Med. Mol. Imaging.* 2003 Feb;30(2):288-95.

[53] Yun M, Lim JS, Noh SH, et al., Lymph node staging of gastric cancer using (18)F-FDG PET: a comparison study with CT. *J. Nucl. Med.* 2005 Oct;46(10):1582-8.

[54] Sohn KM, Lee JM, Lee SY, Ahn BY, Park SM, Kim KM. Comparing MR imaging and CT in the staging of gastric carcinoma. *AJR Am. J. Roentgenol.* 2000 Jun;174(6):1551-7.

[55] Lim JS, Kim MJ, Yun MJ, et al., Comparison of CT and 18F-FDG pet for detecting peritoneal metastasis on the preoperative evaluation for gastric carcinoma. *Korean J. Radiol.* 2006 Oct-Dec;7(4):249-56.

[56] Tian J, Chen L, Wei B, et al., The value of vesicant 18F-fluorodeoxyglucose positron emission tomography (18F-FDG PET) in gastric malignancies. *Nucl. Med. Commun.* 2004 Aug;25(8):825-31.

[57] Kinkel K, Lu Y, Both M, Warren RS, Thoeni RF. Detection of hepatic metastases from cancers of the gastrointestinal tract by using noninvasive imaging methods (US, CT, MR imaging, PET): a meta-analysis. *Radiology.* 2002 Sep;224(3):748-56.

[58] Yoshioka T, Yamaguchi K, Kubota K, et al., Evaluation of 18F-FDG PET in patients with advanced, metastatic, or recurrent gastric cancer. *J. Nucl. Med.* 2003 May;44(5):690-9.

[59] Shoda H, Kakugawa Y, Saito D, et al., Evaluation of 18F-2-deoxy-2-fluoro-glucose positron emission tomography for gastric cancer screening in asymptomatic individuals undergoing endoscopy. *Br. J. Cancer.* 2007 Dec 3;97(11):1493-8.

[60] Coburn N, Seevaratnam R, Paszat L, et al., Optimal Management of Gastric Cancer: Results From an International RAND/UCLA Expert Panel. *Ann. Surg.* 2013 Mar 8.

[61] Dux M, Roeren T, Kuntz C, et al., MRI for staging of gastric carcinoma: first results of an experimental prospective study. *J. Comput. Assist. Tomogr.* 1997 Jan-Feb;21(1):66-72.

[62] Goldberg HI, Thoeni RF. MRI of the gastrointestinal tract. *Radiol. Clin. North Am.* 1989 Jul;27(4):805-12.

[63] Hahn P, Stark D, Glastad K. Biliary system, pancreas, spleen, and alimentary tract. In: Stark D, Bradley WJ, eds. Magnetic resonance imaging, 2nd ed. St. Louis: Mosby; 1992. p. 1838-51.

[64] Halvorsen RA, Jr., Thompson WM. Primary neoplasms of the hollow organs of the gastrointestinal tract. Staging and follow-up. *Cancer.* 1991 Feb 15;67(4 Suppl):1181-8.

[65] Kang BC, Kim JH, Kim KW, et al., Value of the dynamic and delayed MR sequence with Gd-DTPA in the T-staging of stomach cancer: correlation with the histopathology. *Abdom Imaging.* 2000 Jan-Feb;25(1):14-24.

[66] Matsushita M, Oi H, Murakami T, et al., Extraserosal invasion in advanced gastric cancer: evaluation with MR imaging. *Radiology.* 1994 Jul;192(1):87-91.

[67] Paley MR, Ros PR. MRI of the gastrointestinal tract. *Eur. Radiol.* 1997;7(9):1387-97.

[68] Wang CK, Kuo YT, Liu GC, Tsai KB, Huang YS. Dynamic contrast-enhanced subtraction and delayed MRI of gastric tumors: radiologic-pathologic correlation. *J. Comput. Assist. Tomogr.* 2000 Nov-Dec;24(6):872-7.

[69] Werthmuller WC, Margulis AR. Magnetic resonance imaging of the alimentary tube. *Invest Radiol.* 1991 Feb;26(2):195-200.

[70] Tatsumi Y, Tanigawa N, Nishimura H, et al., Preoperative diagnosis of lymph node metastases in gastric cancer by magnetic resonance imaging with ferumoxtran-10. *Gastric Cancer.* 2006;9(2):120-8.

[71] Lim JH, Ko YT, Lee DH. Transabdominal US staging of gastric cancer. *Abdom Imaging*. 1994 Nov-Dec;19(6):527-31.

[72] Suk KT, Lim DW, Kim MY, et al., Thickening of the gastric wall on transabdominal sonography: a sign of gastric cancer. *J. Clin. Ultrasound.* 2008 Oct;36(8):462-6.

[73] Lee DH, Ko YT, Park SJ, Lim JW. Comparison of hydro-US and spiral CT in the staging of gastric cancer. *Clin. Imaging*. 2001 May-Jun;25(3):181-6.

[74] Gimondo P, Mirk P, Messina G, Pizzi C. Abdominal lymphadenopathy in benign diseases: sonographic detection and clinical significance. *J. Ultrasound Med.* 1996 May;15(5):353-9; quiz 61-2.

[75] Metreweli C, Ward SC. Ultrasound demonstration of lymph nodes in the hepatoduodenal ligament ('Daisy Chain nodes') in normal subjects. *Clin. Radiol.* 1995 Feb;50(2):99-101.

[76] Heintz A, Mildenberger P, Georg M, Braunstein S, Junginger T. Endoscopic ultrasonography in the diagnosis of regional lymph nodes in esophageal and gastric cancer--results of studies in vitro. *Endoscopy*. 1993 Mar;25(3):231-5.

[77] Kayaalp C, Arda K, Orug T, Ozcay N. Value of computed tomography in addition to ultrasound for preoperative staging of gastric cancer. *Eur. J. Surg. Oncol.* 2002 Aug;28(5):540-3.

[78] Cohen J, Safdi MA, Deal SE, et al., Quality indicators for esophagogastroduodenoscopy. *Am. J. Gastroenterol.* 2006 Apr; 101(4):886-91.

[79] Voutilainen ME, Juhola MT. Evaluation of the diagnostic accuracy of gastroscopy to detect gastric tumours: clinicopathological features and prognosis of patients with gastric cancer missed on endoscopy. *Eur. J. Gastroenterol. Hepatol.* 2005 Dec;17(12):1345-9.

[80] Puli SR, Batapati Krishna Reddy J, Bechtold ML, Antillon MR, Ibdah JA. How good is endoscopic ultrasound for TNM staging of gastric cancers? A meta-analysis and systematic review. *World J. Gastroenterol.* 2008 Jul 7;14(25):4011-9.

[81] Takemoto T, Yanai H, Tada M, et al., Application of ultrasonic probes prior to endoscopic resection of early gastric cancer. *Endoscopy*. 1992 May;24 Suppl 1:329-33.

[82] Kelly S, Harris KM, Berry E, et al., A systematic review of the staging performance of endoscopic ultrasound in gastro-oesophageal carcinoma. *Gut.* 2001 Oct;49(4):534-9.

[83] Cardoso R, Coburn N, Seevaratnam R, et al., A systematic review and meta-analysis of the utility of EUS for preoperative staging for gastric cancer. *Gastric Cancer*. 2012 Sep;15 Suppl 1:S19-26.

[84] Pollack BJ, Chak A, Sivak MV, Jr. Endoscopic ultrasonography. *Semin Oncol.* 1996 Jun;23(3):336-46.

[85] Kim JH, Song KS, Youn YH, et al., Clinicopathologic factors influence accurate endosonographic assessment for early gastric cancer. *Gastrointest Endosc.* 2007 Nov;66(5):901-8.

[86] Bentrem D, Gerdes H, Tang L, Brennan M, Coit D. Clinical correlation of endoscopic ultrasonography with pathologic stage and outcome in patients undergoing curative resection for gastric cancer. *Ann. Surg.* Oncol. 2007 Jun;14(6):1853-9.

[87] Burke EC, Karpeh MS, Conlon KC, Brennan MF. Laparoscopy in the management of gastric adenocarcinoma. *Ann. Surg.* 1997 Mar;225(3):262-7.

[88] Leake PA, Cardoso R, Seevaratnam R, et al., A systematic review of the accuracy and indications for diagnostic laparoscopy prior to curative-intent resection of gastric cancer. *Gastric Cancer.* 2012 Sep;15 Suppl 1:S38-47.

[89] Sarela AI, Lefkowitz R, Brennan MF, Karpeh MS. Selection of patients with gastric adenocarcinoma for laparoscopic staging. *Am. J. Surg.* 2006 Jan;191(1):134-8.

[90] D'Ugo DM, Pende V, Persiani R, Rausei S, Picciocchi A. Laparoscopic staging of gastric cancer: an overview. *J. Am. Coll. Surg.* 2003 Jun;196(6):965-74.

[91] Karanicolas PJ, Elkin EB, Jacks LM, et al., Staging laparoscopy in the management of gastric cancer: a population-based analysis. *J. Am. Coll. Surg.* 2011 Nov;213(5):644-51, 51 e1.

[92] Society of American Gastrointestinal and Endoscopic Surgeons. Guidelines for Diagnostic Laparoscopy. http://www.sages.org/ publications/guidelines/guidelines-for-diagnostic-laparoscopy/. Available at.

[93] Abe N, Watanabe T, Toda H, et al., Prognostic significance of carcinoembryonic antigen levels in peritoneal washes in patients with gastric cancer. *Am. J. Surg.* 2001 Apr;181(4):356-61.

[94] Creasman WT, Rutledge F. The prognostic value of peritoneal cytology in gynecologic malignant disease. *Am. J. Obstet. Gynecol.* 1971 Jul 15;110(6):773-81.

[95] Moore GE, Sako K, Kondo T, Badillo J, Burke E. Assessment of the exfoliation of tumor cells into the body cavities. *Surg. Gynecol. Obstet.* 1961 Apr;112:469-74.

[96] Bentrem D, Wilton A, Mazumdar M, Brennan M, Coit D. The value of peritoneal cytology as a preoperative predictor in patients with gastric carcinoma undergoing a curative resection. *Ann. Surg. Oncol.* 2005 May;12(5):347-53.

[97] Boku T, Nakane Y, Minoura T, et al., Prognostic significance of serosal invasion and free intraperitoneal cancer cells in gastric cancer. *Br. J. Surg.* 1990 Apr;77(4):436-9.

[98] Leake PA, Cardoso R, Seevaratnam R, et al., A systematic review of the accuracy and utility of peritoneal cytology in patients with gastric cancer. *Gastric Cancer.* 2011 Sep;15 Suppl 1:S27-37.

[99] Badgwell B, Cormier JN, Krishnan S, et al., Does neoadjuvant treatment for gastric cancer patients with positive peritoneal cytology at staging laparoscopy improve survival? *Ann. Surg. Oncol.* 2008 Oct;15(10):2684-91.

[100] Burke EC, Karpeh MS, Jr., Conlon KC, Brennan MF. Peritoneal lavage cytology in gastric cancer: an independent predictor of outcome. *Ann. Surg. Oncol.* 1998 Jul-Aug;5(5):411-5.

[101] Mezhir JJ, Shah MA, Jacks LM, Brennan MF, Coit DG, Strong VE. Positive peritoneal cytology in patients with gastric cancer: natural history and outcome of 291 patients. *Ann. Surg. Oncol.* 2010 Dec;17(12):3173-80.

[102] Vogel I, Kalthoff H. Disseminated tumour cells. Their detection and significance for prognosis of gastrointestinal and pancreatic carcinomas. *Virchows Arch.* 2001 Aug;439(2):109-17.

[103] Lorenzen S, Panzram B, Rosenberg R, et al., Prognostic significance of free peritoneal tumor cells in the peritoneal cavity before and after neoadjuvant chemotherapy in patients with gastric carcinoma undergoing potentially curative resection. *Ann. Surg. Oncol.* 2010 Oct;17(10):2733-9.

[104] Kuramoto M, Shimada S, Ikeshima S, et al., Extensive intraoperative peritoneal lavage as a standard prophylactic strategy for peritoneal recurrence in patients with gastric carcinoma. *Ann. Surg.* 2009 Aug;250(2):242-6.

[105] Yonemura Y, Ninomiya I, Kaji M, et al., Prophylaxis with intraoperative chemohyperthermia against peritoneal recurrence of serosal invasion-positive gastric cancer. *World J. Surg.* 1995 May-Jun;19(3):450-4; discussion 5.

[106] Yu W, Whang I, Suh I, Averbach A, Chang D, Sugarbaker PH. Prospective randomized trial of early postoperative intraperitoneal chemotherapy as an adjuvant to resectable gastric cancer. *Ann. Surg.* 1998 Sep;228(3):347-54.

[107] Goto O, Fujishiro M, Kodashima S, Ono S, Omata M. Outcomes of endoscopic submucosal dissection for early gastric cancer with special reference to validation for curability criteria. *Endoscopy.* 2009 Feb;41(2):118-22.

[108] Gotoda T, Yanagisawa A, Sasako M, et al., Incidence of lymph node metastasis from early gastric cancer: estimation with a large number of cases at two large centers. *Gastric Cancer.* 2000 Dec;3(4):219-25.

[109] Hayashi H, Ochiai T, Mori M, et al., Sentinel lymph node mapping for gastric cancer using a dual procedure with dye- and gamma probe-guided techniques. *J. Am. Coll. Surg.* 2003 Jan;196(1):68-74.

[110] Miwa K, Kinami S, Taniguchi K, Fushida S, Fujimura T, Nonomura A. Mapping sentinel nodes in patients with early-stage gastric carcinoma. *Br. J. Surg.* 2003 Feb;90(2):178-82.

[111] Kim MC, Kim HH, Jung GJ, et al., Lymphatic mapping and sentinel node biopsy using 99mTc tin colloid in gastric cancer. *Ann. Surg.* 2004 Mar;239(3):383-7.

[112] Becher RD, Shen P, Stewart JH, Geisinger KR, McCarthy LP, Levine EA. Sentinel lymph node mapping for gastric adenocarcinoma. *Am. Surg.* 2009 Aug;75(8):710-4.

[113] Cardoso R, Bocicariu A, Dixon M, et al., What is the accuracy of sentinel lymph node biopsy for gastric cancer? A systematic review. *Gastric Cancer.* 2012 Sep;15 Suppl 1:S48-59.

[114] Can MF, Yagci G, Cetiner S. Systematic review of studies investigating sentinel node navigation surgery and lymphatic mapping for gastric cancer. *J. Laparoendosc Adv. Surg. Tech. A.* 2013 Aug;23(8):651-62.

[115] Hirayama R, Seshimo A, Miyake K, Nishizawa M, Kameoka S. Intraoperative diagnosis of lymph node metastasis by transcription-reverse transcription concerted reaction assay in gastric cancer. *Int. J.. Clin. Oncol.* 2013 Jun 14.

[116] Miyashiro I, Hiratsuka M, Sasako M, et al., High false-negative proportion of intraoperative histological examination as a serious problem for clinical application of sentinel node biopsy for early gastric cancer: final results of the Japan Clinical Oncology Group multicenter trial JCOG0302. *Gastric Cancer.* 2013 Aug 10.

[117] Kitagawa Y, Takeuchi H, Takagi Y, et al., Sentinel node mapping for gastric cancer: a prospective multicenter trial in Japan. *J. Clin. Oncol.* 2013 Oct 10;31(29):3704-10.

In: Gastric Cancer
Editor: Jasneet Singh Bhullar

ISBN: 978-1-63117-983-9
© 2014 Nova Science Publishers, Inc.

Chapter 4

Early Gastric Cancer: A Comprehensive View of Management

Wenbo Meng[1,2], Xun Li, M.D., Ph.D.[2,*], Wence Zhou[2], Yan Li[3], Kiyohito Tanaka, M.D., Ph.D.[4,†] and Liang Qiao[5]

[1]Special Minimally Invasive Surgery, the First Hospital of Lanzhou University, Lanzhou, Gansu, China
[2]The Second Department of General Surgery, the First Hospital of Lanzhou University, Hepatopancreatobiliary Surgery Institute of Gansu Province, Clinical Medical College Cancer Center of Lanzhou University, Lanzhou, Gansu, China
[3]Department of Immunology, Cleveland Clinic, Cleveland, OH, US
[4]Department of Gastroenterology, Kyoto Second Red Cross Hospital, Kyoto City, Japan
[5]Storr Liver Unit, Westmead Millennium Institute, Department of Medicine, The University of Sydney at Westmead Hospital, Australia

Abstract

Gastric cancer is one of the most common malignancies worldwide in terms of incidence and mortality. Nearly one million new cases of gastric cancer were diagnosed in 2008, representing 7.8% of all new cancer cases in that year. Most of those diagnosed patients died of this malignancy [1]. Late diagnosis, lack of effective treatment with tumor invasion and distant metastasis, as well as the poor understanding of the molecular mechanisms involved in the development of gastric cancer are among the major factors

---

* Corresponding author: Xun Li, M.D., Ph.D., Professor of Surgery, Department-II of General Surgery, the First Hospital of Lanzhou University, Lanzhou 730000, Gansu Province, China, Hepatopancreatobiliary Surgery Institute of Gansu Province, Lanzhou 730000, Gansu Province, China; Clinical Medical College Anti-Cancer Center of Lanzhou University, Lanzhou 730000, Gansu Province, China. Phone: +86931 8356821; Fax: +86931 8622275. E-mail: drlixun@163.com.
† Kiyohito Tanaka, M.D., Ph.D., Professor of Endoscopy, Department of Gastroenterology, Kyoto Second Red Cross Hospital. Kyoto city, 602-8096, Japan. Phone: +81 75 2315171; Fax: +81 75 212 6128; E-mail: seijin7705@gmail.com.

responsible for poor prognosis and high mortality rate. Advanced gastric cancer is not only associated with poor prognosis, but is also an important source of heavy financial burden and poor quality of life. The witnessed improvement in long-term survival rate of patients with gastric cancer over the past few decades is mainly attributable to improved early diagnosis and radical management [2]. As a comparison, the 5-year survival rate for advanced gastric cancer was reported to be 29% whereas that for early gastric cancer (EGC) was 91.8% [3]. Apparently, early diagnosis and treatment are the key components of effective management of patients with gastric cancer. However, the diagnosis and treatment of EGC remain a great challenge even in the hands of the experienced endoscopic experts.

Pathologically, EGC refers to the carcinoma with invasion depth limited to mucosa or submucosa. EGC can only be reliably diagnosed endoscopically [4]. Over the recent years, many endoscopic diagnostic approaches have been developed, such as endoscopic ultrasound (EUS), chromoscopy, the narrowband imaging zoom endoscope (NBI), confocal laser endomicroscopy, magnifying chromoendoscopy, autoflourescent endoscopy and infrared endoscopy. These newly developed endoscopic procedures have remarkably improved the diagnostic accuracy and enhanced the resection rate of EGC. Endoscopic submucosl dissection (ESD) has great advantages over conventional surgical resection in the management of EGC. As such, this procedure has been adopted as the standard method to treat the patients with EGC [5-7].

Measurement of serum biochemical parameters such as pepsinogen and *Helicobacter Pylori* IgG (HP-IgG) coupled with intelligent dyeing endoscopy (i-scan) has also been shown to greatly improve the detection rates of EGC, and the patients can have the chance to be radically cured at early stage [8].

In this article, we will systematically review the recent development in the endoscopic diagnosis and treatment of EGC. The article would greatly interest the gastroenterologists and surgical endoscopists.

Part A. On Overview of Gastric Cancer, Early Gastric Cancer, Diagnosis and Screening

A1. A Brief Introduction of the Epidemiology for Gastric Cancer

Gastric cancer is the second leading cause of death from malignant diseases worldwide, with especially high mortality rates in East, South, and Central Asia; Central and Eastern Europe; and South America [1, 2]. In 2008 worldwide, approximately 989,000 new cases of gastric cancer were diagnosed and 738,000 deaths recorded of whom approximately 70% were in the economically developing world [3]. In the developed countries/regions, the incidence rates of gastric cancer were reported to be 16.7% for males and 7.3% for females, and the reported death rates were 10.4% for males and 4.7% for females. Higher rates of incidence were reported in developing countries: 21.1% for males, and 7.3% for females. Likewise, higher death rates were reported in developing countries: 10% for males and 8.1% for females. Regardless of the geographic locations, gastric cancer is twice as common in males than in females. Despite a constant reduction in the mortality rate [3, 4], the prognosis of advanced gastric cancer remains poor, and surgery is the only option for cure with a 5-year survival rate of nearly 61%.

A2. Overview of Early Gastric Cancer

Early gastric cancer (EGC) was first defined in 1962 by the Japanese Society of Gastroenterological Endoscopy as the gastric adenocarcinoma confined to the mucosa or submucosa irrespective of lymph node involvement [5, 6].

The precise etiology for gastric cancer including EGC is unknown. Helicobacter pylori (H. pylori) infection has been identified as an essential but not a sole and sufficient causal factor. Host-bacterial interaction in H. pylori infected individuals may lead to different patterns of gastritis which may affect the disease outcomes. Due to the close association between H. pylori infection and the development of gastric cancer, strategies of H. pylori screening and eradication in high-risk populations have been recommended as effective approaches for reducing the incidence of gastric cancer.

Pathologically, EGC has been termed Type 0 gastric cancer, which is subdivided according to the macroscopic appearance of the lesions: 0-I, protruded or polypoid; 0-II, superficial; 0-III, excavated lesion characterized by a deep ulcer-like excavation. Among these sub-types, Type 0-II lesions are most prevalent and are further subdivided into IIa (slightly elevated), IIb (flat), and IIc (slightly depressed) [7, 8]. In EGC, the lymphatic metastasis rate is low, and for mucosa tumor the lymph node metastasis rate was reported to be only 1-3% [9].

EGC is a curable disease in many cases, and a variety of minimal invasive, function-preserving treatment options have been developed. In contrast to advanced gastric cancer, EGC has a much better prognosis, with a 5-year survival rate of 84% to 99% if properly treated [10-13]. However, as EGC hardly has any clinical symptoms, most patients are diagnosed at advanced stages. This has created a critical challenge for gastroenterologists and surgeons. Thus, early detection and treatment constitutes an important pre-requisite for the successful management of gastric cancer. In Japan, significantly reduced mortality rate and much improved survival of the patients with gastric cancer are largely attributable to successful endoscopic screening among the high-risk populations and subsequent effective early detection and treatment. Based on a study involving a 5-year screening for gastric cancer in 3,723 healthy subjects in Japan, it was recommended that endoscopic screening should be conducted on an yearly basis in people at their seventies, once every two to three years in their sixties, once every four years in their fifties, and once every five years in those under fifties [15].

Currently in Japan, the endoscopy based diagnosis rate for EGC reaches 40-50%. This is in sharp contrast to the developing countries where the endoscopic detection rate for EGC is only 8-15%. Several factors are believed to contribute to the low detection rate of EGC in developing countries, including insufficient knowledge of EGC among the endoscopists, lack of enthusiasm, and relatively poorer facilities [6, 16]. Continuous intensive training for endoscopists and constant improvement of the endoscopic equipments are essential for improved diagnostic rate.

A3. Endoscopic Diagnosis of EGC

The digestive endoscopy is an important method for early diagnosis and treatment for EGC. Because most cases of EGC have subtle lesions without typical clinical manifestations, diagnosis is frequently missed or wrongly made. Currently, gastroscopy with biopsy has become the standard, most precise and effective modality for the diagnosis of EGC, with an overall false negative rate of only 0.6%, an accuracy rate of 97.4%, and a specificity of 99.6% [17, 18]. Overall, more than 93.8% of patients with gastric cancer may be correctly diagnosed by endoscopy.

The conventional endoscopic method (so called "white light endoscopy") is still a standard method for diagnosis of EGC. However, in order to improve its low detection rate and inaccuracy in reaching a correct diagnosis, image enhanced endoscopy such as chromoendoscopy (also termed dye endoscopy, or pigment endoscopy), narrow-band imaging endoscopy (NBI), endoscopic ultrasonography (EUS), and confocal endomicroscopy (CLE) have been developed and entered into clinical practice.

Among the image enhanced endoscopic procedures, chromoendoscopy has the advantages of being able to inspect and identify the gastric mucosal lesions through various stains whilst the endoscopy is being performed. More importantly, the stains will help accurately identify the suspicious lesions where biopsy should be taken. When coupled with more accurate tissue sampling, the accuracy of chromoendoscopy in diagnosing cancerous mucosal lesions of the stomach can be improved by 5-10% [19, 20]. The recently developed Flexible spectral imaging color enhancement (FICE) can achieve a diagnostic accuracy and specificity of >90% [21].

NBI endoscopy is another powerful endoscopic procedure for the diagnosis of EGC [22]. With magnifying endoscopy, NBI enables a better visualization of the mucosal morphology and capillary structures, thereby facilitating accurate biopsy and improved detection rate. The diagnostic accuracy and specificity of NBI can achieve >90% [23].

With its magnifying power of 100 times, magnifying endoscopy confocal endomicroscopy can clearly reveal the structures at the cellular and sub-cellular glandular levels, thereby allowing immediate histological diagnosis and targeted biopsy. Data from Japanese studies have shown that the diagnostic accuracy and specificity of magnifying endoscopy for EGC exceed 95% [24]. If combined with chromoendoscopy, the diagnostic power can be further enhanced [25, 26].

EUS offers a unique diagnostic value for EGC in that it can detect the tumor invasion depth [27]. With EUS, it is possible to detect whether regional lymph node metastasis is present.

Confocal laser microendoscope (CLE) is a sophisticated diagnostic tool for EGC. CLE is particularly useful for detecting very small EGC, with a diagnostic accuracy of 89.7%.

In European Gastrointestinal Endoscope Manual, the recommended diagnostic approaches for EGC include magnifying chromoendoscopy, NBI, multiple biopsies (>4 suspicious areas), pathological staging, low serum pepsinogen, and a positive family history [28].

More detailed discussion on the endoscopic features and endoscopic management of EGC are presented in Part B.

A4. Other Diagnostic Approaches for EGC

X-ray barium examination, particularly gastric double contrast (GDC) barium meal was once believed a very useful method of diagnosing EGC. It has an accuracy rate of 50% to

91%, depending on several factors such as the X-ray machine used, the experience of the radiologist, and the quality of the barium meal preparation. The consensus holds that when GDC is combined with gastroscopy and histological examination, the diagnostic accuracy for EGC can reach 95.4% [29].

CT scan has a higher diagnosis value for locating and determining the advanced gastric cancers, but it has little value for diagnosing EGC. Three-stage enhancement spiral CT scan has a low diagnostic rate for EGC, but it has a high accuracy for TNM staging.

The experience of using MRI in the diagnosis of EGC is very limited, and so is its diagnostic value.

A5. A Brief Account on the Screening for EGC

Effective screening program facilitate early diagnosis and treatment of gastric cancer and is believed to reduce the incidence of gastric cancer. The benefit of screening for EGC is probably reflected by the considerable reduction in the mortality rate of gastric cancer in Japan and Korea where nationwide screening program was established in the sixties and nineties, respectively.

The Japanese Cancer Association recommended conducting gastroscopy on the positive patients preliminarily screened by X-ray pneumobarium double contrast. With the development of endoscopy technologies over the past years, endoscopy-based screening program has become more popular compare to the X-ray-based upper gastrointestinal contrast studies and other screening approaches such as serum pepsinogen studies. Precancerous conditions such as atypical hyperplasia or polyps could be safely removed endoscopically, preventing further development into frank gastric cancer.

Presently in Japan, the combination of serum anti-H. pylori antibody (anti-HP-IgG) and the serum level of pepsinogen (PG) is used as a guidance for how frequent an endoscopic based screening for EGC should be exercised. Based on this program, patients can be divided into several groups. Group A (H. Pylori$^-$/PG$^-$), Group B (H. Pylori$^+$/PG$^-$), Group C (H. Pylori$^+$/PG$^+$), and Group D (H. Pylori$^-$/PG$^+$). The recommendation states that endoscopic examination should be performed once every five years for patients in Group A, once every three years for those in Group B, once every two years for those in Group C, and on an yearly basis for those in Group D.

A6. Eradication of H. Pylori Infection as gastric Cancer Prevention

H. pylori infection is by far the most important risk factor for gastric cancer. As such, H. pylori has been classified the Class I carcinogen by the World Health Organization (WHO). In patients with H. pylori infection, eradication therapy can reduce the chances of malignant transformation of the gastric mucosa. Therefore, even in the patients with H. pylori related high-grade intraepithelial neoplasia, eradicating H. pylori is endorsed to reduce the risk of developing gastric cancer [30]. It is recommended that a yearly endoscopic follow-up should be performed in patients with extensive atrophy of the gastric and intestinal mucosa.

Development of drug resistance is a hurdle for effective H. pylori eradication. For example, in China, 60-70% of the H. pylori strains are resistant to metronidazole, 20-38% are resistant to clarithromycin, 30-38% are resistant to levofloxacin, and 1-5% are resistant to amoxicillin, furazolidone, and tetracycline. As such, the traditional standard triple therapy (PPI + amoxicillin + clarithromycin or PPI + clarithromycin + metronidazole) only has an eradication rate of less than 80%, and even after extended course of treatment, the eradication rate could only be raised by 5%.

Consequently, new eradication programs have been developed, such as sequential therapy, accompanying therapy, and lavo-ofloxacin based triple therapy. However, multi-center randomized controlled trials (RCT) in China have revealed that sequential therapy has no advantage over the standard triple therapy. No research data are currently available on the use of "accompanying therapy", which is said to increase the risk of developing adverse reactions of the anti-H. pylori drugs, therefore making the antibiotic selection difficult after unsuccessful treatments. Similarly, RCTs in China have found that lavo-ofloxacin triple therapy has no obvious advantages over other regimens. Clearly, the above "new" therapies are not suitable in China [31].

The Maastricht IV Consensus stated that in the areas where the rate of clarithromycin resistance to H. pylori is high, Bismuth agents (four-outreach program) may be used but if they are not available, sequential therapy and accompanying therapy are recommended. In the areas where the rate of clarithromycin resistance to H. pylori is low, standard triple therapy, sequential therapy and accompanying therapy can all be chosen as the first-line treatments.

The classic Bismuth agents (four-outreach program) consists of bismuth agent + PPI + tetracycline + metronidazole. Alternatively, Bismuth agents may be added into the PPI triple therapy to form new Bismuth agents four outreach program.

Part B. Endoscopic Features of EGC and Various Approaches for Diagnosing EGC

B1. Characteristics and Classification of EGC

A variety of endoscopic features of EGC have been described. These features mainly consist of mucosal color changes (pale redness, or fading of color) and morphological changes (ulceration, erosion, depression, rough, uplift, plaques and nodules). However, these signs are by no means the specific characteristics for EGC. As a result, it is extremely important to screen EGC from the cases showing these non-specific signs.

Based on the classification system by JGCA (Japanese Gastric Cancer Association) [32], the gross morphology of the EGC can be categorized as either superficial or advanced type. Superficial type is typical of T1 tumors while T2-4 tumors usually manifest as advanced types. Viewed from the mucosal surface, gross tumor appearance is further classified into three types as detailed below in the sub-classification of Type 0 (EGC).

1. Type 0-I (protruding): polypoid tumors*.
2. Type 0-II (superficial): Tumors with or without minimal elevation or depression relative to the surrounding mucosa.
   (1) Type 0-IIa (superficial elevated): Slightly elevated tumors*.
   (2) Type 0-IIb (superficial flat): Tumors without elevation or depression.

(3) Type 0-IIc (superficial depressed): Slightly depressed tumors.
3. Type 0-III (excavated): Tumors with deep depression

*: Tumors with less than 3 mm elevation are usually classified as 0-IIa, those elevated more than 3 mm are usually classified as 0-I.

This classification is better illustrated in Figure 1.

Small gastric cancer refers to the pathological changes within the range of 6-10 mm.

If the lesion is less than 5 mm, it is called minute gastric carcinoma. Cancers identified in biopsy specimen under endoscope but not found in surgical pathological examination are called supermicro cancer or a tip cancer.

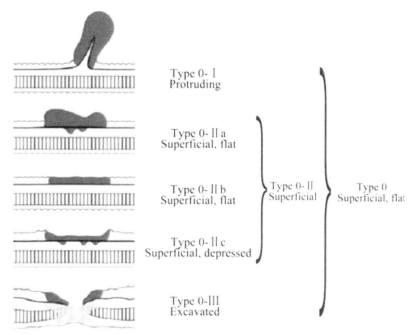

Cited from Japanese Classification of Gastric Carcinoma: 3rd English Edition, Gastric Cancer (2011) 14:101–112. DOI 10.1007/s10120-011-0041-5. [32].

Figure 1. Macroscopic classification of EGC by JGCA (Japanese Gastric Cancer Association).

Under endoscope, the depressed type of EGC mainly present as irregularly depressed erosion or shallow ulcer, with rugged surface mucosa or granular changes. Depressed EGC may also manifest as bulging lesions with surrounding irregular nodular mucosa and interruptions, often with hard texture of tissue creeping through the weakened. The protruding type (0-I and 0-IIa Types) mainly manifest as irregularly shaped bulging lesions, and is usually easy to identify. The flat lesions (0-IIb Type) mainly present as the single congestive erosion, with rough and red mucosa. Gastric mucosa particularly that in the gastric body folds should be carefully inspected if this type of lesions are suspected (Figure 2).

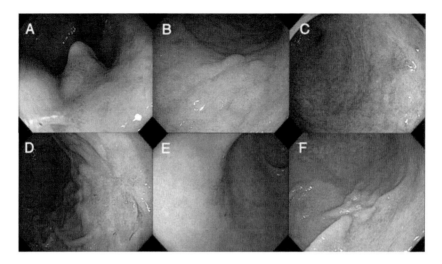

Figure 2. T0 Macroscopic classification of early gastric cancer (EGC). A: 0-I, well-differentiated adenocarcinoma; B: 0-IIa, well-differentiated adenocarcinoma; C: 0-IIb, well-differentiated adenocarcinoma; D: 0-IIc, poorly-differentiated adenocarcinoma; E: 0-IIc + IIb, well-differentiated adenocarcinoma; F: 0-IIc+III, poorly-differentiated adenocarcinoma.

B2. Practical Considerations in Pathological Diagnosis of EGC

It should be noted that there exist some differences between the diagnostic criteria for EGC used in Japan and those used in other Western countries [33]. In Western countries, cancer is diagnosed if the tumor has invaded the submucosa or muscularis mucosae and has at least invaded deeper than the lamina propria mucosae. In Japan, however, cancer is diagnosed based on cellular atypia or structural atypia, regardless of the extent of invasion. Although this discrepancy has lessened since the Vienna Classification was proposed, lesions diagnosed as intramucosal carcinoma in Japan are still classified as high-grade adenoma/dysplasia (Vienna Classification 4.1) in Western countries and often not diagnosed as cancer [34]. More than 40% of lesions classified as equivalent to Vienna Classification 3 or 4.1 on preoperative biopsy are diagnosed as cancer on the post endoscopic resection assessment.

It has been reported that invasion into deeper regions of the submucosa also occurs in a small number of EGC cases [35, 36]. Therefore, when considering a complete cure, it is necessary to proceed carefully in cases with histological diagnosis of neoplastic or dysplastic diseases and, on a case-by-case basis, to consider endoscopic resection [37].

Unlike advanced cancers which are easy to detect endoscopically, EGC often shows subtle changes in the mucosal surface. To avoid missing the diagnosis of a cancer on endoscopy, the characteristics of EGC must be well understood and gastric inspection must be thorough [38]. While diagnosis is based on conventional white light endoscopy findings, the use of other sophisticated endoscopic procedures such as chromoendoscopy, NBI, and EUS has considerably improved the diagnostic value for EGC.

B3. Application of Chromoendoscopy in the Diagnosis of EGC

Chromoendoscopy has been shown to significantly improve the diagnostic accuracy for intestinal metaplasia (IM) and other precancerous conditions, leading to an enhanced diagnostic yield for EGC. Staining dye is typically directly sprayed onto the gastric mucosa via the biopsy channel [39-41]. Commonly used staining methods include *Methylene Blue methods* and *Indigo Carmine methods*.

When 0.5% of Methylene Blue is sprayed onto the gastric mucosa, the dye is absorbed by absorptive mucosal epithelium. The staining patterns will help judge the nature of the lesions. Usually, the abnormal epithelium such as mucosa with intestinal metaplasia and atypical hyperplasia will be stained dark or dark blue, making them easily identifiable under the endoscopy. It was reported that when combined with magnification endoscopy, Methylene Blue staining will detect gastric intestinal metaplasia and dysplasia with 84% and 83% accuracy, respectively. However, false positivity may occur [42-47].

With *Indigo Carmine methods*, gastric mucosa is sprayed with 0.1-0.2% Indigo Carmine via the biopsy forceps channel.

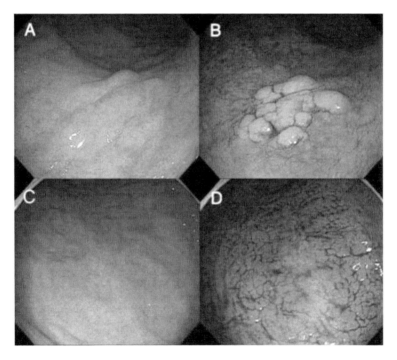

Figure 3. Chromoendoscopy with Indigo Carmine staining. Endoscopic review of protruded lesions (0-IIa) without (A) or with (B) Indigo Carmine staining. Similarly, the depressed lesions (0-IIc) (C) can also be clearly shown by Indigo Carmine staining (D).

Indigo Carmine is not absorbed by the mucosal epithelium, but instead, it highlights the mucosal topography by giving a dark bluish color, making the possible mucosal lesions more readily identifiable. With the assistance of Indigo Carmine staining, EGC especially small gastric cancer of the 0-IIb type may be easily identified.

The diagnostic rate for malignant changes by Indigo Carmine staining exceeds 90% [48-54]. Typical views of EGC identified by Indigo Carmine staining are shown in Figure 3.

B4. Narrow-Band Imaging (NBI)

The first generation of NBI technology, jointly developed by Olympus Corporation and the National Cancer Center East in Japan, aims at enhancing the visibility of the fine capillaries and structures in the mucosal surface in order to improve the diagnostic accuracy of EGC [55-64].

NBI is an image-enhanced endoscopy system that enhances the visibility of the superficial surface structure including vascular architecture of the mucosa by illuminating blue and green narrowband lights (Figures 4 and Figure 5).

Combination of the magnification endoscopy and NBI makes it possible to observe microvascular (MV) and microsurface (MS) patterns of the gastric mucosa in detail. Based on the imaging patterns of the magnifying NBI endoscopy, a diagnostic system termed VS Classification System was developed which combines the endoscopic changes with the presence or absence of a demarcation line [65, 66]. With the conventional white light observation, the NBI magnification endoscopy could reach an excellent diagnostic yield for EGC.

With the use of VS System, the difference between cancer and gastritis can be better distinguished, thereby reducing the number of unnecessary biopsies. NBI magnification system has also proven useful for margin determination when conducting the detailed examination prior to endoscopic therapy [67].

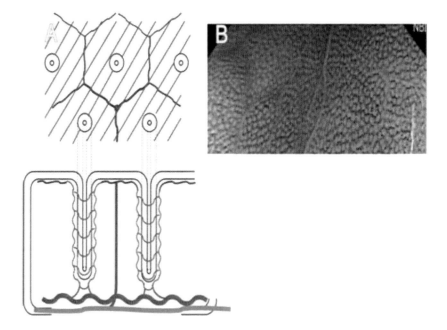

Figure 4. Normal gastric mucosa at gastric body as revealed by NBI. A. Structure of normal gastric mucosa at gastric body. B. True capillaries in gastric body as shown by NBI.

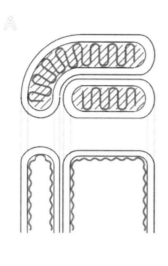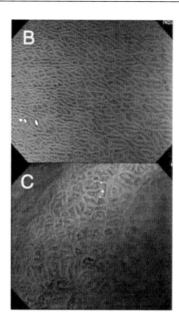

Figure 5. Normal pyloric gland region as shown by NBI. A. Structure of normal pyloric gland; B. polygon-shaped crypt marginal epithelia; C. coil-shaped capillary vessel.

However, it should be noted that NBI is not an all-purpose method. Because of the large size of the gastric lumen and use of narrow band lights darkens the endoscopic image, NBI, therefore, is not suitable for identifying lesions within the stomach. Furthermore, non-magnified NBI has limited utility with undifferentiated cancers because these cancers are often localized to the height of the glandular neck within the lamina propria mucosae, and the tumor surface remains covered with normal crypt epithelium. As such, it is difficult for the conventional NBI to reveal the characteristic irregular MV and MS patterns of cancer. Accordingly, diagnosis of undifferentiated cancers requires negative biopsies in the area surrounding the cancer [68-75].

Magnify NBI is useful in identifying the changes in mucosal microvascular architecture in the course of malignant transformation. The microvascular patterns associated with malignant transformation were classified into three groups: A, fine network; B, corkscrew; and C, unclassified pattern [69]. Under magnifying endoscope, normal mucosa shows the rugular micro-vascular and micro surface patterns. In contrast, malignant ulcers may be associated with some characteristic changes such as alteration in mucosal pattern, loss of subepithelial capillary network, and appearances of tumor angiogenesis. The newly formed blood vessels in tumor may demonstrate irregular size and shape (e.g., dilatation, tortuosity, difference of caliber and variety in shape). Typical views of EGC under the NBI magnifying endoscopy are shown in Figure 6 and Figure 7. Based on the Nakayoshi's Classification, the patterns of the micro-veins in well-differentiated gastric adenocarcinoma are generally regular in 66.1% of cases, whereas in undifferentiated gastric adenocaicnoma, 85.7% of the micro-veins are distorted and irregular [69]. Under the NBI magnification endoscopy, differentiated gastric adenocarcinoma may display grid-like pits and expanded or twisted veins in the fovea, whereas poorly-differentiated or undifferentiated adenocarcinomas usually present with irregularly expanded or twisted small veins, and destroyed or loss of fovea.

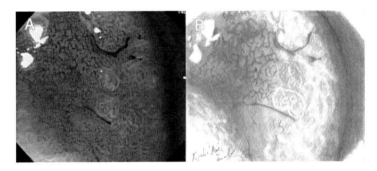

Figure 6. Well-differentiated adenocarcinoma, viewed by magnifying NBI. A. Honey comb like capillaries called "fine network pattern"; B. "fine network pattern" sketch by Dr. K. Tanaka. These vessels are often seen in differentiated adenocarcinoma.

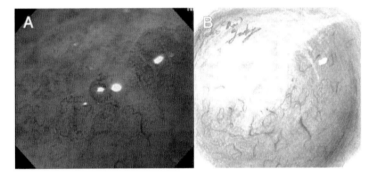

Figure 7. Poorly-differentiated adenocarcinoma, viewed by magnifying NBI. A. Heterogeneous and tortous capillaries called "cork screw pattern"; B. "cork screw pattern" sketch by Dr. K. Tanaka. These vessels are often seen in undifferentiated adenocarcinoma.

Thus, magnifying NBI may help distinguish the differentiated from undifferentiated gastric cancers.

B5. Endoscopic Ultrasound (EUS)

EUS is of particular use in TNM classification as it has a superior value in assessing the penetration depth of gastrointestinal malignancies. EUS is also a powerful tool in the assessment of locoregional lymphadenopathy and involvement of adjacent organs, thereby provide critical guidance on selecting appropriate therapeutic modalities. Depending on the frequencies used and the alternating bright (hyperechoic) and dark (hypoechoic) appearance of the tissues being examined, 5 to 9 layers of the gastric wall can be detected by EUS. Under the EUS, mucosa, muscularis mucosa, submucosa, muscularis propria, and serosa usually show a pattern of "hyper- hypo- hyper- hypo- hyperechoic" (Figure 8). Based on a meta-analysis of 22 studies [76], the sensitivity and specificity of EUS in assessing the tumor penetration were 88.1% and 100% in T1, 82.3% and 95.6% in T2, 89.7% and 94.7 in T3, and 99.2% and 96.7% in T4. In the assessment of T stages, EUS is more accurate in advanced gastric cancers compared to EGC.

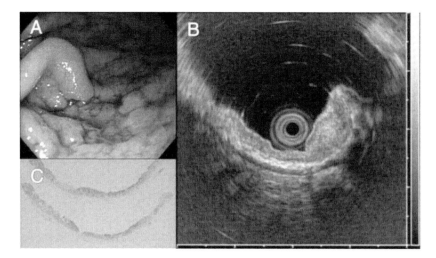

Figure 8. EUS with depth "M" EGC. A. 0-IIc signet ring cell carcinoma, M; B. The invasion depth and the layers of the gastric wall can be clearly distinguished by bright (hyperechoic) and dark (hypoechoic) appearance under EUS. The invasion-related mucosa is shown. C. Pathological view of the corresponding mucosa layers.

Based on a meta-analysis involving 5,601 patients from 54 studies [81], EUS was found to be particularly accurate in distinguishing between the lesions. EUS can be an effective option to accurately evaluate the depth of invasion and predict bleeding if endoscopic procedures. However, in the lesions with ulcer or fibrosis, the accuracy of the depth of invasion may be under estimated by EUS [77-82].

B6. FICE

FICE is based on a spectral estimation technology initially invented by Professor Yoichi Miyake of the Chiba University. An image captured by the Fujifilm electronic scope is processed with the Spectral Estimation Matrix processing circuit. Various pixilated spectrums of the image were estimated. Since the spectrums by pixels are estimated, it is possible to implement imaging on a single wavelength. Such single wavelength images are randomly selected, and assigned to R (Red) G (Green) and B (Blue) respectively to build and display a FICE enhanced color image. The expected advantage of this new digital processing system is a dramatic enhancement in the detection and identification of pathologic changes. The FICE system is expected to enable doctors to make more accurate clinical diagnosis.

B7. Confocal Laser Endomicroscopy (CLE)

Confocal laser endomicroscopy (CLE) is a novel endoscopic procedure combining the on-site microscopy of the gastrointestinal mucosa with fluorescence. Since its first description in 2004, the number of diseases studied with this technique has steadily increased [83]. CLE can enhance the biopsy accuracy by means of "intravital microscopy", and its indications have extended from the upper and lower gastrointestinal tract to the hepatobiliary system. The intravital microscopy makes CLE an ideal tool to study the pathophysiological events dynamically in their natural environment in patients. The observation depth of mucosal surface and submucosal surface can be 250 μm, which is the distance between the mucosal surface and submucosa.

The CLE can provide high quality pictures of the tumor cells and normal mucosal cells in digestive tract. The histopathology obtained by CLE is highly consistent with that obtained by H&E staining in the biopsy tissues. CLE is said to have a high sensibility and specificity for diagnosing EGC. Under the CLE, normal mucosa shows smooth nucleolus whereas gastric cancer cells may display irregular nucleolus [84]. Furthermore, CLE has tremendous advantages for distinguishing the micro-vein images between normal and malignant tissues. The characteristic features of differentiated gastric cancer under CLE include loss of normal gastric pits, disorganization of gastric glands, and deeply stained glandular epithelial cells with inhomogeneity.

In contrast, loss of normal gastric pits, loss of gastric glands, and appearance of black non-conventional cell clusters suggest undifferentiated gastric cancers.

B8. The Laser-Induced Fluorescence (LIFE)

Laser-induced fluorescence (LIFE) is a new diagnostic technology combining primary fluorescence with gastroscopy. With this technology, it is possible to differentiate tumor tissues from non-tumor tissues [85]. Therefore, LIFE can more precisely guide the biopsy and enhance the diagnostic accuracy. As such, LIFE is regarded by the international community as the fifth most useful diagnostic tool for tumors after X-ray, ultrasonography, CT scan, and MRI.

LIFE offers two diagnostic modes: imaging diagnostics and spectrum diagnostics. Under the LIFE endoscopy, normal smooth mucosal surface show bright green fluorescence, whereas atypical hyperplasia or cancer mucosa show red or purple fluorescence. Moreover, the surface veins in the tumor marginal region can absorb light to display blue color (because of the hemoglobin), this can be considered a sign for cancer tissues. In the wavelength of 400-550 nm, the intrinsic fluorescence intensity of cancer tissues is lower than that of the non-tumorous mucosa. Thus, LIFE is a very useful tool for enhancing the biopsy accuracy.

Part C. Endoscopic Management of EGC by Endoscopic Mucosal Resection (EMR) and Endoscopic Submucosal Dissection (ESD)

Diagnostic accuracy for EGC has considerably improved owing to the constant improvement of the endoscopic technologies (Figure 9). Enhanced diagnostic efficiency for EGC means an increased cure rate and improved patient survival.

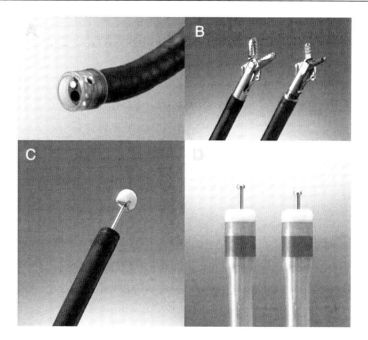

Figure 9. ESD instruments. A. Normal in-viewing endoscope with transparent cap; B. Electric cauterization using forceps such as Coagrasper; C. IT2 knife; D. Dual knife.

It is now believed that EGC is a curable disease in many cases. A variety of less invasive, function-preserving treatment options are increasingly used in the management of patients with EGC. At the present time, the most commonly used endoscopic approaches for the treatment of EGC are endoscopic mucosal resection (EMR) and endoscopic submucosa dissection (ESD). In East Asian countries, such as Japan, Korea, and China, EMR and ESD have become the standard treatment for EGC [86].

C1. A Brief Introduction of Endoscopic Mucosal Resection (EMR)

EMR is a widely accepted minimally invasive treatment for EGC with little risk of lymph node metastasis [87]. Since its first report by Tamoto Tada et al. in 1984, more than 3,000 cases of EMR have been reported in Japan alone [88].

At present, EMR is indicated for gastric cancers if they are: (a) confined to mucosa, (b) less than 2 cm in size, (c) histologically confirmed differentiated type, and (d) without ulcer or ulcer scar in the lesion [89]. Different techniques may be used to perform EMR, including injection-assisted, cap-assisted, and ligation-assisted techniques. Regardless of what techniques are used in a given case of EMR, the basic procedures are identification and demarcation of the lesions, submucosal injection to lift the lesion, and endoscopic snare resection. Due to its overall safety and efficacy in appropriately selected patient populations, EMR has become firmly integrated in the diagnostic and treatment algorithms of superficial malignancies of the gastrointestinal tract.

However, EMR is associated with high frequency of residual disease and recurrence, making this procedure inferior to surgical therapy. With the continuous development of endoscopy technologies and operation equipment, another powerful endoscopic procedure termed "endoscopic submucosa dissection (ESD)" has been developed, which gradually replaces EMR in many cases in the past few years [90].

C2. A Brief Introduction of Endoscopic Submucosa Dissection (ESD)

ESD was developed in late 1990 for the complete removal of the gastric dysplasia and cancer regardless of their size and location. Presently, ESD is indicated for EGCs if they are: Indication: A differentiated-type adenocarcinoma without ulcerative findings (UL(-)), of which the depth of invasion is clinically diagnosed as T1a and the diameter is≤2 cm. Expanded indication (investigational treatment): Tumors clinically diagnosed as T1a and: (a) of differentiated-type, UL(-), but>2 cm in diameter; (b) of differentiated-type, UL(+), and≤3 cm in diameter; (c) of undifferentiated-type, UL(-), and≤2 cm in diameter [89].

ESD uses a specialized needle knife or equipment to dissect the lesions from the wall, assisted by a long-lasting submucosal fluid cushion. The major advantage of ESD is that it offers significantly larger *en bloc* resection of tumor than EMR. Gotoda et al. analyzed more than 5,000 EGC patients who underwent gastrectomy with meticulous D2 level lymph node dissection [89]. They have observed that the intramucosal differentiated gastric cancers (well- and moderately-differentiated tubular adenocarcinoma and papillary adenocarcinoma) without lymphatic and vascular involvement had a nominal risk of lymph node metastasis.

However, ESD also has several disadvantages compared to EMR in that ESD is technically demanding, requires longer time to perform, and carries higher risk of complications. Nevertheless, ESD is still believed to be an effective method to treat EGC [91-96]. Currently, the International Gastric Cancer Association has expected to listed ESD as the standard curative method for T1 stage gastric cancer. As revealed by a retrospective cohort study for the treatment of EGC, the 3-year survival rate following ESD was 94.6%, and that for radical resection was 89.7%. Furthermore, ESD was found to be superior to radical resection in terms of operation time, complications, and length of hospital stay [97].

In the *en bloc* resection, it is crucial to ensure that no cancer cells are detectable in the incisional margin, and no basal layer and vascular invasion are present.

Preoperative comprehensive assessment is essential. If the guideline criteria are strictly adhered to, ESD should yield long-term outcomes comparable to the gold standard radical gastrectomy.

C3. The Procedures for EMR and ESD

C3.1. Equipment and Agents

The following items/materials should be available: normal in-viewing endoscope (automatic water jet systems of endoscopy for ESD), various types of knife, local injection needles, snare, transparent caps, epinephrine, saline, Indigo Carmine, Methylene Blue, and high-frequency and electrosurgical generator.

The injection solution for EMR: glycerol and fructose solution (10% glycerol + 50 K fructose + saline). The injection solution for ESD: 10% glycerol fructose (200 ml) + Indigo Carmine (0.5 ml) + adrenaline (2 ml) + hyaluronic acid.

C3.2. Basic Operation

1. Define the lesion range: the distance from the therapeutic focus to surrounding tissues is 5 mm. Multiple points can be burned along the whole boundary by coagulating current.
2. Local injection: hypertonic saline, epinephrine, glycerol and fructose solution are mixed with Methylene Blue. The mixture is injected from remote end to make focus bulge.

It should be noted that the preoperative preparation and intraoperative management for both EMR and ESD are the same except that ESD requires longer operating time than EMR, and proper anesthesia should be arranged.

C3.3. Procedures for EMR

In 1984, strip biopsy was described as a part of the endoscopic snare polypectomy [98]. This technique used a double channel endoscope. After submucosal injection around the lesion, a grasper was inserted through one channel to lift the lesion, and then a snare was inserted through the other channel to resect the lesion.

In 1988, another EMR technique (with circumferential pre-cutting, EMR-P) using hypertonic saline mixed with diluted epinephrine solution was introduced. In this procedure, after hypertonic saline is injected into the submucosal layer, a needle knife is used to cut the lesion around the injection line and the lesion is removed by a snare [99].

In 1992, transparent cap-assisted EMR (EMR-C) technique was developed and has since been used to treat early esophageal cancer and EGC [100]. This technique uses a transparent hood that is connected to the tip of a standard endoscope. Following the submucosal injection, the lesion is sucked into the cap while a specialized crescent-shaped snare located at the tip of the cap is closed. (Figure 10, Figure 11). Later, EMR with ligation (EMR-L) was introduced [101]. This technique uses a standard endoscopic variceal ligation device to capture the lesion. The EMR-C and the EMR-L are simple and effective methods for small cancers; however, they are unsuitable for lesions larger than 20 mm. EMR has limited usefulness for *en bloc* resections.

Supplemental resection: after resection, if there are still mark spots left, injection should be done again and supplemental resection should be conducted.

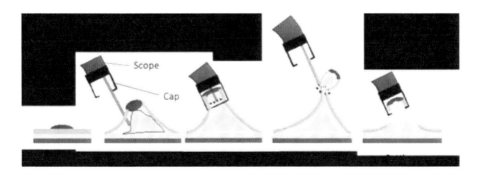

Figure 10. Illustration of EMR-C.

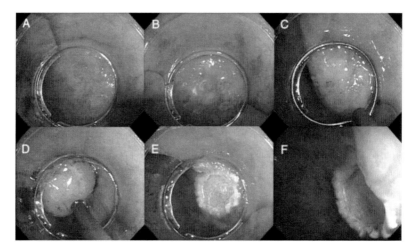

Figure 11. The procedure of EMR-C for EGC. A. Find the EGC and focus; B. Submucosal injection around the lesion; C. Using hypertonic saline mixed with diluted epinephrine solution; D. Snare was inserted and enclosed the lesion; E. Resect the lesion; F. The lesion was removed.

If the residual tissue is little, the boundary should be remediated by APC electrical burn. Exposed veins in the resection stump should be properly treated with electrocoagulation.

Broken muscle layer should be properly sewed with chin clips to prevent possible perforation. The resected specimens should be appropriately treated as discussed in Part D.

C3.4 Procedures for ESD

1. *Mark the target lesions.* Usually, the morphology of the lesions particularly small lesions in the gastric lumen is not clear. Thus, Indigo Carmine staining should be used to highlight the lesions to be resected. Alternatively, hydrogen knife or needle knife can be used to burn out white dots alongside the lesion (3-5 mm away from the lesion) so that the target lesion is clearly visible.
2. *Local injection and mucosa incision*: sufficient glycerin fructose solution containing Indigo Carmine and adrenaline is injected into submucosa so that the mucosal lesion is sufficiently uplifted. The needle knife or knife IT is then used to cut alongside but 5 mm away from the marked points with soft pressure on uplift parts. If uplifted properly, small lesions can be cut completely.

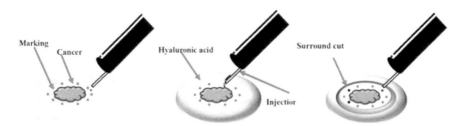

Figure 12. Illustration of ESD procedures.

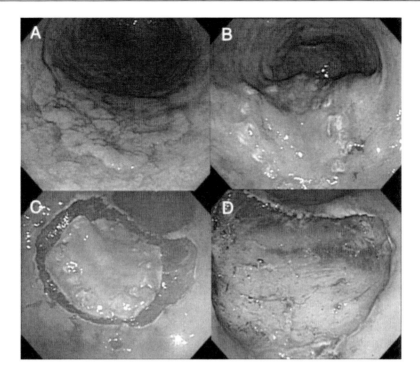

Figure 13. The procedures of ESD. A. Find the EGC using Chromoendoscopy Indigo Carmine method; B. Mark the lesion; C. Hypertonic saline mixed with diluted epinephrine solution injection; D. Resect the lesion.

The submucosal dissection: IT or hook knife should be used to strip mucosa. If the mucosa including lesions is fully uplifted, the mucosa can be completely detached. Snare can be used to completely trap the mucosa with electric coagulation and to remove the resected tissues. Alternatively, endoscopic front-end transparent cap can be used to remove the tissues. If the lesion stripping turns out to be difficult, the mucosa can be partitioned into several pieces in order to prevent severe complications (Figure 12, Figure 13).

3. *Post-resection processing*: The stripped surface should be completely flushed to exam if bleeding occurs. Hemostatic forceps, clips, or electrocautery unit should be used when necessary. In case of serious bleeding that can not be managed endoscopically, surgery should be performed.
4. *Processing of the resected specimens*: please refer to Part D.

C4. Management of Residual Tumor

It is very rare to have the residual tumors after EMR or ESD. A positive margin is defined as the distance between tumor and incisional margin being less than 1 mm, and/or tumor cells can be seen along the incisional margin. Poor prognosis is indicated if the tumors invade the submucosa, have already invaded into the blood vessels and lymphatic ducts, and positive incisional margins are identified. If a positive margin is identified on follow up, repeat EMR may be performed. The residual lesion may be burnt with microwave or laser. If necessary, partial stomach resection can be considered.

If tumor infiltration to SM_1 with vessel invasion or infiltration to under SM_2 is identified, additional surgical procedure of stomach is needed, and lymph node resection should be conducted.

C5. The Advantages of Endoscopic Resection (ER)

Compared with traditional laparotomy, ER has many advantages, such as better safety profile, minimal invasion, fewer complications, and a better tolerability. ER can provide intuitive information for postoperative and academic discussion. In case of ESD, the procedure can be conducted in multiple positions in one treatment session, and one patient can accept repeated treatments on multiple occasions. Most importantly, with ESD, complete pathological specimens can be obtained, making the clinical diagnosis more accurate and treatment more desirable [102].

C6. The Complications of EMR and ESD and the Management

ER may be associated with various complications, most notably pain, bleeding, gastric perforation, and stenosis.

C6.1. Pain

The pain after endoscopic resection is generally mild and can be easily controlled by proton pump inhibitors and opioids.

C6.2. Bleeding

Bleeding is the most common complication of EMR and ESD [103]. On average, 10% (ranging from 1% to 45%) of the patients underwent EMR or ESD will experience excessive bleeding [104, 105]. Bleeding can occur immediately in the procedures, or after the procedures are completed (delayed bleeding).

According to the National Cancer Center in Japan, EMR has a hemorrhage rate of 6%, and the majority of bleeding cases occurred intraoperatively or within 24 hours postoperatively.

ER related hemorrhage is closely related to the tumor site and size. Immediate bleeding (defined as bleeding occurred within 24 hours of the procedures) frequently occurs with the resection of tumors located in the upper third of the stomach because of the rich blood supply and the presence of many large blood vessels in this region.

Delayed bleeding (defined as hematemesis or melena at 0 to 30 days after the procedure) occurs more commonly in patients underwent ESD, with the reported rate of 7-13.9% [106, 107] . In Korea, the reported rate of bleeding after ESD ranges from 1.8% to 15.6% [108]. A slightly higher bleeding rate of 18% was reported in Western countries [109].

Immediate bleeding during ESD can be treated by electrocautery or endoscopic clipping, depending on the degree of bleeding. Slight oozing can be controlled by the electrocautery using cutting devices, such as an IT tool, hook, double knife (KD -611 L, KD 620LR, or KD -

650 L, Olympus Medical Systems Corp), or SAFEKnifeV or FlushKnife BT (DK2618JB DK2518DV, Fuji Photo Film Co).

Electric cauterization using forceps such as Coagrasper (FD-410LR, Olympus Medical Systems Corp) or hot biopsy forceps (Boston Scientific) may be used to treat the artery bleeding.

The key step to achieve a good hemostasis effect is to precisely identify the bleeding point and rinse with water. Endoscopic water jet system has recently become a useful tool for bleeding control during the ER procedures.

Some studies have suggested that use of acid suppressive agents such as proton pump inhibitors (PPIs) after ESD could help the healing and prevent delayed bleeding, whereas other studies showed no benefit of using PPIs or H2 receptor antagonists after ESD [110-113].

C6.3. Perforation

Perforation is another common and serious complication. ESD was reported to be associated with a higher rate of perforation than EMR (4-10% vs 0.3-0.5%) [114-122].

Perforations are divided into micro-perforation or frank perforation depending on the size, and immediate or delayed, depending on the onset. Two endoscopic clipping methods have been reported, including "single sealing method" and "omentum patch method" (HX-610-090, HX-610-090L, Olympus Medical Systems Corp). Generally, a small perforation of the stomach is managed with "single sealing method" without needing a surgery, as the stomach during endoscopic resection is considered clean due to fasting and gastric acid [123, 124].

Larger perforation may be sealed with omental patch method. If a severe pneumoperitoneum develops after perforation, decompression must be performed using a 14-G puncture needle to prevent the deterioration of breathing and/or neurogenic shock. Large perforations require urgent salvage surgery to prevent peritonitis.

The possible mechanism of ESD-induced perforation include accidental injury of muscular propria, and this is likely caused by inadequate or false gastric submucosal injection. A sufficient amount of solution should be injected into the submucosa to avoid perforation. Injection of solutions containing hyaluronic acid and glycerol have previously been shown to effectively uplift mucosa during prolonged ESD. Indigo Carmine in the injection solution could help better recognize the injection sites.

C6.4. Stenosis

Stenosis has been reported after removal of gastric (pre-pyloric) lesions. Strictures frequently occur at the cardia and pylorus, especially with lesions around 1 cm of the gastroesophageal junction and pylorus, 3/4 circumferential resection of the lumen and/or longitudinal dissection of more than 5 cm in size [125]. The strictures can be successfully treated by endoscopic dilation.

However, it should be noted that balloon dilatation have the risk of perforation. Benign biodegradable esophageal stenting has been reported to effectively prevent the cardiac and pyloric stenosis following ESD [126].

C7. Perioperative Care

1. *Preoperative evaluation*. Before the ER procedures, patients should be thoroughly evaluated for psychological status, cognition of endoscopic operation, and experience of endoscopic examination. Patient's physical status, such as heart and lung diseases, hypertension, diabetes, history of drug allergy, and asthma history should be evaluated. Clotting time, prothrombin time and history of recent use of anticoagulant drugs should also be evaluated [127-133]. Effective communication with patients in terms of the process of the procedure is essential so that patients can actively cooperate during the procedure.
2. *Patients*: In order to prevent the intraoperative aspiration, patients should start fasting 12 hours prior to the procedures, and nothing to drink 4 hours prior. Patients should stop smoking 2 weeks prior to the procedure in order to reduce the respiratory tract secretion and respiratory depression following anesthesia. Informed written consents should be obtained with the patients and family members fully made aware of the risks and complications of the procedures [134-136].
3. *Establishing venous access for patients*: Intravenous injection access should be established. Raceanisodamine should be given to the patient to reduce intraoperative gastrointestinal peristalsis. Oral lidocaine (10 ml) and nasal catheter oxygen (2-4 L /min) should also be given. The patient should put into left lateral decubitus position, with the legs bent into the natural state. Fixed mouth pad should be applied to prevent irritable prolapse or lockjaw in the operation. After effective anaesthesia is initiated (indicated by soft limbs, disappearance of eyelash reflex), the endoscopic procedure may start. An effective cooperation between the nurses and endoscopists is very important.

C8. Observation after the Procedure

Patients should be closely monitored for mental status, ECG, heart rate, pulse rate, respiration rate, blood pressure, and oxygen saturation. Patients should also be closely monitored for chest pain, breathing difficulty, subcutaneous emphysema, abdominal distention, hematemesis, melena, and signs of perforation [137, 138].

Prompt management should be initiated if the patient develops any of the above signs and symptoms.

The critical role of nurses in the post-operative care of the patients underwent ER procedures can not be stressed enough.

C9. Follow up Endoscopy

The endoscopic follow-up should be conducted once every three months in the first year, once every six months in the second year and once a year after two relapse-free years. The overall recurrence rate is around 0.2%, (ESD 1/421), 4.2 %, (EMR 15/359), if the resection stump is negative [139].

Part D. Processing of Endoscopic Specimens for Pathological Diagnosis

The specimens from EMR and ESD are crucial components in making correct diagnosis and rendering appropriate management of patients with gastric cancer. Highly professional processing of these specimens is essential.

Once resected, the mucosal surface of the gastric tissues should be immediately unbent without excessive extension. Tissues should be fixed with pins in all sides on a corkboard, and promptly fixed with 10% formaldehyde solution at room temperature for a minimum of six hours but no more than 48 hours [140-144]. Ample amount of fixative (approximately 10 time in excess of the tissue volume) should be used to ensure proper fixation.

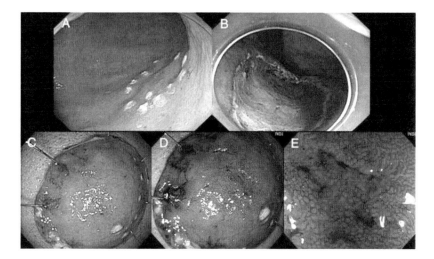

Figure 14. Proper handling of EMR specimen. A. Mark the lesion; B. Resect the lesion; C and D. Unbend the mucosal surface is fixed all sides on the cork board with pins; E. Recheck by NBI mode.

Important information regarding the resected tissue specimens as listed below must be recorded.

a. The basic information of patients and submission information;
b. Macroscopic tumor type, tumor size (mm×mm), histological type, depth of invasion [mucosal (M), sub-mucosal 1 (SM1), and sub-mucosal 2 (SM2)], ulceration status, presence or absence of lymphatic and vascular invasion. A diagram with appropriate orientation marks and annotation should be drawn.
c. Resection stumps: inspect the status of the peripheral stumps (side edges) and bottom ends to check if they are positive or negative. The distance between lesions and lateral margin (mm) should be recorded. If positive, report the amount of slices on the positive ends.
d. The contents of the pathology report should be recorded. An appropriately prepared pathological report of the biopsy specimens should include the following:
   (1) Patient information, submission details;
   (2) For intraepithelial tumor (dysplasia), proper classification should be given;

(3) For suspicious infiltration, information on the repeated biopsy materials should be recorded. Data on the appropriate immunohistochemistry studies for tumor markers should be obtained

(4) For early invasive carcinoma, the depth of invasion must be recorded. (Figure 14).

Part E. Laboratory Studies for EGC

Overall, there are no specific tumor markers for gastric cancer. Nevertheless, the following markers are frequently used in clinical practice in the diagnosis and management of gastric cancer, each with different value and applications.

E1. Commonly Used Serum Tumor Markers for Gastric Cancer

(1) *Carcino-embryonic antigen (CEA).* The normal serum level of CEA in healthy adults is <5ng/ml. Increased serum level of CEA can be found in approximately 19-56.1% of patients with gastric adenocarcinoma. The reported specificity of serum CEA in the diagnosis of gastric cancer varies in the range of 50% to 92% [145].

(2) *Carbohydrate antigen (CA).* The serum level of CA is closely related to the staging of gastric cancer, with a dramatic decline after excision of cancer tissues. The CA-class antigens used in the management of patients with gastric cancer include (1) CA199. It is produced by gastric adenocarcinoma cells, and increased serum level of CA199 was found in 26.3-69.0% of patients with gastric cancer, with a specificity of 52-95%. (2) CA724. The serum level of CA724 reflects the tumor load. Increased serum level of CA724 is present in approximately 31.4-84.2% of patients with gastric cancer, with a specificity of 92-95.9%. The detection rate of gastric cancer with single use of CA724 is higher than that with CA199 or CEA. Thus, CA724 appears to be an ideal tumor maker for diagnosing gastric cancer at the present time. (3) CA242. This is a newly identified tumor antigen related to mucoprotein. CA242 is a sialyl sphingolipids antigen. Its presence in the serum has no obvious correlation with the histological type of gastric cancer.

(3) *MG7 antigen.* The serum level of this gastric cancer-related antigen correlates with tumor differentiation status and pathological stage. MG7 is different from other known gastrointestinal tumor-related antigens in its physical and chemical properties.

(4) *Pepsinogen (PG)* It is mainly expressed by the chief cells at the bottom of the stomach, and is the precursor of pepsin. Once secreted into the gastric lumen, PG is activated in the acid environment and is converted into bioactive pepsin. According to its biochemical and immunological characteristics, PG can be divided into PGI and PGII [146].

E2. Tumor Markers in Gastric Juice

Apart from being present in the serum of patients with gastric cancer, some of the above tumor markers are also detectable in the gastric juice, and therefore may be used in the diagnosis of gastric cancer. For example, highly increased levels of CEA, CA199 and CA724 have been found in the gastric juice in patients with gastric cancer. If combined, the positive diagnostic rate of these three markers for gastric cancer reaches 94.4% [147].

E3. Joint Detection of Tumor Markers in Serum and Gastric Juice

Combined detection of MG7 antigen, PGI and PGII in the serum of gastric cancer patients using the enzyme-linked immunosorbent assay (ELISA) revealed a positive rate of 93.55% [148]. By using the electrochemical luminescence (ECL) to detect the levels of CEA, CA199 and CA724 in the serum and gastric juice of patients with gastric cancer, it was revealed that the positive rate of these three markers in gastric juice was higher than that in the serum.

Using the newly developed multi-tumor-marker protein chips, 12 tumor markers can be simultaneously detected, and simultaneous positivity of CEA, CA125, CA199, CA242, AFP, and neuron-specific enolase (NSE) has a diagnostic rate of 88.4% for gastric cancer.

E4. Genetic Analysis of Gene Expression

Detection of the tumor suppressor gene mutation has become an integral part of cancer diagnosis. For example, mutation of the tumor suppressor gene p53 occurs in approximately 50% of gastric cancer cases, and identification of p53 mutation in gastric cancer patients forms a part of the diagnostic workup [149]. Apart from p53, the expression level and the methylation status of the promoter of RUNX3 have been found to be related to the presence of lymphatic metastasis, a newly recognized feature of EGC [150]. Detection of the p16 gene methylation in serum is also a useful molecular tool for the diagnosis of EGC.

Acknowledgment

We are extremely grateful to Professor Noriya Uedo at the Department of Gastrointestinal Oncology, Osaka Medical Center for Cancer and Cardiovascular Diseases, Osaka, Japan (Email: uedou-no@mc.pref.osaka.jp) for his extensive revision of this manuscript.

References for Abstract

[1]   GLBOCAN 2008. http://globocan.iarc.fr/.
[2]   Ahmedin J, et al. Global Cancer Statistics. *CA CANCER J. CLIN*. 2011; 61:69-90.

[3] Suzuki H, et al. Is endoscopic submucosal dissection an effective treatment for operable patients with clinical submucosal invasive early gastric cancer? *Endoscopy* 2013; 45:93-7.

[4] Dohi O, et al. Recognition of endoscopic diagnosis in differentiated-type early gastric cancer by flexible spectral imaging color enhancement with indigo carmine. *Digestion.* 2012; 86:161-70.

[5] Gotoda T, et al. Endoscopic resection (endoscopic mucosal resection/ endoscopic submucosal dissection) for early gastric cancer. *Dig. Endosc.* 2013; 25 (Suppl 1):55-63.

[6] Lian J, et al. A meta-analysis of endoscopic submucosal dissection and EMR for early gastric cancer. *Gastrointest. Endosc.* 2012; 76: 763-70.

[7] Takizawa, et al. A phase II clinical trial of endoscopic submucosal dissection for early gastric cancer of undifferentiated type: Japan Clinical Oncology Group study JCOG1009/1010. *Jpn. J. Clin. Oncol.* 2013; 43: 87-91.

[8] Watanabe M, et al. Development of gastric cancer in nonatrophic stomach with highly active inflammation identified by serum levels of pepsinogen and Helicobacter pylori antibody together with endoscopic rugal hyperplastic gastritis. *Int. J. Cancer* 2012; 131: 2632-42.

References

[1] Parkin DM, Bray F; Ferlay J, Pisani P. Global cancer statistics, 2002. *CA Cancer J. Clin.* 2005; 55(2): 74-108.

[2] Shiratori Y, Nakagawa S; Kikuchi A, Ishii M. Significance of a gastric mass screening survey. *Am. J. Gastroenterol.* 1985; 80(11): 831-4.

[3] Ferlay J, Shin HR; Bray F, Forman D. et al. Estimates of worldwide burden of cancer in 2008: GLOBOCAN 2008, *Int. J. Cancer.* 2010; 15; 127(12): 2893-2917.

[4] Takahashi T, Saikawa Y; Kitagawa Y. Gastric cancer: current status of diagnosis and treatment. Cancers (Basel). 2013; 16;5(1): 48-63.

[5] Murakami T. Pathomorphological diagnosis, definition and gross classification of early gastric cancer. *Gann. Monogr. Cancer Res.* 1971; 11: 53–66.

[6] Ono H. Early gastric cancer: diagnosis, pathology, treatment techniques and treatment outcomes. *Eur. J. Gastroenterol. Hepatol.* 2006; 18(8): 863-6.

[7] The Paris endoscopic classification of superficial neoplastic lesions: esophagus, stomach, and colon. *Gastrointest Endosc.* 2003; 58 (6 Suppl): S3-43.

[8] Clemente I. Early Gastric Cancer: An Overview and Future Perspective. *J. Gastroint. Dig. Syst.* 2013; S12: 45-67.

[9] Adachi Y, Shiraishi N; Kitano S. Modern treatment of early gastric cancer: review of the Japanese experience. *Dig. Surg.* 2002; 19(5):333-9.

[10] Hamashima C, Shibuya D, Yamazaki H, Inoue K. et al. The Japanese guidelines for gastric cancer screening. *Jpn. J. Clin. Oncol.* 2008; 38(4): 259-67.

[11] Japanese Gastric Cancer Association Registration Committee, Maruyama K, Kaminishi M, Hayashi K. et al. Gastric cancer treated in 1991 in Japan: data analysis of nationwide registry. *Gastric Cancer.* 2006; 9(2): 51-66.

[12] Uedo N, Takeuchi Y, Ishihara R. Endoscopic management of early gastric cancer: endoscopic mucosal resection or endoscopic submucosal dissection: data from a Japanese high-volume center and literature review. *Annals of Gastroenterology*. 2012; 25;281-290.

[13] Ono H, Kondo H; Gotoda T, Shirao K. et al.Endoscopic mucosal resection for treatment of early gastric cancer. *Gut.* 2001; 48(2):225-9.

[14] Uedo N, Iishi H; Tatsuta M, Ishihara R. et al. Long term outcomes after endoscopic mucosal resection for early gastric cancer. *Gastric Cancer.* 2006; 9(2): 88-92.

[15] Kobayashi D, Takahashi O; Arioka H, Fukui T. The optimal screening interval for gastric cancer using esophago-gastro-duodenoscopy in Japan. *BMC Gastroenterol.* 2012; 17; 12: 144.

[16] Costamagna G, Cesaro P. Early gastric cancer: detection and endoscopic treatment. *Ann. Ital. Chir.* 2012; 83(3): 183-91.

[17] Ince AT, Senates E; Bahadir O, Coşgun S. Conventional video-gastroscopes for the recognition of early gastric cancers. *Hepatogastroenterology.* 2011; 58(107-108): 1081-5.

[18] Catalano F, Trecca A;Rodella L, Lombardo F. et al. The modern treatment of early gastric cancer: our experience in an Italian cohort. *Surg. Endosc.* 2009; 23(7): 1581-6.

[19] Canto MI. Staining in Gastrointestinal Endoscopy: The Basics. *Endoscopy.* 1999; 31 (6): 479–486.

[20] Toshihisa TAKEUCHI, Eiji UMEGAKI; Satoshi TOKIOKA. Development of a new contrast endoscopic method With Techno Color blue P. *Bulletin of the Osaka Medical College.* 2007; 53(1): 45-55.

[21] Liu YX, Huang LY, Bian XP, Cui J. et al. Fuji Intelligent Chromo Endoscopy and staining technique for the diagnosis of colon tumor. *Chin. Med. J.* (Engl). 2008; 121(11): 977-82.

[22] Gheorghe C. Narrow-band imaging endoscopy for diagnosis of malignant and premalignant gastrointestinal lesions. *J. Gastrointestin. Liver Dis.* 2006; 15(1): 77-82.

[23] Maki S, Yao K, Nagahama T, Beppu T, et al. Magnifying endoscopy with narrow-band imaging is useful in the differential diagnosis between low-grade adenoma and early cancer of superficial elevated gastric lesions. *Gastric Cancer.* 2013; 16(2): 140-6.

[24] Kawahara Y, Takenaka R, Okada H, Kawano S. et al. Novel chromoendoscopic method using an acetic acid-indigocarmine mixture for diagnostic accuracy in delineating the margin of early gastric cancers. *Dig. Endosc.* 2009; 21(1): 14-9.

[25] Isomoto H, Uehara R; Hayashi T, Shiota J. Magnifying Endoscopic Findings Can Predict Clinical Outcome during Long-Term Follow-Up of More Than 12 Months in Patients with Ulcerative Colitis. *Gastroenterol. Res. Pract.* 2013; 2013: 671576.

[26] *Yagi K, Saka A; Nozawa Y,* Nakamura A. Prediction of submucosal gastric cancer by narrow-band imaging magnifying endoscopy. *Dig. Liver Dis.* 2013; 21. S1590-8658(13)00549-5.

[27] Bohle W, Scheidig A; Zoller WG. Endosonographic tumor staging for treatment decision in resectable gastric cancer. *J. Gastrointestin. Liver Dis.* 2011; 20(2): 135-139.

[28] Dinis-Ribeiro M, Areia M; de Vries A, Marcos-Pinto R. et al. European Society of Gastrointestinal Endoscopy; European Helicobacter Study Group; European Society of Pathology; Sociedade Portuguesa de Endoscopia Digestiva. Management of precancerous conditions and lesions in the stomach (MAPS): guideline from the

European Society of Gastrointestinal Endoscopy (ESGE), European Helicobacter Study Group (EHSG), European Society of Pathology (ESP), and the Sociedade Portuguesa de Endoscopia Digestiva (SPED). *Endoscopy.* 2012; 44 (1): 74-94.

[29] Ono S, Kato M, Suzuki M, Ishigaki S. et al. Frequency of Helicobacter pylori -negative gastric cancer and gastric mucosal atrophy in a Japanese endoscopic submucosal dissection series including histological, endoscopic and serological atrophy. *Digestion.* 2012; 86(1): 59-65.

[30] Fock KM, Talley N; Moayyedi P, Hunt R.Asia–Pacific consensus guidelines on gastric cancer Prevention. *J. Gastroenterol. Hepatol.* 2008; 23(3): 351-65.

[31] Chen Y, Wu LH, He XX. Sequential therapy versus standard triple therapy for Helicobacter pylori eradication in Chinese patients: a metaanalysis. *World Chinese Journal of Difestology.* 2009; 17(32): 3365-3369.

[32] Japanese Gastric Cancer Association. Japanese classification of gastric carcinoma: 3rd English edition. Gastric Cancer. 2011; 14(2): 101-12

[33] Schlemper RJ, Itabashi M; Kato Y, Lewin KJ. et al. Differences in diagnostic criteria for gastric carcinoma between Japanese and western pathologists. *Lancet.* 1997; 14; 349(9067): 1725-9.

[34] Schlemper RJ, Riddell RH; Kato Y, Borchard F. et al. The Vienna classification of gastrointestinal epithelial neoplasia. *Gut.* 2000; 47(2): 251-5.

[35] Kato M, Nishida T; Tsutsui S, Komori M. et al. Endoscopic submucosal dissection as a treatment for gastric noninvasive neoplasia: a multicenter study by Osaka University ESD Study Group. *J. Gastroenterol.* 2011; 46(3): 325-31.

[36] Miwa K, Doyama H; Ito R, Nakanishi H. et al. Can magnifying endoscopy with narrow band imaging be useful for low grade adenomas in preoperative biopsy specimens? *Gastric Cancer.* 2012; 15(2): 170-8.

[37] Yada T, Yokoi C; Uemura N. The current state of diagnosis and treatment for early gastric cancer. *Diagn. Ther. Endosc.* 2013; 2013: 241320.

[38] Sugano K, Sato K; Yao K. New diagnostic approaches for early detection *Dig. Dis.* 2004; 22(4): 327-33.

[39] Okabayashi T, Gotoda T; Kondo H, Ono H. et al. Usefulness of indigo carmine chromoendoscopy and endoscopic clipping for accurate preoperative assessment of proximal gastric cancer. *Endoscopy.* 2000; 32(10): S62.

[40] Zhang J, Guo SB; Duan ZJ. Application of magnifying narrow-band imaging endoscopy for diagnosis of early gastric cancer and precancerous lesion. *BMC Gastroenterol.* 2011; 14; 11:135.

[41] Trivedi PJ, Braden B. Indications, stains and techniques in chromoendoscopy. *QJM.* 2013; 106(2): 117-31.

[42] Niveloni S, Fiorini A; Dezi R, Pedreira S. et al. Usefulness of video duodenoscopy and vital dye staining as indicators of mucosal atrophy of celiac disease: assessment of inter observer agreement. *Gastrointest. Endosc.* 1998; 47(3): 223-9.

[43] Fennerty MB, Sampliner RE; McGee DL, Hixson LJ. et al. Intestinal metaplasia of the stomach: identification by a selective mucosal staining technique. *Gastrointest. Endosc.* 1992; 38(6): 696-8.

[44] Ida K, Hashimoto Y; Takeda S, Murakami K. et al. Endoscopic diagnosis of gastric cancer with dye scattering. *Am. J. Gastroenterol.* 1975; 63(4): 316-20.

[45] Tatsuta M, Iishi H; Okuda S, Taniguchi H. Diagnosis of early gastric cancers in the upper part of the stomach by the endoscopic Congo red-methylene blue test. *Endoscopy.* 1984; 16(4): 131-4.

[46] Suzuki S, Murakami H; Suzuki H, Sakakibara N. et al. An endoscopic staining method for detection *Int. Adv. Surg. Oncol.* 1979; 2: 223-41.

[47] Dinis-Ribeiro M, da Costa-Pereira A, Lopes C, Lara-Santos L. et al. Magnification chromoendoscopy for the diagnosis of gastric intestinal metaplasia and dysplasia. *Gastrointest. Endosc.* 2003; 57(4): 498-504.

[48] Fennerty MB. Tissue staining. *Gastrointest. Endosc. Clin. N. Am.* 1994; 4(2): 297-311.

[49] Stevens PD, Lightdale CJ; Green PH, Siegel LM. et al. Combined magnification endoscopy *Gastrointest. Endosc.* 1994; 40(6): 747-9.

[50] Siegel LM, Stevens PD; Lightdale CJ, Green PH. et al. Combined magnification endoscopy with chromoendoscopy in the evaluation of patients with suspected malabsorption. *Gastrointest. Endosc.* 1997; 46(3): 226-30.

[51] Axelrad AM, Fleischer DE; Geller AJ, Nguyen CC. et al. High-resolution chromoendoscopy for the diagnosis of diminutive colon polyps: implications for colon cancer screening. *Gastroenterology.* 1996; 110(4): 1253-8.

[52] Kudo S, Kashida H; Nakajima T, Tamura S. et al. Endoscopic diagnosis and treatment of early colorectal cancer. *World J. Surg.* 1997; 21(7): 694-701.

[53] Jaramillo E, Watanabe M; Slezak P, Rubio C. Flat neoplastic lesions of colon and rectum detected by high-resolution video endoscopy and chromoscopy (see comments). *Gastrointest. Endosc.* 1995; 42: 114–122.

[54] Ikeda K, Sannohe Y; Araki S, Inutsuka S. Intra-arterial dye method with vasomotors (PIAD method) applied for the endoscopic diagnosis of gastric cancer and the side effects of indigo carmine. *Endoscopy.* 1982; 14(4): 119-23.

[55] Gheorghe C. Narrow-band imaging endoscopy for diagnosis of malignant and premalignant gastrointestinal lesions. *J. Gastrointestin. Liver Dis.* 2006; 15(1): 77-82.

[56] Taiiri H, Masuda K; Fujisaki J. *What can we see with the endoscopy? Present status and future perspectives. Digestive Endoscopy.* 2002; 14: 131-137.

[57] Kara MA, Peters FP; Rosmolen WD, Krishnadath KK. et al. High-resolution *Endoscopy.* 2005; 37(10): 929-36.

[58] Sambongi M, Igarashi M; Obi T. Analysis of spectral reflectance of mucous membrane for endoscopic diagnosis. *Med. Phys.* 2000; 27: 1396-1398.

[59] Kiesslich R, Jung M. Magnification endoscopy: does it improve mucosal surface analysis for the diagnosis of gastrointestinal neoplasias? *Endoscopy.* 2002; 34(10): 819-22.

[60] The Paris endoscopic classification of superficial neoplastic lesions: esophagus, stomach, and colon : November 30 to December 1, 2002. *Gastrointest. Endosc.* 2003; 58(6 Suppl): S3-43.

[61] Kudo S, Rubio CA; Teixeira CR, Kashida H. et al. Pit pattern in colorectal neoplasia: endoscopic magnifying view. *Endoscopy.* 2001; 33(4): 367-73.

[62] Sharma P, Weston AP; Topalovski M, Cherian R. Magnification chromoendoscopy for the detection of intestinal metaplasia and dysplasia in Barrett's oesophagus. *Gut.* 2003; 52(1): 24-7.

[63] Paris Workshop on Columnar Metaplasia in the Esophagus and the Esophagogastric Junction, Paris, France, December 11-12, 2004. *Endoscopy.* 2005; 37(9): 879-920.

[64] Kuznetsov K, Lambert R; Rey JF. Narrow-band imaging: potential and limitations. *Endoscopy.* 2006; 38(1): 76-81.

[65] Yao K. How is the VS (vessel plus surface) classification system applicable to magnifying narrow-band imaging examinations of gastric neoplasias initially diagnosed as low-grade adenomas? *Gastric Cancer.* 2012; 15(2): 118-20.

[66] Maki S, Yao K; Nagahama T, Beppu T. Magnifying endoscopy with narrow-band imaging is useful in the differential diagnosis between low-grade adenoma and early cancer of superficial elevated gastric lesions. *Gastric Cancer.* 2013; 16(2): 140-6.

[67] Yasutoshi Ochiai, Shin Arai; Masamitsu Nakao. Diagnosis of boundary in early gastric cancer. *World J. Gastrointest. Endosc.* 2012; 4(3): 75-79.

[68] Gono K, Obi T; Yamaguchi M, Ohyama N. Appearance of enhanced tissue features in narrow-band endoscopic imaging. *J. Biomed. Opt.* 2004; 9(3): 568-77.

[69] Kaise M, Kato M; Urashima M, Arai Y. et al. Magnifying endoscopy combined with narrow-band imaging for differential diagnosis of superficial depressed gastric lesions. *Endoscopy.* 2009; 41(4): 310-5.

[70] Nakayoshi T, Tajiri H; Matsuda K, Kaise M. Endoscopy. *Magnifying endoscopy combined with narrow band imaging system for early gastric cancer: correlation of vascular pattern with histopathology* (including video). 2004; 36(12): 1080-4.

[71] Sakaki N. Magnifying endoscopic observation on the effect of a proton pump inhibitor on the healing process of gastric ulcer. *Nihon Rinsho.* 1992; 50(1): 86-93.

[72] Yao K, Oishi T; Matsui T, Yao T. et al. Novel magnified endoscopic findings of microvascular architecture in intramucosal gastric cancer. *Gastrointest. Endosc.* 2002 ; 56(2): 279-84.

[73] Mouri R, Yoshida S; Tanaka S, Oka S. et al. Evaluation and validation of computed virtual chromoendoscopy in early gastric cancer. *Gastrointest. Endosc.* 2009; 69(6): 1052-8.

[74] Osawa H, Yoshizawa M; Yamamoto H, Kita H. et al. Gastrointest Endosc. *Optimal band imaging system can facilitate detection of changes in depressed-type early gastric cancer.* 2008; 67(2): 226-34.

[75] Pohl J, May A; Rabenstein T, Pech O. et al. Computed virtual chromoendoscopy: a new tool for enhancing tissue surface structures. *Endoscopy.* 2007; 39(1): 80-3.

[76] Puli SR, Batapati Krishna; Reddy J, Bechtold ML, et al. How good is endoscopic ultrasound for TNM staging of gastric cancers? A meta-analysis and systematic review. *World J. Gastroenterol.* 2008; 14: 4011-4019.

[77] Hwang SW, Lee DH; Lee SH, Park YS. et al. Preoperative staging of gastric cancer *J. Gastroenterol. Hepatol.* 2010; 25(3): 512-8.

[78] Meyer L, Meyer F; Schmidt U, Gastinger I. et al. Endoscopic ultrasonography (EUS) in preoperative staging of gastric cancer--demand and reality. *Pol. Przegl. Chir.* 2012; 84(3): 152-7.

[79] Polkowski M, Palucki J; Wronska E, Szawlowski A. Endosonography versus helical computed tomography for locoregional staging of gastric cancer. *Endoscopy.* 2004 ; 36(7): 617-23.

[80] Habermann CR, Weiss F; Riecken R, Honarpisheh H. Preoperative staging of gastric adenocarcinoma: comparison of helical CT and endoscopic US. *Radiology.* 2004; 230(2): 465-71.

[81] Repiso A, Gómez-Rodríguez R; López-Pardo R, Lombera MM. et al. Usefulness of endoscopic ultrasonography in preoperative gastric cancer staging: diagnostic yield and therapeutic impact. *Rev. Esp. Enferm. Dig.* 2010; 102(7): 413-20.

[82] Potrc S, Skalicky M; Ivanecz A. Does endoscopic ultrasound staging allow individual treatment regimens in gastric cancer. *Wien Klin Wochen.* 2006; 118, Suppl 2: 48-51.

[83] Li Z, Zuo XL, Yu T, Gu XM. et al. Confocal laser endomicroscopy for in vivo detection of gastric intestinal metaplasia: a randomized controlled trial. *Endoscopy.* 2014; 28.

[84] Gheorghe C, Iacob R, Becheanu G, Dumbrav Abreve M. Confocal endomicroscopy for in vivo microscopic analysis of upper gastrointestinal tract premalignant and malignant lesions. *J. Gastrointestin. Liver Dis.* 2008; 17(1): 95-100.

[85] Balcerzyk A, Baldacchino G. Implementation of laser induced fluorescence in a pulse radiolysis experiment - a new way to analyze resazurin-like reduction mechanisms. *Analyst.* 2014; 139(7): 1707-12.

[86] Gotoda T, Jung HY. Endoscopic resection (endoscopic mucosal resection/ endoscopic submucosal dissection) for early gastric cancer. *Dig. Endosc.* 2013; 25 Suppl 1: 55-63.

[87] Soetikno R, Kaltenbach T; Yeh R, Gotoda T. Endoscopic mucosal resection for early cancers of the upper gastrointestinal tract. *J. Clin. Oncol.* 2005; 23(20): 4490-8.

[88] Tada M, Shimada M, Murakami F. Development of stripoff biopsy. *Gastroenterol. Endosc.* 1984; 26: 833–9.

[89] Japanese Gastric Cancer Association, Japanese gastric cancer treatment guidelines 2010 (ver. 3). *Gastric Cancer.* 2011; 14:113–123.

[90] Costamagna G, Cesaro P. Early gastric cancer: detection and endoscopic treatment. *Ann. Ital. Chir.* 2012; 83(3): 183-91.

[91] Yamamoto H, Kawata H; Sunada K, Sasaki A. et al. Successful en-bloc resection of large superficial tumors in the stomach and colon using sodium hyaluronate and small-caliber-tip transparent hood. *Endoscopy.* 2003; 35(8): 690-4.

[92] Oyama T, Tomori A; Hotta K, Morita S. et al. Endoscopic submucosal dissection of early esophageal cancer *Clin. Gastroenterol. Hepatol.* 2005; 3(7 Suppl 1): S67-70.

[93] Yahagi N, Fujishiro M; Kakushima N. Endoscopic sub-mucosal dissection for early gastric cancer using the tip of an Electro surgical snare(thin type). *Digestive Endoscopy.* 2004; 16(1): 34–38.

[94] Yokoi C, Gotoda T; Hamanaka H, Oda I. et al. Endoscopic submucosal dissection allows curative resection of locally recurrent early gastric cancer after prior endoscopic mucosal resection. *Gastrointest. Endosc.* 2006; 64(2): 212-8.

[95] Gotoda T, Yanagisawa A; Sasako M, Ono H. et al. Incidence of lymph node metastasis from early gastric cancer: estimation with a large number of cases at two large centers. *Gastric Cancer.* 2000; 3(4): 219-225.

[96] Hirasawa T, Gotoda T; Miyata S, Kato Y. et al. Incidence of lymph node metastasis and the feasibility of endoscopic resection for undifferentiated-type early gastric cancer. *Gastric Cancer.* 2009; 12(3): 148-52.

[97] Chiu PW, Teoh AY; To KF, Wong SK. Endoscopic submucosal dissection (ESD) compared with gastrectomy for treatment of early gastric neoplasia: a retrospective cohort study. *Surg. Endosc.* 2012; 26(12): 3584-91.

[98] De Melo SW Jr, Cleveland P, Raimondo M, Wallace MB. et al. Endoscopic mucosal resection with the grasp-and-snare technique through a double-channel endoscope in humans. *Gastrointest. Endosc.* 2011; 73(2): 349-52.

[99] Lee DW, Lee HS, Jung MK, Kim SK. et al. A switch to endoscopic mucosal resection after precutting following gastric perforation during endoscopic submucosal dissection: a simple and useful technique. *Endoscopy.* 2012; 44(3): 293-6.

[100] Kume K, Yamasaki M, Tashiro M, Santo N. et al. Endoscopic mucosal resection for early gastric cancer: comparison of two modifications of the cap method. *Endoscopy.* 2008; 40(4): 280-3.

[101] Kim GH, Kim JI, Jeon SW, Moon JS. et al. Korean College of Helicobacter and Upper Gastrointestinal Research. Endoscopic resection for duodenal carcinoid tumors: a multicenter, retrospective study. *J. Gastroenterol. Hepatol.* 2014 ;29(2): 318-24.

[102] Lian J, Chen S; Zhang Y, Qiu F. A meta-analysis of endoscopic submucosal dissection and EMR for early gastric cancer. *Gastrointest. Endosc.* 2012; 76(4):763-70.

[103] Larghi A, Waxman I. State of the art on endoscopic mucosal resection and endoscopic submucosal dissection. *Gastrointest. Endosc. Clin. N Am.* 2007; 17(3): 441-69.

[104] Kodama M, Kakegawa T. Treatment of superficial cancer of the esophagus: a summary of responses to a questionnaire on superficial cancer of the esophagus in Japan. *Surgery.* 1998; 123(4): 432-9.

[105] Rembacken BJ, Gotoda T; Fujii T, Axon AT. Endoscopic mucosal resection. *Endoscopy.* 2001; 33(8): 709-18.

[106] Iishi H, Tatsuta M; Iseki K, Narahara H. et al. Endoscopic piecemeal resection with submucosal saline injection of large sessile colorectal polyps. *Gastrointest. Endosc.* 2000; 51(6): 697-700.

[107] Lee SH, Park JH;Park do H, Chung IK. et al. Clinical efficacy of EMR with submucosal injection of a fibrinogen mixture: a prospective randomized trial. *Gastrointest. Endosc.* 2006; 64(5): 691-6.

[108] Kang KJ, Kim KM; Min BH, Lee JH. et al. Endoscopic submucosal dissection of early gastric cancer. *Gut. Liver.* 2011; 5(4):418-26.

[109] Chaves DM, Maluf Filho F; de Moura EG, Santos ME. et al. Endoscopic submucosal dissection for the treatment *Clinics* (Sao Paulo). 2010; 65(4): 377-82.

[110] Goto O, Fujishiro M; Kodashima S, Minatsuki C. et al. Short-term healing process of artificial ulcers after gastric endoscopic submucosal dissection. *Gut. Liver.* 2011; 5(3): 293-7.

[111] Uedo N, Takeuchi Y; Yamada T, Ishihara R. et al. Effect of a proton pump inhibitor or an H2-receptor antagonist on prevention of bleeding from ulcer after endoscopic submucosal dissection of early gastric cancer: a prospective randomized controlled trial. *Am. J. Gastroenterol.* 2007; 102(8): 1610-6.

[112] Kato T, Araki H, Onogi F, Ibuka T, Sugiyama A.et al. Clinical trial: rebamipide promotes gastric ulcer healing by proton pump inhibitor after endoscopic submucosal dissection--a randomized controlled study. *J. Gastroenterol.* 2010; 45(3): 285-90.

[113] Inaba T, Ishikawa S; Toyokawa T, Ishikawa H. et al. Basal protrusion of ulcers induced by endoscopic submucosal dissection (ESD) during treatment with proton pump inhibitors, and the suppressive effects of polapre zinc. *Hepatogastroenterology.* 2010; 57(99-100): 678-84.

[114] Tanaka S, Oka S; Kaneko I, Hirata M.et al. Endoscopic submucosal dissection for colorectal neoplasia: possibility of standardization. *Gastrointest. Endosc.* 2007; 66(1): 100-7.

[115] Oka S, Tanaka S; Kaneko I, Mouri R. et al. Advantage of endoscopic submucosal dissection compared with EMR for early gastric cancer. *Gastrointest. Endosc.* 2006 ; 64(6): 877-83.

[116] Kato M. Endoscopic submucosal dissection (ESD) is being accepted as a new procedure of endoscopic treatment of early gastric cancer. *Intern. Med.* 2005 ; 44(2): 85-6.

[117] Fujishiro M, Kodashima S; Goto O, Ono S. et al. Dig Endosc. *Endoscopic submucosal dissection for esophageal squamous cell neoplasms.* 2009 ; 21(2): 109-15.

[118] Gotoda T. A large endoscopic resection by endoscopic submucosal dissection procedure for early gastric cancer. *Clin. Gastroenterol. Hepatol.* 2005; 3(7 Suppl 1): S71-3.

[119] Ono H. Early gastric cancer: diagnosis, pathology, treatment techniques and treatment outcomes. *Eur. J. Gastroenterol. Hepatol.* 2006; 18(8): 863-6.

[120] Fujishiro M, Yahagi N; Nakamura M, Kakushima N. et al. Endoscopic submucosal dissection for rectal epithelial neoplasia. *Endoscopy.* 2006; 38(5): 493-7.

[121] Inoue H. Endoscopic mucosal resection for esophageal and gastric mucosal cancers. *Can. J. Gastroenterol.* 1998; 12(5): 355-9.

[122] Yokoi C, Gotoda T; Hamanaka H, Oda I. Endoscopic submucosal dissection allows curative resection of locally recurrent early gastric cancer after prior endoscopic mucosal resection. *Gastrointest. Endosc.* 2006; 64(2): 212-8.

[123] Fujishiro M, Yahagi N; Nakamura M, Kakushima N. et al. Successful outcomes of a novel endoscopic treatment for GI tumors: endoscopic submucosal dissection with a mixture of high-molecular-weight hyaluronic acid, glycerin, and sugar. *Gastrointest. Endosc.* 2006; 63(2): 243-9.

[124] Kim HS, Lee DK; Jeong YS, Kim KH. Successful endoscopic management of a perforated gastric dysplastic lesion after endoscopic mucosal resection. *Gastrointest. Endosc.* 2000; 51(5).

[125] Takeuchi Y, Uedo N; Iishi H, Yamamoto S. et al.Endoscopic submucosal dissection with insulated-tip knife for large mucosal early gastric cancer: a feasibility study (with videos). *Gastrointest. Endosc.* 2007; 66(1): 186-93.

[126] Mizutani T, Tadauchi A, Arinobe M, Narita Y, Kato R, Niwa Y, Ohmiya N, Itoh A, Hirooka Y, Honda H, Ueda M, Goto H. Novel strategy for prevention of esophageal stricture after endoscopic surgery. *Hepatogastroenterology.* 2010; 57(102-103): 1150-6.

[127] Kim SH, Moon JS; Youn YH, Lee KM. et al. Management of the complications of endoscopic submucosal dissection. *World J. Gastroenterol.* 2011; 21; 17(31): 3575-9.

[128] Fujishiro M, Yahagi N; Kakushima N, Kodashima S. et al. Successful nonsurgical management of perforation complicating endoscopic submucosal dissection of gastrointestinal epithelial neoplasms. *Endoscopy.* 2006; 38(10): 1001-6.

[129] Seong BJ, Lee IS, Cho JW. A case of successful nonsurgical management of iatrogenic gastric perforation with fluid collection after endoscopic mucosal resection. *Korean J. Gastrointest. Endosc.* 2007; 34: 43-46

[130] Oka S, Tanaka S; Kaneko I, Mouri R. et al. Advantage of endoscopic submucosal dissection compared with EMR for early gastric cancer. *Gastrointest. Endosc.* 2006; 64(6): 877-83.

[131] Jeong G, Lee JH; Yu MK, Moon W. Non-surgical management of microperforation induced by EMR of the stomach. *Dig. Liver Dis.* 2006; 38(8): 605-8.

[132] Kakushima N, Yahagi N; Fujishiro M, Kodashima S. et al. Efficacy and safety of endoscopic submucosal dissection for tumors of the esophagogastric junction. *Endoscopy.* 2006 ; 38(2): 170-4.

[133] Yang JC, Park EH; Lee JH. Successful conservative management of perforation in stomach caused by endoscopic mucosal resection (EMR). *Korean J. Med.* 2004; 66: 526-531.

[134] Tanaka M, Ono H; Hasuike N, Takizawa K. Endoscopic submucosal dissection of early gastric cancer. *Digestion.* 2008; 77, Suppl 1: 23-8.

[135] Tsunada S, Ogata S; Ohyama T, Ootani H. et al. Endoscopic closure of perforations caused by EMR in the stomach by application of metallic clips. *Gastrointest. Endosc.* 2003; 57(7): 948-51.

[136] Abe S, Oda I; Suzuki H, Nonaka S.et al. Short- and long-term outcomes of endoscopic submucosal dissection for undifferentiated early gastric cancer. *Endoscopy.* 2013; 45(9): 703-7.

[137] Tsunada S, Ogata S;Ohyama T, Ootani H. et al. Endoscopic closure of perforations caused by EMR in the stomach by application of metallic clips. *Gastrointest. Endosc.* 2003; 57(7): 948-51.

[138] Lee JH, Kim JJ. Endoscopic mucosal resection of early gastric cancer: Experiences in Korea. *World J. Gastroenterol.* 2007; 21; 13(27): 3657-61.

[139] Tanabe S, Ishido K, Higuchi K, Sasaki T. et al. Long-term outcomes of endoscopic submucosal dissection for early gastric cancer: a retrospective comparison with conventional endoscopic resection in a single center. *Gastric Cancer.* 2014; 17(1): 130-6.

[140] Wilfred weinstein. *Tissue sampling, specimen handing, and chromoendoscopy.* 3rd Edition. Elsevier Science , Holland. 2008.

[141] Kim CG. Tissue Acquisition in Gastric Epithelial Tumor Prior to Endoscopic Resection. *Clin. Endosc.* 2013; 46(5): 436-440.

[142] Sharma P, Misra V; Singh PA, Misra SP.et al. A correlative study of histology and imprint cytology in the diagnosis of gastrointestinal tract malignancies. *Indian J. Pathol. Microbiol.* 1997; 40(2): 139-46.

[143] Fustar-Preradović L, Coha B; Pajić-Penavić I. A correlative study of histology and imprint cytology of gastric mucosa biopsy in the diagnosis gastric cancer. *Coll. Antropol.* 2010 ; 34(2): 355-8.

[144] Kang MS, Hong SJ; Han JP, Seo JY. et al. Endoscopic submucosal dissection of a leiomyoma originating from the muscularis propria of upper esophagus. *Korean J. Gastroenterol.* 2013; 25; 62 (4):234-7.

[145] Wu JT. Clinical applications. In: Human Circulating Tumor Markers: Current Concepts and Clinical Applications. *Am. Soc. Clin. Pathol.,* 1998; 44(4): 21-24.

[146] Uedo N, Yao K, Ishihara R. Screening and Treating Intermediate Lesions to Prevent Gastric Cancer. *Gastroenterol. Clin. N. Am.* 2013; 42: 317–335.

[147] Chen XZ, Zhang WK, Yang K, Wang LL. et al. Correlation between serum CA724 and gastric cancer: multiple analyses based on Chinese population. *Mol. Biol. Rep.* 2012; 39(9): 9031-9.

[148] Yuan Y. A survey and evaluation of population-based screening for gastric cancer. *Cancer Biol. Med.* 2013; 10(2): 72-80.

[149] Salih BA, Gucin Z; Bayyurt N. A study on the effect of Helicobacter pylori infection on p53 expression in gastric cancer and gastritis tissues. *J. Infect. Dev. Ctries.* 2013; 16; 7(9): 651-7.

[150] Zhang YW, Eom SY; Yim DH, Song YJ. Evaluation of the relationship between dietary factors, CagA-positive Helicobacter pylori infection, and RUNX3 promoter hypermethylation in gastric cancer tissue. *World J. Gastroenterol.* 2013; 21; 19(11): 1778-87.

In: Gastric Cancer
Editor: Jasneet Singh Bhullar

ISBN: 978-1-63117-983-9
© 2014 Nova Science Publishers, Inc.

Chapter 5

Advancements in Murine Models of Human Gastric Cancer

Jasneet Singh Bhullar, M.D., M.S., Neha Varshney, M.D. and Vijay K. Mittal, M.D., FACS
Department of Surgery, Providence Hospital & Medical Centers,
Southfield, MI, USA

Abstract

Murine models of gastric carcinogenesis are an in vivo tool essential for understanding the mechanisms of pathogenesis and search of better treatments. Over the years considerable changes in the understanding of the murine models of human gastric cancer have resulted in numerous models being reported in the literature. The gastric cancer transgenic mice and human xenograft heterotopic murine models were reported initially. These were followed by orthotopic tumor models which were found to be more relevant in portraying the human disease process as opposed to heterotopic models. Over time many techniques for making orthotopic gastric murine models were reported, each trying to overcome the drawbacks of the previously reported models. Although all of these models have their advantages and limitations, the latest orthotopic murine models seem to more accurately represent and replicate the human disease process.

We discuss the different human gastric cancer murine models, their background, the techniques of creating them along with their advantages and limitations. Some of the studies in which human gastric murine models have been used are also briefly discussed. This extensive overview and details of an array of different resources in this field offer researchers a wide choice to choose a model which is more applicable to the type of study being planned.

Keywords: Animals; therapeutic use; diagnostic use;chemoprevention; gastric neoplasms; prevention and control; diet disease models; mice; mouse; murine; mutant strains; animal model; diet; chemoprevention; gastric cancer-carcinogenesis; min-mice; gastric cancer; stomach cancer; xenograft; heterotopic model; orthotopic model; murine model; Her2/neu receptor

Background

Gastric cancer is one of the most common tumors after lung, breast and colon cancer. It remains the second leading cause of cancer-related mortality in the world despite a sharp decline of its incidence [1]. Infection with *Helicobacter pylori*, intestinal metaplasia [associated with Barrett's esophagus], atrophic gastritis and dysplasia have been identified as important steps in the pathogenesis of gastric adenocarcinoma [2]. The incidence of this cancer in white males increased more than 3.5- fold between 1974 and 1994 in the United States, which is more than that of any other malignancy.Similar observations have been made in other Western countries as well [3, 4]. It is difficult to determine whether these cancers are gastroesophageal junction tumors or distal esophageal malignancies, though they are usually treated in the same manner in clinical trials for advanced disease.

Surgical resection is the mainstay of treatment and can cure patients with early-stage cancer. There has been a significant amount of research to study pathogenesis and epidemiological factors. Despite all these advances and the development and the use of new treatment strategies such as perioperative chemotherapy [5] or adjuvant chemo radiation, the survival rate with advanced resectable gastric or gastro esophageal junction cancers has still not improved substantially. It is mainly due to its delayed diagnosis when the cancer becomes inoperable. Moreover, recurrent tumors are often detected later, even after curative surgery. For these patients, systemic chemotherapy is the main treatment option. To further decrease the mortality rate in high risk individuals, screening programs for high risk individuals in some countries have been started recently [6].

Currently, there is no internationally accepted standard therapy; uncertainty still remains regarding the choice of the chemotherapy regimen. Hence, many newer areas are being explored [7]. Recent modalities like immunotherapy and targeted therapies are under evaluation and are currently the subject of aggressive research [8].

For a better understanding of the pathogenesis and to further evaluate therapeutic and preventive measures, murine gastric cancer models have been developed as an important tool in gastric cancer research.

In this chapter, emphasis is given on different human gastric murine models, their background, the technique of creating them and various studies done on these models. Also, the advantages and limitations have been discussed.

Introduction to Murine Cancer Models

The laboratory mouse (*Mus musculus*) has become one of the best animal model species in biomedical research today because of: 1) the availability of genetic/genomic information 2) precise and well-established mutagenesis techniques to construct transgenic and knockout mice and 3) chemical mutagenesis technologies [9].

The nude mouse is the prototype of experimental rodents that display congenital thymic aplasia, T - lymphocyte related immune deficiency and hairlessness [10-12]. Despite the absence of the thymus, the mouse is not immunologically neutral, and can produce immunoglobulins as well as display NK-cell reactivity. Changes in phenotypic characteristics have been noted on some tumors transplanted into these animals. Susceptibility to infection requires special housing facilities and strict separation from immunocompetent rodents [13]. These considerations must be taken into account by the investigator planning to use this mouse for their research.

These mice have been used extensively in animal cancer research. Additionally, these mice have been used for investigations in immunology, pathology, genetics, virology, parasitology, endocrinology, dermatology, diabetes, allergy and many other areas [13].

Murine cancer models are very useful to study the morphologic, biologic and biochemical characteristics of various cancer types [14]. They are very important in understanding the mechanisms of pathogenesis, investigation of potential therapeutic and preventive measures. They are considered a very essential part of the ongoing oncology research, which includes studies on the mechanisms and characteristics of tumor development, growth, metastasis, and treatment.

It has been found that rodents and humans have many similar biological functions. Moreover, rodents are invaluable for toxicity tests. Rodent studies should be conducted in the chemoprevention area, because epidemiological studies do not lead to firm conclusions as confounding factors cannot be fully eliminated. Thus, the hypotheses generated by epidemiology must be tested in controlled experiments, ideally in a human population [15]. However this is a very long and costly process, with moral and ethical complications, and it could jeopardize the health of the volunteers. Thus, animal trials should ideally precede human trials of innovations in treatment and prevention of any disease, gastric cancer in this case.

Major differences between rodents and humans in lifespan, body weight, intestinal morphology (e.g., cecum), gut microflora, way of eating and digestion (e.g., meals, chewing, coprophagia), and gene regulation may change the outcome of dietary interventions.

Both basic science studies and clinical trials are essential components of the cancer drug discovery process. Trial drugs found to be significantly better than no treatment or standard therapies (i.e., active) in preclinical laboratory cancer models or compounds with novel chemotypes and equivalent effectiveness to standard treatments are advanced to confirmatory testing in early (Phase I and II) clinical trials. A favorable response rate in Phase II trials advances a drug into additional clinical testing and is considered a prerequisite of drug success in the clinic setting [16].

Advancement of a trial drug from preclinical testing in the laboratory to testing in Phase II clinical trials is based on the assumption that drug activity in cancer models translates into at least some efficacy in human patients, *i.e.,* that cancer laboratory models are clinically predictive.

The use of preclinical cancer models for selection of potential cancer therapeutics was pioneered by the National Cancer Institute (NCI) in the United States in the mid-1950s. Subsequently, in 1990, the NCI introduced a disease-oriented *in vitro* Human Tumor Cell Line Screen comprised of 60 cell lines from the most common adult tumors [17-19]. The screen was designed so that each tumor type was represented by a panel of cell lines, selected on the basis of different sub-histological features, and common drug resistance profiles. It was hoped that this screen would help identify drug leads with high potency and/or selective activity against particular tumor types.

The NCI had examined various studies. The results from these studies have shown that *in vitro* cell lines {in the context of the NCI Human Tumor Cell Line Screen} and appropriate panels of the human xenograft model have significant advantages over the murine allograft model in drug development [20].

Murine cancer models can also allow the study of mechanisms to help identify new biomarkers and novel target genes. Mechanisms can be studied because invasive procedures and the use of toxic compounds pose less ethical problems in rodents than in humans. Moreover, less time and money are required to test a hypothesis in rodents than in humans [21]. Once biomarkers and novel genes are identified in mice, they can subsequently be detected in humans. For example, targets were identified in human tumors on the basis of evidence collected from transcriptional profiles in Min mice [22].

Keeping in mind all of the extensive studies on murine cancer models, it is obvious that human beings will not be able to find new ways to prevent cancer without the help of animal models. Extensive research has been done towards the understanding of various cancers using animal models.

Gastric Cancer Cell Lines

A wide range of gastric cancer cell lines are commercially available to the researchers. These stomach cancer cell lines have been isolated from both primary and metastatic sites. Each culture contains genomic mutations in one or more of the following genes according to the Sanger COSMIC database: CDKN2A, TP53, SMAD4, CDH1, CTNNB1, KRAS, MLH1 and PIK3CA [www.atcc.com].

Evolution of Murine Cancer Models

Heterotopic Models

Transplants of human tumors in nude mice have shown a progressive increase during the last 15 years as an experimental model for cancer research. The most widely described technique for creating human cancer xenograft (graft from human) murine models, including gastric cancer, has been subcutaneous injection (heterotopic) of tumor cells in immune-compromised mice. The frequency of tumor 'take' varies according to tumor origin, tumor type, inoculation site, age and conditioning of the mouse host, and a variety of other factors. Manipulation of these variables has led to successful propagation of almost every known variety of human malignancy. It offers great interest as a model for the in-vivo study of metastasis.

Successful transplantation of human tumors to nude mice was first reported by Rygaard and Povlsen in 1969 [14] and tumor growth resulting from inoculation of cultured human cells was published 3 years later [23]. Successful transplantation was observed for approximately 50 % of all the tumors derived from several tissues and organs including soft tissues, bone, lung, kidney, germ cell, head and neck region, female genital tract, breast and gastrointestinal tract. Many variables have been identified that affect the frequency and speed of growth of tumor transplants, including tumor origin, age, sex and genetic background of the mouse strain, the site of tumor inoculation, and other factors. Depending upon the researcher's choice, either BALB/c nude (*nu/nu*) mice or NOD SCID mice are preferred. Sometimes females are used more often than males for the convenience of housing the animals, as female mice can be housed together in a single cage while males usually need to be housed individually.

The subcutaneous xenograft heterotopic model is made by injection of 1×10^6 tumor cells/site within the subcutaneous tissues of flank/hind leg of the mouse. The preferred volume of injection is 0.1 ml. Different suspension media can be used to suspend the tumor cells for injection. The commonly used solutions are 10% Fetal Bovine Serum [FBS] [24] and Matrigel. The use of Matrigel as a suspension solution has been helpful because it has shown improved tumor implantation. Matrigel is a liquid when kept in low temperature and acquires a gel form when exposed to body temperature. Matrigel contains extracellular matrix components [such as laminin and collagen IV], tumor growth factors [such as transforming growth factor beta], fibroblast growth factor, and tissue plasminogen activator. These components aid in implantation of the human tumor cells [25].

The resultant tumor can be followed easily and the growth can be monitored accurately with calipers as the tumor is on the outside of the mouse's body (Figure 1- showing a medium sized tumor on flank of a mouse). Also the tumor can grow to a substantial size without causing much discomfort to the animal.

Making a heterotopic model may be easy, but it has multiple drawbacks. The use of these models is limited by the fact that it does not mimic the human disease process because of its extra - anatomic site of tumor growth. Also, the absence and irregularity of metastasis from the subcutaneous site renders the model inappropriate for investigating the spontaneous metastatic process [24].

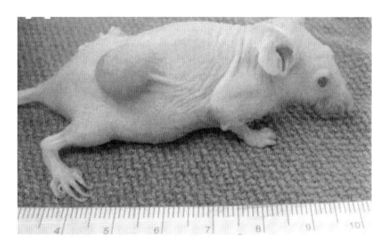

Figure 1. Picture showing the heterotopic tumor on the flank of the mouse.

In 1988, Yamashita T, successfully transplanted gastric cell lines into the subcutis of nude mice and stomach wall and compared them. The human gastric cancer cell line G/F was derived from a poorly differentiated carcinoma in the stomach of a 72 year old man as described by Matsuda et al. The biological properties of human gastric cancer cell line G/F implanted into either the subcutis or the stomach wall of nude mice were compared. The G/F tumor in the stomach wall showed a slower growth rate than that in the subcutis. The level of carcinoembryonic antigen in serum was greater when the tumor was in the stomach wall than when it was in the subcutis. The tumor in the stomach wall had invaded the surrounding tissues and metastasized to the regional lymph nodes and distant organs such as the lung and the liver in 27 of the 43 mice [68%]. In contrast, the tumor in the subcutis was highly capsulated and metastasis to other organs was not observed. These findings indicate that the stomach wall might provide a suitable microenvironment for G/F gastric cancer to exert its intrinsic properties. Human tumor xenograft in the gastric wall of athymic nude mice closely resembles the original tumors in morphological, biological and biochemical characteristics. Therefore, implantation of human gastric cancer into the stomach wall of nude mice may provide a useful model to study the intrinsic characteristics of human cancer as well the effectiveness of experimental chemotherapy [26].

In 1990, Teruo et al. established a human cancer xenograft which, when inoculated into nude mice, showed a positive correlation between tumor growth and the serum level of carcinoembryonic antigen [CEA]. CEA production was associated with the proliferative activity of gastric cancer cells. The CEA positivity of cells tended to increase with tumor growth, and indeed a correlation between CEA localization in cancer cells and serum CEA has been reported [27]. This study suggested that human gastric cancer xenografts in mice are a good model for investigating the biological role of CEA, and that serum CEA can be a marker of tumor growth.

One of the present uses of the heterotopic model is as a step for making the orthotopic model. The subcutaneously grown tumor is resected after euthanizing the animal and small parts of the tumor are then implanted in the colon to make the orthotopic model [28].

Kubota, in 1994, devised a metastatic model of human gastric cancer xenograft in the nude mouse using orthotopic transplantation. Tumors used for this experiment were human stomach cancer xenograft lines St-40, H-111, and SC-1-NU. The experimentally grown tumors were removed, cut into pieces and placed on the serosal surface in the middle of the greater curvature of the stomach through para-median incision. Some tumor cell suspension was made and was injected into the middle of the greater curvature of the stomach. The mice were observed daily for 12 weeks after transplantation and 24weeks after inoculation of a single cell suspension. Local tumor growth of the gastric xenograft was observed in all mice, after orthotopic transplantation of the intact-tissue, while only 50% of the mice developed localtumor growth after single cell suspension injection. Liver metastasis was observed in 18 of 26 animals [70%], after orthotopic transplantation of intact tissue, while no hepatic metastases were found after single-cell suspension injection [29].

Orthotopic Models

By improving on the drawbacks of the heterotopic gastric cancer murine models, the orthotopic model was created [30]. It was reported that the implantation of tumor cells into the same organ provided a suitable microenvironment for the cancer to exert its intrinsic properties. The role of animal models of human cancers for oncologic research has been well established. The use of these models has contributed to the development of treatment strategies in the laboratory in in-vivo settings. For gastric cancer, numerous approaches have been used to implant the tumor cells into the recipient immunocompromised mice. Orthotopic models, in which the tumor tissue is implanted into the organ of origin, have been demonstrated to produce a superior model of human tumor development, particularly regarding metastatic growth [30]. By definition, in a true orthotopic human gastric cancer murine model the tumor growth should start from the intraluminal mucosal surface, which subsequently grows to involve the deeper gastric layers.

In the orthotopic xenograft model, the cancer cells were implanted into the murine stomach layers, which were shown by numerous studies to be an effective technique. For gastric cancer in particular, the superiority of orthotopic models over heterotopic models has been established [26].

The superiority of orthotopic models over heterotopic models are that the heterotopic tumor models lack metastasis because of the extra-anatomic location of these tumors on the flank or hind limb of the mouse. As the implanted tumor cells often become encapsulated, which renders them incapable of regional or distant metastasis. However, orthotopic models can successfully result in metastasis. Furukawa et al. in 1993 reported the application of this intact tissue orthotopic implant technique to stomach cancer resulting in the formation of metastasis in 100% of the mice with extensive primary growth to the regional lymph nodes, liver, and lung [30]. In contrast, when cell suspensions were used to inject stomach cancer cells at the same site, metastases occurred in only 6.7% of the mice with local tumor formation, emphasizing the importance of using intact tissue to allow full expression of metastatic potential. Injuring the serosa similar to that occurring in intact tissue transplantation did not increase the metastatic rate after orthotopic injection of cell suspensions of stomach tumor cells.

In recent years, numerous methods have been reprorted for creating human gastric cancer orthotopic models, including gastric wall seeding of tumor cell suspension [31], in which cancer cells are implanted on the serosal surface; intra-gastric wall transplantation of histologically intact tissue secured by suturing [32]; "gastric bursa method" [33]; or OB glue paste technique [34]. The site of transplantation is usually between the serous and seromuscular layer of the greater curvature of stomach. The "suture method" or the "gastric bursa method" has many practical difficulties and disadvantages in establishing the model of transplantation. For example, the tumor tissue may readily fall off postoperatively, manipulation is complex and needs relatively high skills, there may be significant blood loss during suturing, and mortality is relatively high.

An attempt was made by Shi J et al. to produce an orthotopic model in 2008 using OB glue paste. This present study used OB glue paste technique to establish two tumor strain orthotopic transplantation models. OB glue is biologic glue and has been used widely in surgery owing to its secure wound adhesion. *In vitro* tumor cells were collected and resuspended at 1×10^7/mL. Each nude mouse was injected subcutaneously with 0.2 mL tumor cells under the skin. When the implanted tumor grew to about 1cm diameter, it was removed from the mouse. The tumor was cut into 1 mm × 1 mm × 2 mm pieces after scraping off the surrounding fibrous capsule, and implanted directly under the skin of the nude mice. Each inter-mouse passage used two mice.The third generation of subcutaneously transplanted tumor was used as the source for orthotopic transplantation in this study. Observations showed that although different tumor strains grewat different rates, infiltrative growth and multi-organ metastases were common features of the two models, and these features were similar to the clinical presentation nof invasive metastasis. Chromosomal identification also demonstrated that both orthotopic and metastatic tumors were derived from the implanted human gastric cancer. This technique is an ideal means of model establishment owing to its easier manipulation, shorter operating time, less blood loss, quicker postoperative recovery, and higher survival of experimental animals and avoidance of tumor falling off.

The success rate was not 100% in both cases. Anatomy of the mice that failed to bear tumors showed that there was local organ adhesion arising from manipulation, and part of the transplanted tumor tissues stops growing. The following factors might have affected the success rate: [1] The amount of glue should be appropriate, 1-2 drops are enough, too much glue would envelope the implant, halting its growth; [2] It is best to wait for 10 seconds or so before closing the abdomen so that the glue can coagulate sufficiently; or it may cause extensive adhesion of the surrounding tissues; [3] It is preferable to use the seromuscular layer near the antrum of the greater curvature, because rich blood flow there facilitates tumor growth and metastasis; [4] Rupture of the seromuscular layer should not be too superficial, and bleeding is the hallmark. In addition, the tumor tissue to be implanted should be placed into the ruptured site before dropping OB glue. Smooth forceps can be used to push the rupture inward to form a denture before implanting the tumor tissues, if necessary [5]. Also it is preferred not to leave too much suture outside the abdomen to avoid suturing failure due to fierce biting between animals.

The different reported techniques have been used with varying degrees of success for producing metastatic gastric cancer models. However, all of these models have many limitations that have prevented their widespread application. They all require an open surgical technique, which entails opening of the peritoneum and implantation or injection of tumor cells/tissue on the serosal surface of the stomach or between stomach layers from the serosal side. The resultant tumor grows outward and never from the intraluminal mucosal surface, as is seen in human gastric cancer. Therefore, the reported models do not replicate of the human disease process and are not true orthotopic models. Also, the disruption of the surgical planes during the surgery makes the metastasis unpredictable and unreliable. These models cannot be used to accurately evaluate the role of different dietary components or the effects of intraluminal agents and therapies. The existing models do not produce tumors from the intraluminal mucosal surface or metastatic patterns similar to the human disease process, which limits their reliability and applicability in research [34].

There appeared to be a need for a better murine model for human gastric carcinoma that would be reliable, easy to create, and would replicate the human disease process. The reported orthotopic models for gastric cancer involving surgical implantation of tumor cells do not meet this definition and, therefore, they have many limitations. There were no true orthotopic models in use that applied nonsurgical techniques to transplant tumor cells onto the intraluminal surface of the stomach. A true Orthotopic gastric cancer murine model using electrocoagulation was reported by Bhullar et al. [35]. They used minimally invasive technique which had also been used in past to create murine models of human bladder [36, 37] and colon cancer [25, 38]. This orthotopic murine model of human gastric cancer represents an important in vivo tool for testing chemotherapeutic agents and for studying intraluminal factors. Non operative procedure was used and the resultant tumor grew from the stomach's mucosal surface and mimiced the human disease process. A low-dose gastric mucosal coagulation was done transorally in the body of stomach using a specially designed polyethylene catheter in 16 female immune compromised mice. This was followed by the instillation of SNU-16 human gastric cancer tumor cells (1×10^6 cells). Five mice each were euthanized at 1 and 2 months, and 6 mice were euthanized at 3 months. Three control mice underwent electrocoagulation alone and 3 mice underwent cell line instillation alone and were the control group. Tumors were detected in 11 of 16 experimental mice, but not in the control mice. Tumors were noted in mice at 1 month. Over time, there was an increase in tumor growth and metastasis to lymph nodes and surrounding organs. Histopathologic evaluation showed that the tumors grew from the gastric mucosa. Thus, they showed that a true orthotopic gastric cancer murine model using a transoral technique that would overcome the limitations of the models currently available.

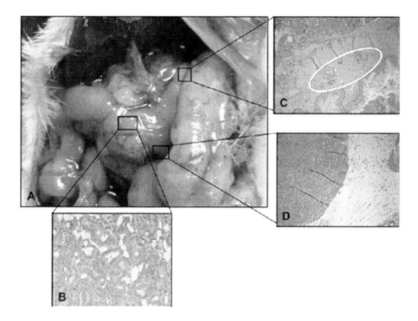

Figure 2. (A) Gross picture of a dissected mouse showing the orthtopic human gastric tumor with omental metastasis at the end of 3 months. (B) Hematoxylin and eosin (H&E) 100, the gastric antral tumor shows poorly differentiated gastric cancer with focal neoplastic glands. (C) H&E 100, the gastric cancer invading the gastroesophageal junction between the stomach muscle layers (oval white marker). (D) H&E 40, the gastric cancer invading the perigastric fat.

(The figures are reproduced from the personal collection of the authors).

In this model, low-dose electrocoagulation of the mucosal surface provided a non-ischemic bed for viable tumor cells to implant and grow. As reported previously, low-dose electrocoagulation applied to the gastrointestinal tract of immune compromised mice produced superficial injury, sparing the deeper layers and avoiding complete bowel perforation. The dosage of electrocoagulation in their study was 10 W, which was more than the 5W they had reported for the orthotopic colon cancer model. The 10-W Bovie setting was derived after different settings were evaluated in pilot mice. As the mouse stomach mucosa is thicker than the mouse colonic mucosa, a higher Bovie setting was required to be effective. Contrary to earlier beliefs of colleagues, the use of disaggregated tumor cells in suspension did not change the nature and biologic behaviour of the tumor or limit its metastatic capability for lymph node metastases.

The design of the gastric lavage tube was very important in the success of the procedure, as the tube was required to be flexible and yet robust enough to with stand the rodent chewing on the tube. The length of the tube was determined by evaluating tubes of different length in pilot mice by in situ dissections of the mice with the tube in place to determine the exact length that would be appropriate for a mouse weighing 16 to 18 g. For the procedure, a polyethylene gavage catheter [25F and 8cm long] was designed and is not commercially available. It can be made by using a 25F polyethylene tube, which is cut at 8 cm and the end is rounded by slightly warming the end of the tube close to a burner flame. After placement of the tube, the tactile sensation of the tube not moving confirmed the location of the tube in the stomach, along with correlating it with the length of the tube inserted. The predetermined length of the tube makes the placement technique reproducible and the tactile sensation of the tube not moving forward ensures that the tube is in contact with the stomach wall.

Although the electrocautery was performed in a blind manner in the stomach, the precise anatomic location of mucosal injury was assumed to be in the stomach antrum, as revealed by the histopathologic analysis of the euthanized mice. The complete insertion of the tube along with the tactile sensation of the tube not moving further made the technique easy and reproducible. This was essential in achieving standard electrocoagulation of the gastric mucosa and implantation of gastric carcinoma cells in every study animal. Also, keeping the mouse lightly sedated was helpful for the transoral insertion of the gavage tube, as active swallowin gby the mouse helped in the safe and smooth insertion of the tube. The low-dose electrocoagulation of the stomach creates a superficial injury of the gastric layers. The evaluation of the pilot mice had revealed that superficial gastric layers undergo coagulative necrosis after the electrocoagulation injury. In the pilot mice, it was noted that, overtime, this injury healed in a manner similar to gastric erosion or a superficial ulcer, which was confirmed by histopathologic evaluation. Post procedure, the mice did not show any different behaviour as compared with pre-procedure. None of the pilot or study mice revealed any signs of an early or late perforation as a result of the electrocoagulation injury. The gastric perforation resulting from the electrocoagulation procedure was a theoretical possibility and that is the reason a low-dose bovie setting [10W] was used. The evaluation of different bovie settings in the pilot mice had revealed that bovie setting of 10W injures the superficial gastric layers only and spares the deeper gastric layers, reducing the possibility of a perforation.

The carcinomatosis and peritoneal metastases were noted at the end of 3rd month in the study mice, and was representative of the late stage of the disease. Although there is a theoretical possibility of a micro-perforation or a near perforation caused by the initial injury, it would have resulted in peritonitic signs in the mouse and early widespread peritoneal metastasis, which were not noted in any of the study mice. It was their experience in the orthotopic colorectal cancer murine model using the similar electrocoagulation injury that a perforation leads to early widespread peritoneal metastasis, which was not noted in any of the mice in this study. There was an initial problem of the gastric secretions damaging the tumor cells through either digestion or dilution of the instilled tumor cell suspension in the pilotmice. The instillation of tumor cells was done using 10% fetal bovine serum as the suspending agent in the pilotmice. To overcome this problem of tumor cell damage, Matrigel was used as the suspending agent. The use of Matrigel as a suspension solution has been helpful because it has shown improved tumor implantation. Matrigel is a liquid when kept at low temperature and acquires a gel form when exposed to body temperature. It provides protection to the tumor cells from the gastric secretions and allows increased time for contact between the tumor cells and the mucosal injury site. They postulated that because Matrigel acquires a gel form in the stomach after instillation, it stayed in the stomach longer compared with fetal bovine serum, resulting in increased contact time between the tumor cells and the injury site. Matrigel also contains extracellular matrix components [laminin and collagen IV] and tumor growth factors [transforming growth factor beta, fibroblast growth factor, and tissue plasminogen activator]. These components aid in implantation of human tumor cells.

The Coloview-mouse colonoscope (Karl Storz) had been used to follow-up the colorectal tumors in the mice, but such an endoscope does not currently exist for evaluating the esophagus and stomach in mice. The euthanization of the study mice at predetermined intervals was done to evaluate tumor growth characteristics. Although local and distant metastases were noted in the study mice, no metastases were found in the liver. In their study, they evaluated only the SNU-16 gastric cancer cell line, so the lack of liver metastasis could be because of the metastatic behaviour of the particular cell line or the limitation of the model. Because the mouse is a rodent with different dietary habits, the stomach anatomy is different compared with that of humans. The difference in anatomy and blood supply might account for the metastatic pattern. Evaluation of more gastric cancer cell lines in this model is ongoing and results from the different cell lines would determine whether the tumor take rate and this metastatic pattern are inherent to cell line SNU-16 or the model itself.

This orthotopic gastric cancer implantation model is unique because it avoids open surgery; tumor growth starts on the mucosa and spreads in the submucosal direction, mimicking early gastric cancer progression in humans. It also replicates metastasis and the biologic behaviour of human gastric cancer The high tumor implantation rate after mucosal injury with electrocoagulation seen in bladder and colon cancer previously has posed the question of whether these findings might explain local recurrence rates after endoscopic resections, an idea that could also be extrapolated to early gastric cancer therapy. With endoscopic mucosal resections of early gastric cancer increasing in application, future research should aim to address this important question at this early stage of its use. This model is easy to create, does not require open surgery, is replicable, and overcomes the limitations of the existing models. This is a true orthotopic gastric cancer murine model, as the tumor arises from the stomach's mucosal layer and replicates the human disease in terms of morphology and biologic behaviour. This model represents a better model for advanced research on gastric cancer and opens new doors for additional studies that were not possible earlier.

Role of Murine Cancer Models in the Development of Chemotherapy for Gastric Cancer

Some studies on murine models have led to better understanding of the action of drugs in gastric cancer hence helping in development of effective chemotherapy for gastric cancer.

A few studies have been briefly described below -

- Role of Monoclonal Antibody [Traztuzumab] targeting Her2/neu receptor in gastric cancer inxenograft model. Her2/neu overexpression is increasingly recognized as a frequent molecular abnormality in gastric cancer, driven as in breast cancer by gene amplification [39]. There is a strong evidence of the role of Her2/neu overexpression in patients with gastric cancer, and it has been solidly correlated to worse outcomes and a more aggressive disease. Preclinical data are showing significant antitumor efficacy of anti-Her2/neu therapies [particularly monoclonal antibodies directed towards the protein] in-vitro and in in-vivo models of gastric cancer. Several studies as detailed below have demonstrated antitumor activity of Traztuzumab in overexpressing Her2/neu human gastric cancer cell lines or xenograft models.

- One such study was reported by Gravalos and Jimeno [40] in 2008 Most of the experiments used the NCI-N87 and/or 4-1ST gastric cancer cell lines, which show Her2/neuexpression by Immuno histochemistry [IHC] and gene amplification by Fluorescence in situ hybridization [FISH]. Tanner et al. [41] studied the sensitivity of the N87 gastric cancer cell line to Traztuzumab and compared its sensitivity with that of the breast cancer cell line with Her2/neu amplification [SKBR-3]. In-vitro, Traztuzumab inhibited the growth of N87 and SKBR-3 at about equal efficacy. Growth inhibition of N87 cells when using a 5 mg/kg weekly dose of trastuzumab was also verified in vivo in N87 xenograft tumors. Matsui et al. used four human gastric cancer cell lines with various expression levels of Her2/neu protein [N87, MKN45P, Kato-III, and MKN-1] to study the association between the expression of Her2/neuprotein and the sensitivity to Trastuzumab. Their experiment showed that Trastuzumab suppressed the growth of human gastric cancer with Her2/neu overexpression in vitro and in vivo and improved the survival of mice with peritoneal dissemination and ascites of gastric cancer [42].

- Another similar study was carried out by Fujimoto-Ouchi et al. in 2006. The goal of this study was to clarify the antitumor activity of Trastuzumab and its potential as an effective treatment for gastric cancer patients. In this study, it was investigated whether Trastuzumab would be useful for the treatment of Her2/neu over expressing human gastric cancer in cell culture and xenograft models as an indication of its use fulness for treating clinical gastric cancer. Efficacy of Trastuzumab was examined as a single agent or in combination with chemotherapeutic agents widely used clinically for gastric cancers. The result was that two of nine human gastric cancer xenograft models, NCI-N87 and 4-1ST, showed overexpression of Her2/neu mRNA and protein by IHC [HercepTest] and Her2/neu gene amplification by FISH [Pathvysion]. HER2 protein showed potent staining in peripheral membranes, similar to the staining pattern of breast cancer. FISH scores were also comparable to those of breast cancer models. Trastuzumab as a single agent inhibited the tumor growth in both of the Her2/neu over expressing models but not in the Her2/neu negative models, GXF97 and MKN-45. In any combination with Capecitabine, Cisplatin, Irinotecan, Docetaxel, or Paclitaxel, Trastuzumab showed more potent antitumor activity than the anticancer agents alone. A three-drug combination of Capecitabine, Cisplatin, and Trastuzumab showed remarkable tumor growth inhibition. For NCI-N87 in-vitro, Trastuzumab showed direct anti-proliferative activity according to cell count or crystal violet dying, and showed indirect antitumor activity such as antibody-dependent cellular cytotoxicity. Therefore, it is clear that Trastuzumab, even in combination therapy, should only be used for Her2/neu positive gastric cancers. The antitumor activity of Trastuzumab observed in human gastric cancer models warrants consideration of its use in clinical treatment regimens for human gastric cancer as a single agent or in a combination drug with various chemotherapeutic agents [43].

- In study by Kasprzyk et al. (1992), they reported on combination chemotherapy with docetaxel [TXT] and S-1 in metastatic gastric carcinoma by modulating the expression of metabolic enzymes of 5-fluorouracil in human gastric cancer cell lines [3]. It had been demonstrated in a Phase I/II study that combination chemotherapy with TXT and S-1 was active against metastatic gastric carcinomas. To elucidate the mechanisms underlying the synergistic effects of these drugs, both the growth inhibitory effects and the expression profiles of enzymes involved in fluorouracil [5-FU] metabolism were examined in vitro and in vivo. TXT alone and in combination with 5-FU inhibited the growth of each of the 5 gastric cancer cell lines that were examined [TMK-1, and MKN-1, -28, -45 and -74], in a time and dose dependent manner. Moreover, striking synergistic effects were observed in TMK-1 cells in vitro. Furthermore, in TMK-1 xenograft, 5-FU/TXT co-treatments exhibited synergistic antitumor effects. The combination of S-1 and TXT, however, exhibited greater growth inhibitory effects than the 5-FU/TXT co-treatments. The mechanisms underlying these synergistic effects of S-1 and TXT were examined by expression and activity analyses of the 5-FU metabolic enzymes. The expression of thymidylate synthase [TS], and dihydropyrimidine dehydrogenase [DPD] were decreased 50 and 73% of control levels, respectively, and that of orotate phosphorybosyl transferase [OPRT] was increased by 3.9-fold at the protein level. These findings suggested that biochemical modulation by 2 drugs had occurred, which was further confirmed by the results of the activity assays. These data strongly indicate that combination chemotherapy of TXT and S-1 was effective against gastric carcinomas and is therefore a good candidate as a standard chemotherapeutic strategy in treating these tumors [44].

Conclusion

The recent advancements in murine models of human gastric cancer have been exciting and broaden the scope of research that can be done using them. Minimally invasive methods have been used to create the orthotopic models which are more replicative of the human disease process. It remains to be seen if advancements in imaging modalities would support such tumors to be followed up *in situ*.

The chapter was reviewed and edited by Dr. Jeff Flynn Ph.D., Department of Patient Care Research, Providence Hospital & Medical Centers, Southfield, MI, USA.

References

[1] Kelley JR, Duggan JM. Gastric cancer epidemiology and risk factors. *J. Clin. Epidemiol.* 2003; 56: 1–9.

[2] Montgomery E, Goldblum JR, Greenson JK et al. Dysplasia as a predictive marker for invasive carcinoma in Barrett's esophagus. A follow-up study based on 138 cases from a diagnostic variability study. *Hum. Pathol.* 2001; 32:379–388.

[3]   Powell J, McConkey CC: The rising trend in oesophageal adenocarcinoma and gastric cardia. *Eur. Cancer Prev.*1992; 1: 265-269.

[4]   Lord RV, Law MG, Ward RL, et al: Rising incidence of esophageal adenocarcinoma in men in Australia. *J. Gastroenterol. Hepatol.* 1998; 13: 356-362.

[5]   Cunningham D, Allum WH, Stenning SP et al. Perioperative chemotherapy versus surgery alone for resectable gastroesophageal cancer. *New Eng. J. Med.* 2006; 355(1): 11–22.

[6]   Macdonald JS, Smalley SR, Benedetti J et al. Chemoradiotherapy after surgery compared with surgery alone for adenocarcinoma of the stomach or gastroesophageal junction. *N. Eng. J. Med.* 2001; 345(10): 725–730.

[7]   Wagner AD, Grothe W, Haerting J et al. Chemotherapy in advanced gastric cancer: a systematic review and meta-analysis based on aggregate data. *J. Clin. Oncol.* 2006; 24: 2903–2909.

[8]   Ouchi KF, Sekiguchi F, Yasumo H, et al. Antitumor activity of transtuzumab in combination with chemotherapy in human gastric cancer xenograft models. *Cancer Chemotherapy Pharmacology.* 2007; 59:795-805.

[9]   Taketo MM, Edelmann W. Mouse models of colon cancer. *Gastroenterology.* 2009; 136: 780–798.

[10] Fogh J, Giovanella BC: *The Nude Mouse in Experimental and Clinical Research.* Academics Press, New York, 1978.

[11] Houchens DP, Ovejera AA: Proceedings of the Symposium on the Use of Athymic (Nude) *Mice in Cancer Research.* Gustav Fischer, New york, 1978.

[12] Sordat B: Immune Deficient Animals: *4ᵗʰ International workshop on Immune-Deficient Animals in Experimental Research.* S. Karger, Basel, 1984.

[13] Sharkey EF, Fogh J: Considerations in the use of nude mice for cancer research. *Cancer Metastasis Reviews.* 1984; 3: 341-360.

[14] Rygaard J, Povlsen C. Heterotransplantation of a human malignant tumor to 'nude' mice. *Acta Pathol. Microbiol. Scand.* 1969; 77:758-760.

[15] Hawk ET, Levin B. Colorectal cancer prevention. *J. Clin. Oncol.* 2005, 23(2), 378–391.

[16] Theodora Voskoglou-Nomikos, Joseph L. Pater, and Lesley Seymour. Clinical Predictive Value of the *in Vitro* Cell Line, Human Xenograft, and Mouse Allograft Preclinical Cancer Models. *Clinical Cancer Research.* Vol. 9, 2003; 4227–4239.

[17] Shoemaker, R. H., Monks, A., Alley, M. C., Scudiero, D. A., Fine, D. L., McLemore, T. L., Abbott, B. J., Paull, K. D., Mayo, J. G., and Boyd, M. R. Development of human tumor cell line panels for use in disease-oriented drug screening. *Prog. Clin. Biol. Res.*1988; 276: 265–286.

[18] Skehan, P., Storeng, R., Scudiero, D., Monks A., McMahon, J., Vistica, D., Warren, J. T., Bokesch, H., Kenney, S., and Boyd, M. R. New colorimetric cytotoxicity assay for anticancer drug screening. *J. Natl. Cancer Inst.* (Bethesda).1990; 82: 1107–1112.

[19] Rubinstein, L. V., Shoemaker, R. H., Paull, K. D., Simon, R. M., Tosini, S., Skehan, P., Scudiero, D., Monks, A., and Boyd, M. R. Comparison of *in vitro* anticancer drug screening data generated with a tetrazolium assay *versus* a protein assay against a diverse panel of human tumor cell lines. *J. Natl. Cancer Inst.* (Bethesda). 1990; 82: 1113–1118.

[20] Johnson, J. I., Decker, S., Zaharevitz, D., Rubinstein, L. V., Venditti, J. M., Schepartz, S., Kalyandrug, S., Christin, M., Arbuck, S., Hollingshead, M., and Sausville, E. A.

Relationships between drug activity in NCI preclinical *in vitro* and *in vivo* models and early clinical trials. *Br. J. Cancer*. 2001; 84: 1424–1431.

[21] Denis E. Corpet, Fabrice Pierre. How good are rodent models of carcinogenesis in predicting efficacy in humans? A systematic review and meta-analysis of colon chemoprevention in rats, mice and men. *European Journal of Cancer* 41. 2005; 1911–1922.

[22] Reichling T, Goss KH, Carson DJ, et al. Transcriptional profiles of intestinal tumors in Apc (Min) mice are unique from those of embryonic intestine and identify novel gene targets dysregulated in human colorectal tumors. *Cancer Res*. 2005; 65(1): 166–176.

[23] Giovanella BC, Yim SO, Stehlin JS, Williams LJ: Development of invasive tumors to 'nude' mouse after injection of cultured human melanoma cells. *JNCI*. 1972; 48:1531-1533.

[24] Flatmark K, Maelandsmo GM, Martinsen M, Rasmussen H, Fodstad O. Twelve colorectal cancer celllines exhibit highly variable growth and metastatic capacities in an orthotopic model in nude mice. *Eur. J. Cancer*. 2004 Jul; 40(10):1593-8.

[25] Bhullar JS, Subhas G, Silberberg B, Tilak J, Andrus L, Decker M, Mittal VK. A novel nonoperative orthotopic colorectal cancer *J. Am. Coll. Surg*. 2011 Jul; 213(1):54-60.

[26] Yamashita. T. Manifestation of metastatic potential in human gastric cancer into the stomach wall of nude mice. *Jpn. J. Cancer Res*. 1988; 79: 945-951.

[27] Teruo K, Masahika O, Akira T, Keigo N et al. Changes in serum and Tissue Carcinoembryonic Antigen with Growth of a Human Gastric Cancer Xenograft in Nude Mice. *Jpn. J. Cancer Res*. 1990 Jan 81;58-62.

[28] Pocard M, Tsukui H, Salmon RJ, et al. Efficiency of orthotopic xenograft models for human colon cancers. In Vivo. 1996; 10, 463–469.

[29] Kubota T. Metastatic models of human cancer xenografted in the nude mouse: the importance of orthotopic transplantation. *J. Cell Biochem*. 1994; 56:4-8.

[30] Furukawa T, Fu X, Kubota T, et al. Nude mouse metastatic models of human stomach cancer constructed using orthotopic implantation of histologically intact tissue. *Cancer Res*. 1993; 53:1204-1208.

[31] Yamaguchi K, Ura H, Yasoshima T, et al. Liver metastatic model for human gastric cancer established by orthotopic tumor cell implantation. *World J. Surg*. 2001; 25:131-137.

[32] Mori T, Fujiwara Y, Yano M, et al. Prevention of peritoneal metastasis of human gastric cancer cells in nude mice by S-1,a novel oral derivative of 5-fluorouracil. *Oncology* 2003; 64:176-182.

[33] Nishimori H, Yasoshima T, Denno R, et al. A novel experimentalmouse model of peritoneal dissemination of human gastric cancer cells: different mechanisms in peritoneal dissemination and hematogenous metastasis. *Jpn. J. Cancer Res*. 2000; 91:715-722.

[34] Shi J, Pin-Kang W, Zhang S, et al. OB glue paste technique for establishing nude mouse human gastric cancer orthotopic transplantation models. *World J. Gastroenterol*. 2008; 14: 4800-4804.

[35] Bhullar JS, Makarawo T, Subhas G, Alomari A et al. A true orthotopic gastric cancer murine model using electrocoagulation. *J. Am. Coll. Surg*. 2013 Jul; 217(1):64-70.

[36] Solloway MS, Masters S. Urothelial susceptibility to tumor cell implantation, influence of cauterization. *Cancer*. 1980; 46:1158-1163.

[37] Gunther JH, Jurczok A, Wulf T, et al. Optimizing syngeneic orthotopic murine bladder cancer (MB49). *Cancer Res.* 1999; 59:2834-2837.

[38] Donigan M, Norcross LS, Aversa J, et al. Novel murine model for colon cancer: non-operative trans-anal rectal injection. *J. Surg. Res.* 2009; 154: 299-303.

[39] Slamon DJ, Clark GM, Wong SG, Levin WJ, Ullrich A,McGuire WL Human breast cancer: correlation of relapse and Survival with amplification of the HER-2/neuoncogene. *Science.* 1987; 235: 177–182.

[40] Gravalos C, Jimeno A. HER2 in gastric cancer: a new prognostic factor and a novel therapeutic target. *Ann. Oncol.* 2008 Sep; 19(9): 1523-9.

[41] Tanner M, Hollmen M, Junttila TT, Kapanen AI, Tommola S, Soini Y et al. AmpliWcation of HER-2 in gastric carcinoma: association with Topoisomerase II- gene ampliWcation, intestinal type, poor prognosis and sensitivity to trastuzumab. *Ann. Oncol.* 2005; 16:273–278.

[42] Matsui Y, Inomata M, Tojigamori M, Sonoda K, Shiraishi N, Kitano S. Suppression of tumor growth in human gastric cancer with HER2 overexpression by an anti-HER2 antibody in a murine model. *Int. J. Oncol.* 2005; 27(3): 681–685.

[43] Fujimoto-Ouchi K, Sekiguchi F, Yasuno H, Moriya Y, Mori K, Tanaka Y.Antitumor activity of trastuzumab in combination with chemotherapy in human gastric cancer xenograft models. *Cancer Chemother. Pharmacol.* 2007 May; 59(6): 795-805.

[44] Kasprzyk PG, Song SU, Di Fiore PP, King CR.Therapy of an animal model of human gastric cancer using a combination of anti-erbB-2 monoclonal antibodies. *Cancer Res.* 1992 May 15; 52(10): 2771-6.

In: Gastric Cancer
Editor: Jasneet Singh Bhullar

ISBN: 978-1-63117-983-9
© 2014 Nova Science Publishers, Inc.

Chapter 6

Adjuvant Treatment Modalities for Gastric Cancer

Leyla Kilic[1], M.D. and Cetin Ordu[2]†, M.D.*

[1] Firat University Hospital, Department of Medical Oncology, Elazig, Turkey
[2] Bilim University, Avrupa Florence Nightingale Hospital, Department of Medical Oncology, Istanbul, Turkey

Abstract

Gastric cancer is a leading cause of cancer-related death and thus represents a significant global health concern. Surgical resection remains the only effective curative treatment of gastric cancer. Less than 40% of cases will be able to be cured with complete surgical resection of tumor. In patients with advanced T3–4 tumors and/or tumor-positive lymph nodes the relapse and death rates from recurrent cancer exceed 70-80%. Because of high incidence of locoregional recurrence, adjuvant and neoadjuvant treatment modalities are crucial.

Following the results of Intergroup trial (INT-0116) twelve years ago and the update of ten years outcome of study with still improvement of overall survival (OS) and disease free survival (DFS), chemoradiotherapy became standart adjuvant treatment modality in operated gastric cancer. Alternative trials have been reproduced without direct comparison to the approach established by INT-0116. The Japanese ACTS-GC (Adjuvant Chemotherapy Trial of S-1 for Gastric Cancer) study demonstrated a 33% improvement in OS for patients receiving 1 year of postoperative adjuvant *S*-1, an oral fluoropyrimidine. In South Korea, Japan, and Taiwan, the CLASSIC (Adjuvant Capecitabine and Oxaliplatin for Gastric Cancer After D2 Gastrectomy) study reported a 44% improvement in DFS for patients randomly assigned to postoperative capecitabine and oxaliplatin (XELOX) when compared with observation. Both ACTS-GC and CLASSIC limited enrollment to patients who had undergone a D2 lymph node dissection which is a common technique for gastric cancer surgery in Asia. However, limited D0 or D1dissections are more widespread in the United States. Thus, the benefit of radiotherapy

---

* e-mail: leylahmet@gmail.com; +90 505 455 97 60; +90 424 248 50 53.
† e-mail: cetinordu@hotmail.com; +90 505 772 53 08.

in the adjuvant setting for D0 and D1 dissections is a subject of debate. According to current guidelines, adjuvant chemotherapy is an option for only D2 lymph node dissections.

Two recently completed trials have directly compared different postoperative adjuvant regimens. The ARTIST (Adjuvant Chemoradiation Therapy in Stomach Cancer) trial compared postoperative capecitabine and cisplatin (XP) to chemoradiotherapy (XP plus radiotherapy with capecitabine) in patients with curative gastrectomy with D2 dissection. Although the addition of radiotherapy to postoperative chemotherapy did not significantly improve DFS among all enrolled subjects, in subgroup analyses, patients with node-positive disease did experience a superior DFS.

Ultimately, beyond the primary objectives of these proposed and ongoing trials, we must continue to identify new prognostic and predictive factors, such as human epidermal growth factor receptor 2 overexpression or diffuse histology in adjuvant setting, that may serve as the basis for more effective, tailored therapeutic approaches in patients with gastric adenocarcinoma.

Introduction

Gastric cancer is the second cause of cancer related death worldwide, with 988,000 new cases and 736,000 deaths per year [1]. Despite decreasing frequency of worldwide, the high incidence of gastric cancer is a still major health concern in Eastern countries such as Korea and Japan.

It's well known that D2 lymph node dissection is considered as standard treatment for early gastric cancer in Japan and Korea. In 1981, the Japanese Society for Research in Gastric Cancer (JSRGC) had standardized gastric resections and the extent of regional lymphadenectomy in accordance with specific rules based on the location of the tumour and the respective regional node drainage [2]. Large retrospective series from Japan of radical gastrectomy with D2 lymph node dissection have shown impressive 5-year survival rates, certainly much higher than experienced in the West [3,4]. Although some non-Japanese centres have reported favourably on D2 resections the benefit of D2 over conventional D1 resections had not been tested prospectively until the randomized Medical Research Council (MRC) and Dutch Gastric Cancer Group trials in 1999 [5-8]. The MRC ST01 trial conducted in United Kingdom randomized 400 patients with gastric adenocarcinoma to D1 resection (removal of regional perigastric nodes) and D2 resection (extended lymphadenectomy to include level 1 and 2 regional nodes) [7]. The 5-year survival rates were 35% for D1 resection and 33% for D2 resection with no statistical difference between the two arms [Hazard Ratio (HR) = 1.10, 95% CI 0.87–1.39]. The Dutch Gastric Cancer Group trial also failed to show a survival advantage for D2 dissection compared with D1 dissection [8]. Besides patients in the D2 group had a significantly higher rate of complications than did those in the D1 group (43 % vs. 25 %, p<0.001), and more postoperative deaths (10 % vs. 4 %, p=0.004). Five-year survival rates were similar in the two groups: 45 % for the D1 group and 47 % for the D2 group, respectively. The mortality reported for the D1 and D2 arms of the MRC ST01 study was virtually identical to that of the equivalent Dutch trial, but undoubtedly higher than that reported by the Japanese trials. The discrepancy in terms of survival difference between the Asian and Western results were not clearly defined either. The patients in both of these trials had not received any adjuvant chemotherapy in contrast to Japanese studies which is supposed to contribute to the difference in survival. Besides, stage migration might be one of the reasons for the discrepancy between the long-term results of surgery for gastric cancer in Japan and the results in the West, because additional information on lymph nodes is available only for patients with D2 dissection. Factors such as experience born of sustained caseload, surgical skill, quality of post-operative care and case selection may also have contributed for this difference. However 15-year follow-up results of the Dutch trial supported D2 dissection as a better option for locoregional control of gastric cancer patients [9]. Overall gastric-cancer-related death rate was significantly higher in the D1 group compared with the D2 group (48% vs 37%, p=0.001), whereas death due to other diseases was similar in both groups. Locoregional recurrences were also higher among D1 group (for local and regional recurrence 22 % vs 12 %.and 19 % vs 13%, respectively). Meanwhile, it was reported that D2 lymphadenectomy can also be done safely in Western Europe and the USA, without increased morbidity and mortality and after an adequate learning period, when routine pancreatico-splenectomy is avoided [10,11]. Wu et al. [12] from Taiwan also demonstrated the benefit of D2 lymph node dissection for gastric cancer in their randomized study. These studies supported rationale for the D2 dissection of gastric cancer worldwide when D2 surgery is done by experienced surgeons.

A review of data from the National Cancer Data Base on 50,169 patients in the United States who underwent gastrectomy between 1985 and 1996 found a 10-year survival rate of 65% among patients with stage IA disease (tumor confined to the gastric mucosa), but the 10-year survival rates among those with more advanced disease ranged from 3 % to 42 percent, despite the struggle on surgical techniques [13]. Thus, the high rate of both locoregional and distant relapse after resection makes it mandatory to optimize adjuvant treatment modalities for patients with stomach cancer.

I. Adjuvant Chemotherapy

Timing, sequence, adjuvant/neoadjuvant strategies and combination of modalities have been questioned in numerous phase II and phase III trials. Fairly large number of studies were undertaken to detect the role of adjuvant chemotherapy for resectable gastric cancer. Some previous phase III trials did not clearly show benefit of adjuvant chemotherapy. However, these studies usually did not enroll large datasets and generally included early stage patients [14-16]. Until the Adjuvant Chemotherapy Trial of S-1 for Gastric Cancer (ACTS-GC) study, there were no well designed, phase III studies with large number of patients that show a significant benefit of adjuvant chemotherapy for gastric cancer patients with D2 lymph node dissection. The ACTS-GC study group demonstrated that one year adjuvant chemotherapy with an oral fluoropyrimidine, S-1, showed a significant survival benefit for stage II and III gastric cancer patients who underwent gastrectomy with extended (D2) lymph node dissection [17]. Adjuvant chemotherapy without radiation for gastric cancer has become the standard of care in Japan after the publication of the results of the ACTS-GS trial reporting on S-1 but not in Europe or the United States.

Many studies have been performed with adjuvant chemotherapy in resectable gastric cancer. These studies have been part of several meta-analyses, which could demonstrate no, or at the most a modest survival benefit for adjuvant chemotherapy [18-22]. Hermans et al.

[21] found no significant benefit of adjuvant chemotherapy comparing surgery alone [Odds ratio (OR) 0.88, 95% confidence interval (CI) 0.72-1.08]. However, a study by Earle and Maroun [23] yielded a significant benefit in terms of survival for adjuvant chemotherapy versus surgery alone among western population (OR 0.8, 95% CI 0.66-0.97). The Global Advanced/ Adjuvant Stomach Tumor Research International Collaboration (GASTRIC) group published results of meta-analysis of individual patient data with median follow up exceeding seven years [24]. Based on the individual data of 3838 patients from 17 different trials and updated follow-up, a modest but statistically significant survival advantage was associated with adjuvant chemotherapy after curative resection of gastric cancer. The mortality hazard was reduced by about 18% and an absolute improvement of about 6% in OS was observed after 5 years. This improvement was maintained at 10 years. An 18% reduction in the risk of relapse, second primary, or death was also observed. This treatment benefit was maintained in three of the four investigated groups of fluorouracil-based regimens, with reductions in the risk of death ranging from 20% to 40% (nonstatistically significant heterogeneity). Only one of the nineteen trials that enrolled 134 patients investigated a non–fluoropyrimidine-based regimen. Sensitivity analysis excluding this trial revealed similar results. This metaanalysis pointed out that adjuvant fluorouracil-based chemotherapy, even as monotherapy, is associated with improvement in overall survival and combination chemotherapy of 5-fluorouracil, mitomycin with/without anthracyclin could be recommended for patients who have not received perioperative treatments. However the analysis could not conclude on the type of optimal chemotherapeutic regimen, schedule, and duration of treatment for adjuvant chemotherapy of gastric cancer.

Previously, large scaled phase III Japanese trial with mitomycin C, fluorouracil, and followed by oral UFT, a combination of tegafur, a prodrug of 5-fluorouracil (5-FU) and uracil treatment did not exhibit significant survival advantage compared with surgery alone [25]. The investigators considered that this result was due to high proportion of pT1 gastric cancer patients included in the trial for whom surgery alone may yield a good prognosis and there seemed to be no requirement for adjuvant therapy. The authors concluded that patients with pT1 gastric cancer should be excluded from further adjuvant chemotherapy trials. In the light of this finding, following trials usually excluded such early stage patients (i.e., $\leq$ stage Ib).

Similarly, neoadjuvant chemotherapy trials have emphasized the benefit of initiating the adjuvant treatment as early as possible. The combination regimen of epirubicin, cisplatin, and infusional fluorouracil (ECF) has achieved response rates between 49 % and 56 % in randomized trials of locally advanced gastric cancer [26,27]. ECF regimen improves survival and response rates among patients with advanced esophagogastric cancer when compared to combination of fluorouracil, doxorubicin, and methotrexate (FAMTX), and the side-effect profile is acceptable [26,28]. Findings of a meta-analysis have also revealed that for advanced disease, epirubicin and cisplatin have synergistic effect [29]. The combination of adjuvant with neo-adjuvant chemotherapy has proven its value in two randomized trials. As the pioneer study of perioperative chemotherapy for gastric cancer, British Medical Research Council Adjuvant Gastric Infusional Chemotherapy (MAGIC) trial have shown significant downstaging of the primary tumour, 10% higher resectability rate with a survival benefit of 13% at 5 years [30]. The potential advantages of administering ECF preoperatively are increasing the likelihood of curative resection by downstaging of the tumor, eliminating micrometastases, rapidly improving tumor-related symptoms, and predicting the tumor sensitivity to chemotherapy. The primary end point of the trial was overall survival;

secondary end points were progression-free survival, surgical and pathological assessments of down-staging (i.e., tumor diameter, tumor stage, and nodal status), the assessments by the surgeons about whether the surgery was curative, and quality of life. In this randomized trial, the investigators initially planned to combine their results with those of the Dutch Gastric Cancer Group study which randomly assigned patients with operable gastric adenocarcinoma to four cycles of FAMTX before surgery or to surgery alone [31]. This study was terminated after accrual of 59 patients due to an interim analysis which showed inadequate rates of curative resection in the chemotherapy group. The median survival at the time of reporting was 18 months in the group receiving chemotherapy plus surgery and 30 months in the group undergoing surgery alone (P = 0.17). One of the major conclusions driven from these trials was the inferiority of FAMTX regimen when compared with the ECF regimen in patients with advanced disease [26,28]. A possible limitation of MAGIC trial was that only 42 % of patients in the perioperative-chemotherapy group completed all protocol treatment; 34 % of patients who completed preoperative chemotherapy and surgery could not receive postoperative chemotherapy, predominantly owing to early disease progression, patient request or postoperative complications. Besides there is no data about D2 dissection rate in MAGIC trial. Nevertheless, patients assigned to perioperative chemotherapy had a significant survival advantage over those who underwent surgery alone. Because this trial evaluated perioperative treatment, it is not possible to attribute the favorable outcome to preoperative or postoperative chemotherapy. In summary, MAGIC trial results showed that perioperative chemotherapy with a regimen of ECF improves overall and progression-free survival among patients with resectable adenocarcinoma of the stomach, lower esophagus, or gastroesophageal junction, as compared with surgery alone.

Due to the high incidence of gastric cancer in Japan, developing an effective regimen for adjuvant chemotherapy has been a considerable goal. S-1 is an orally active combination of tegafur (a prodrug that is converted by cells to fluorouracil), gimeracil (an inhibitor of dihydropyrimidine dehydrogenase, which degrades fluorouracil), and oteracil (which inhibits the phosphorylation of fluorouracil in the gastrointestinal tract, thereby reducing the gastrointestinal toxic effects of fluorouracil) in a molar ratio of 1:0.4:1.12,13. The rate of response to treatment with S-1 alone exceeded 40% in two late phase II trials involving patients with advanced or recurrent gastric cancer [32,33]. The pharmacokinetics of the fluorouracil that is derived from S-1 is not influenced by gastrectomy [34]. A pilot study by ACTS-GC group reported the results of a large-scale trial including patients with stage II or III gastric cancer treated with S-1 following complete resection [17]. After a median follow-up of 2.9 years, the overall survival in S-1 group (n=530) was 33% higher than the surgery-only group (n=529). Adverse events of grade 3 or grade 4 occurred in less than 5% of patients in the S-1 group, except for anorexia (which occurred in 6% of patients), and S-1 treatment was well-tolerated The overall survival rate at 3 years after surgery was 80.5% in the S-1 group and 70.1% in the surgery-only group. Thus, S-1 was approved as an effective option for adjuvant chemotherapy after curative surgery in patients with gastric cancer.

Increased acceptance of D2 gastrectomy raises new questions about the optimal adjuvant therapy for patients with operable gastric cancer. The Capecitabine and Oxaliplatin Adjuvant Study in Stomach Cancer (CLASSIC) study was designed to compare the effect of adjuvant capecitabine plus oxaliplatin after D2 gastrectomy with surgery alone on disease-free survival in patients with stage II or III gastric cancer [35]. Although several phase II trials had shown the efficiency of capecitabine and oxaliplatin in advanced gastric cancer, phase III data advocating this regimen as an adjuvant treatment was lacking since the establishment of CLASSIC trial results (33–36). Among 1,035 resected gastric cancer patients in South Korea, Japan, and Taiwan, the CLASSIC study reported 44% improvement in disease-free survival (DFS) for patients randomly assigned to postoperative capecitabine and oxaliplatin (XELOX) when compared with observation. Chemotherapy reduced the relative risk of disease recurrence, new disease occurrence, or death compared with surgery alone. Moreover, a subgroup analysis suggested that adjuvant capecitabine and oxaliplatin was beneficial for all disease stages (II, IIIA or IIIB). The overall survival data from this study are not yet mature; however, the data suggest an improvement in overall survival with capecitabine and oxaliplatin compared with surgery alone. The investigators of CLASSIC trial defined 3-year DFS as the primary endpoint because most relapses occur within 3 years of surgery for gastric cancer. Although 3 year disease-free survival has not yet been formally validated as a surrogate measure, preliminary data from the Global Advanced/Adjuvant Stomach Tumor Research International Collaboration (GASTRIC) group indicate that 3 year disease-free survival is strongly correlated with 5 year overall survival, the benchmark for judging effectiveness of adjuvant therapy in gastric cancer. The clinical relevance of disease-free survival in gastric cancer is supported by the GASTRIC group meta-analysis of 17 trials [24].

The discrepancy regarding the surgical technique, type of adjuvant chemotherapeutics utilized in trials and different overall survival rates in similar studies has led to the generation of different adjuvant treatment protocols in distinct parts of the world. The recommended adjuvant treatment is chemoradiotherapy in the USA; perioperative chemotherapy in the United Kingdom (UK) and parts of Europe; and adjuvant chemotherapy in Japan. These recommendations are based on the US Intergroup-0116 and UK MAGIC (26) trials, which showed survival benefits with postoperative chemoradiotherapy and perioperative chemotherapy, respectively, compared with surgery alone [37,38]. However, the benefits were evident only after limited dissection of regional lymph nodes in both studies which evoked questions about the need for postoperative radiotherapy or perioperative chemotherapy after D2 gastrectomy. Both ACTS-GC and CLASSIC clearly showed the benefit of adjuvant chemotherapy compared to surgery alone in Japan and Korea, where the D2 dissection in standart for gastrectomy in resected gastric cancer patients, which contrasts to the limited D0 or D1 dissections more widespread in the United States. Thereafter, the extrapolation of data obtained from both ACTS-GC and CLASSIC trials for patients undergoing a D0 or D1 dissection is not convincing enough. Moreover, the striking epidemiologic differences in gastric cancer between Asian and Western populations further confound the application of these Asian trials to Western patient populations. However, it's assumed that, if adequate D2 dissection was performed, treatment outcomes in Western countries would be similar to those in Japan.

And there is a question; could results of CLASSIC trial be adapted to geographical regions where disease management practices might differ? The CLASSIC trial had good patient outcomes; the 3 year overall survival rate in the surgery only group was substantially higher than that in the US Intergroup-0116 and UK MAGIC populations (78% in CLASSIC *vs* 30–40% in Intergroup-0116 and MAGIC). Although patient population in CLASSIC trial had fewer T3 and T4 lesions than did US and European gastric cancer populations (44% in CLASSIC *vs* 68% in Intergroup-0116 *vs* 64% in MAGIC), node-positive disease was more frequent (90% *vs* 85% *vs* 72%). The difference in outcomes seems unlikely to be due to prognostic disparities, although the possibility of intrinsic biological differences in gastric cancer by region has been suggested [39]. Whereas, it is suggested that the favourable outcomes in this study were a result of the consistent use of D2 surgery and the high quality of that surgery (ensured by prospectively defined standard operating procedures and sampling of at least 15 lymph nodes). Now that D2 gastrectomy is standard of care in both Europe and the USA, the findings of this study could be highly significant and might be generalized to the other regions where D2 surgery is accomplished by experienced surgeons. On the basis of CLASSIC findings, it is assumed that a trial of capecitabine and oxaliplatin plus trastuzumab after D2 gastrectomy in patients with human epidermal growth factor receptor (HER)-2 positive operable disease is warranted. Such a study would build on the ToGA trial, which showed improved overall survival with trastuzumab plus chemotherapy in patients with HER-2-positive advanced disease [40]. The future of adjuvant treatment for gastric cancer is supposed to rely on the utilization of novel agents in conjunction with the classic fluorouracil backbone, in the light of biomarkers and genetic tests which predict response to specific treatment protocols.

II. Adjuvant Chemoradiotherapy

Even after gastric resection with curative intent local or regional recurrence in the gastric or tumor bed, the anastomosis, or regional lymph nodes occurs in 40 to 65 percent of patients [41]. According to the reoperative analysis of 107 evaluable patients in the University of Minnesota, 80% had later evidence of relapse. Locoregional failure occurred as the only evidence of relapse in 29% of the 86 patients with relapse (23% of the 107 evaluable patients at risk) and as any component of relapse in 88% (69% of evaluable patients at risk). Locoregional relapse occurred in three major locations: (1) gastric bed (organs and structures in proximity to the primary tumor), (2) regional nodes, and (3) gastric remnant, anastomoses and duodenal stump [42]. Thus, radiotherapy is supposed to be an essential adjunct of postoperative treatment in gastric cancer patients.

Two randomized trials have compared surgery alone to surgery plus RT in patients with gastric cancer. In the first trial conducted by the British Stomach Cancer Group, 436 patients were randomized to undergo surgery alone or surgery followed by RT or chemotherapy with mitomycin, doxorubicin, and fluorouracil [43]. Of note, 40% of patients on this trial had gross or microscopic residual disease following surgery. At 5-year follow-up, no survival benefit was seen for patients receiving postoperative RT or chemotherapy compared with those who underwent surgery alone. The 5-year survival for surgery alone was 20%, for surgery plus radiotherapy 12%, and for surgery plus chemotherapy 19%. However, there was a significant reduction in locoregional recurrence with the addition of RT to surgery (27% with surgery vs. 10% for surgery plus RT and 19% for surgery plus chemotherapy). The second trial by Zhang et al. [44] randomized 370 patients to preoperative RT or surgery alone. There was a significant improvement in survival with preoperative RT (30% vs. 20%, p = 0.0094). Resection rates were also higher in the preoperative RT arm (89.5%) compared to surgery alone (79%). The causes of failure were local uncontrol and recurrence in 38.6% vs. 51.7% (p < 0.025), regional lymph node metastasis 38.6% vs. 54.6% (p < 0.005) suggesting that preoperative RT improves local control, but not the frequency of distant metastasis (24.3% vs.

24.7%). While encouraging, this trial included only cardiac lesions, and it is unknown if these results can be generalized to include distal lesions.

In a systematic review of randomized clinical trials (RCTs) in which radiotherapy, (preoperative, postoperative and/or intraoperative), was compared with surgery alone or surgery plus chemotherapy in resectable gastric cancer revealed that radiotherapy had a significant impact on 5-year survival [45]. However external-beam RT (45 to 50.4 Gy) as a single modality has minimal value in patients with locally unresectable gastric cancer and does not improve survival. Wieland and Hymmen [46] used radiotherapy alone in patients with unresectable gastric cancer. The radiation dose was 60 Gy when feasible, in 1.5 to 2.0 Gy fractions. They noted an 11% 3-year and 7% 5-year survival. Abe and Takahashi [47] reported a 14.7% 5-year survival rate with intraoperative radiation therapy (28 to 35 Gy) in a group of 27 patients with stage IV disease. In the same study, there were no 5-year survivors in the stage IV patients randomized to a surgery-alone control arm. These quite low survival rates have eliminated radiotherapy as a single adjuvant modality in the treatment of resected gastric cancer.

Due to the high rates of local and distant failure after radiotherapy-alone protocols, the investigators tested for combined chemoradiotherapy (CRT) schemes in both adjuvant and neoadjuvant settings. The landmark trial in the combined modality treatment of gastric cancer in the U.S. is Intergroup 0116 study [37]. A total of 556 patients with resected adenocarcinoma of the stomach or gastroesophageal junction (stage IB through IVM0) disease were randomly assigned to surgery plus postoperative chemoradiotherapy with or surgery alone. The adjuvant treatment consisted of two cycles of 5-FU and leucovorin followed by two more cycles of chemotherapy concurrent with radiation therapy. Patients received 45 Gy of radiation in 25 fractions to the preoperative tumor volume, surgical bed, and regional lymph nodes. In the Intergroup 0116 trial, 2D radiation therapy with an anterior-posterior (AP) and a posterior- anterior (PA) radiation beam was utilized. The majority of patients on this trial had advanced disease (66% were T3/4 and 85% were node positive). The median overall survival in the surgery only group was 27 months, as compared with 36 months in the chemoradiotherapy group; the hazard ratio for death was 1.35 (95 % CI: 1.09 - 1.66; p=0.005). The hazard ratio for relapse was 1.52 (95 % CI: 1.23 - 1.86; p<0.001). An important issue regarding the surgical procedure was the extent of surgery in this trial. Although an extensive (D2) lymph-node dissection was recommended, only 10 percent of the patients underwent a D2 dissection, 36 percent had a D1 dissection, and 54 percent had a D0 lymphadenectomy (a resection in which not all of the N1 nodes were removed). This situation had raised the question of whether chemoradiation was simply compensating for inadequate surgery. Besides, toxicity was significantly higher with chemoradiation, with nearly three-quarter of patients experiencing grade 3/4 toxicity, and 17% of patients were unable to complete radiation due to toxicity. Among the 281 patients assigned to the chemoradiation group only 64% of patients completed treatment and 17% discontinued treatment due to toxicity. However, treatment related mortality was low (1% on the chemoradiation arm versus 0% on the surgery alone arm) and overall chemoradiation appeared tolerable in light of its benefits. Updated analysis of this trial with more than 10-year median follow-up has reinforced the persistant benefit of adjuvant CRT [48]. The overall survival (OS) and recurrence-free survival (RFS) data demonstrated continued strong benefit from postoperative radiochemotherapy. Hazard ratios were virtually unchanged since the original report.

The major limitation for global acceptance of the INT-0116 (or MacDonald's) regimen as an adjuvant treatment modality has been the inadequate lymph node dissection (D0 or D1) in 90 % of patients included in the trial. In Asian and European centers where D2 lymph node dissection is routinely performed, addition of further radiotherapy has been questioned due to the high morbidity rates and poor tolerance. However, another observational study involving Korean gastric cancer patients with D2 lymph node dissection has advocated chemoradiotherapy as an adjunct to surgery, with acceptable toxicities and good tumor control [49]. Kim et al. randomized a total of 990 patients to postoperative chemoradiotherapy protocol similar to Intergroup trial or surgery without further adjuvant treatment. The median duration of overall survival was significantly longer in the CRT group than in the comparison group (95.3 months vs. 62.6 months). But this strategy still has little popularity outside the USA.

One of the most criticized aspects of the Intergroup trial was the toxicity profile of the FU/LV regimen, thus alternative postoperative chemoradiation regimens containing infusional fluorouracil or capecitabine have been evaluated by other investigators. In a pilot study by Lee et al. [50] postoperative chemoradiation with fluorouracil and cisplatin before and after capecitabine and concurrent RT was administered to patients with completely resected stage III-IV (M0) gastric cancer. All patients had undergone extensive D2 lymph node dissection. A total dose of 4500 cGy in 25 fractions over five weeks was delivered to the target volume that included the gastric bed, anastomosis, stump, and regional lymph nodes areas similar to the INT-0116 trial. This study demonstrated a 3-year disease free and overall survival of 82.7 % and 83.4 %, respectively with the use of adjuvant chemoradiotherapy. Compared with the results from postoperative chemoradiotherapy with D2 lymph node dissection study for gastric cancer, if adjusted for stage, this study showed superior 3-year survival in patients with advanced gastric cancer [51].

Although response rates have been higher in general, prospective randomized studies have not consistently demonstrated a significant improvement in survival for patients receiving cisplatin-containing regimens when compared to other combination or single agent [52,53]. Nevertheless, there has been a substantial interest in the use of cisplatin-containing regimens in the adjuvant setting. Leong et al. [54] reported that postoperative chemotherapy with epirubicin, cisplatin, and 5-FU (ECF) before and after concurrent chemoradiation with infusional fluorouracil was safe and effective in patients with completely resected gastric adenocarcinoma. Radiotherapy was delivered using multiple-field, three-dimensional conformal techniques. At a median follow-up of 36 months, the estimated 3-year OS rate was 61.6 %. A similar regimen with ECF before and after radiation with infusional fluorouracil has been compared to INT-0116 regimen in a randomized phase III trial (CALGB 80101) [55]. Although the ECF regimen had a more favourable toxicity profile compared to bolus fluorouracil and leucovorin there was no significant improvement in survival.

The benefit of adjuvant RT has long been debated in D2 resected gastric cancer based on the hypothesis that D2 resection alone may be adequate to control locoregional recurrence.

One prospective study comparing adjuvant CRT with FU and cisplatin versus chemotherapy in D2 resected gastric cancer was terminated early because of poor patient accrual. A total of 61 patients with stage IIIA, IIIB and IV (M0) were enrolled. The median follow-up duration was 77.2 months and no significant difference in 5- year DFS or OS was reported (76.7 vs 59.1%, p= 0.222 and 70.1 vs 70.0%, p= 0.814, for DFS and OS, respectively) [56]. Several retrospective studies including ours have assessed the feasibility and efficacy of adjuvant CRT in D2 resected gastric cancer. In our study including completely resected pN3 (M0) gastric cancer patients with D2 lymph node dissection, no significant improvement in DFS or OS was deteceted with the addition of radiotherapy [57]. The results of the recently completed phase III trial (ARTIST) trial further showed that postoperative chemoradiation with capecitabine and cisplatin (XP) did not significantly reduce recurrence after D2 lymph node dissection in patients with curatively resected gastric cancer [58]. The study was designed to compare six cycles of XP chemotherapy with two cycles of XP followed by concurrent chemoradiotherapy followed by two additional cycles of XP in patients with gastric cancer after D2 dissection. Anterior-posterior parallel opposing fields were used for RT, and the RT dose was 45 Gy, with 1.8-Gy daily fractions administered over 5 weeks. Patients with T2a, N0 tumors, microscopically positive resection margin, involvement of M1 lymph node or distant metastases and those who had undergone gastrectomy with D1 lymph node dissection were excluded from this study. Treatment was completed as planned by 75.4% of patients in the chemotherapy arm and 81.7% in the CRT arm. The most common nonhematologic grade 3 to 4 adverse events were vomiting, stomatitis, hand and foot syndrome and diarrhea, each of which occurred in 1% to 12% of patients in both arms. The rate of grade 3 and 4 neutropenia was 39 % in the CT arm and 48% in the CRT arm, however the rate of febrile neutropenia was quite low in both arms (< 1%). This study also demonstrated that postoperative treatment with capecitabine and cisplatin is feasible following a D2 lymph node dissection. In the ARTIST trial the addition of CRT to XP regimen did not significantly prolong DFS after a median follow-up of 53 months (p=0.08, 3-year DFS rates 78.2 vs 74.2 % for CRT and CT arms, respectively). However, the subgroup of patients with pathologic lymph node metastasis assigned to CRT, experienced superior DFS when compared with those who received CT alone (77.5 % vs 72 %, p=0.03). The major limitation of the study, inadequacy of events is supposed to contribute to further conclude about the efficacy of CRT after D2 dissection. Approximately 60 % of the patients in both arms had relatively early stage disease (Ib and II), thus the planned number of events have not occurred in a fairly better prognostic group. The investigators assumed that 8 years of additional follow-up time after the completion of accrual is required for final analysis. However, the subgroup analysis regarding the beneficial effect of CRT in patients with lymph node metastasis has emerged the establishment of a subsequent trial (ARTIST II) in patients with lymph node involvement.

Technology has evolved over time to allow increasingly conformal radiation therapy, potentially sparing normal tissues and decreasing toxicity and/or allowing dose escalation to the target volume. Radiation using anterior–posterior opposed fields inevitably damages normal organs, resulting in increased radiotherapy side effects and decreased tolerance. Three- dimensional conformal radiotherapy reduces the damage to normal tissues to some extent, and it is superior to radiation with anterior–posterior opposed fields [59]. IMRT is a more advanced radiotherapy technique, with high geometrical accuracy as well as capabilities of delivering a high dose to a targeted area. Recent studies show that IMRT for gastric cancer is dosimetrically superior to conventional therapy, as IMRT reduces the radiation dose to normal organs while ensuring the targeted radiation dose to specified areas [60,61]. The most recent phase III trial comparing CRT with chemotherapy alone investigated the role of intensity-modulated radiotherapy (IMRT) with concomitant CT in gastric cancer patients with D2 lymph node dissection [62]. The experimental arm (IMRT plus CT) was feasible and well tolerated with improvement in relapse-free survival, however this trial also failed to show an OS difference like the previous comparative studies.

Another issue regarding the availibility of CRT is the neoadjuvant setting. Since the results of the MAGIC trial, perioperative chemotherapy has been widely accomplished in European countries. The Intergroup study has already demonstrated the survival benefit for operated gastric cancer in the adjuvant setting. The important question that needs to be answered is whether postoperative chemoradiotherapy improves survival as compared to postoperative chemotherapy in patients who are treated with neoadjuvant chemotherapy followed by gastric resection. CRITICS trial (ChemoRadiotherapy after Induction chemoTherapy In Cancer of the Stomach) has been designed to respond to this question [63]. In this phase III multicentre study, patients with resectable gastric cancer are treated with three cycles of preoperative ECC (epirubicin, cisplatin and capecitabine), followed by gastrectomy and adequate lymph node dissection with a minimum of 15 lymph nodes, and then either another three cycles of ECC or concurrent chemoradiation (45 Gy, cisplatin and capecitabine). The primary endpoint is overall survival, secondary endpoints are disease-free survival, toxicity and health-related quality of life. The investigators are also planning to assess the risk of recurrence and response through genomic and expression profiling. The results of this trial is expected to elucidate remarkable questions regarding adjuvant treatment of gastric cancer.

Conclusion

The high rates of both locoregional and distant metastasis following surgery with even extended lymph node dissection for gastric cancer has deemed adjuvant treatment necessary. The selection of appropriate protocol with the most effective chemotherapeutical agent(s) and the least side effect profile constitutes the compulsive side of 'chemotherapy' aspect. Whether new radiation techniques should be adjunct to the systemic chemotherapy is still a subject of debate in some parts of the world although it is a standard adjuvant treatment modality elsewhere. The future is supposed to rely on trials which will be designed on patients specified according to pathologic (lymph node involvement, histological subtype, HER-2 expression) or even genomic profiles.

References

[1] Ferlay J, Shin HR, Bray F, Forman D, Mathers C, Parkin DM.GLOBOCAN 2008, Cancer Incidence and Mortality Worldwide: IARC CancerBase No. 10. Lyon, France: International Agency for Research on Cancer; 2010. Available from: http://globocan.iarc.fr/ factsheets/cancers/stomach.asp (accessed Oct 12, 2011).

[2] Kajitani T. (1981). Japanese Research Society for Gastric Cancer. The general rules for the gastric cancer study in surgery and pathology. *Jpn J Surg* 11: 127–139.

[3] Maruyama K, Okabayashi K and Kinoshita T. (1987) Progress in gastric cancer surgery and its limits of radicality. *World J Surg* 11: 418–426.

[4] Nakajima T and Nishi M. (1989). Surgery and adjuvant chemotherapy for gastric cancer. *Hepatogastroenterology* 36: 79–85.

[5] Siewert JR, Bottcher K, Roder JD, Busch R, Hermanek P and Meyer HJ. (1993). Prognostic relevance of systematic node dissection in gastric carcinoma. *Br J Surg* 80: 1015–1018.

[6] Mendes de Almeida JC, Bettencourt A, Santos Costa C and Mendes de Almedida JM. (1995). Impact of distal pancreatectomy and splenectomy in D2 dissection for gastric cancer. In First International Gastric Cancer Congress 1995, vol 2, pp. 1165–1169. Monduzzi Editore SpA: Bologna.

[7] Cuschieri A, Weeden S, Fielding J, et al. (1999). Patient survival after D1 and D2 resections for gastric cancer: long-term results of the MRC randomized surgical trial. *Br J Cancer* 79:1522-30.

[8] Bonenkamp JJ, Hermans J, Sasako M, van de Velde CJH. (1999). Extended lymph-node dissection for gastric cancer. *N Engl J Med* 340:908-14.

[9] Songun I, Putter H, Kranenbarg EM, Sasako M, van de Velde CJ. (2010). Surgical treatment of gastric cancer: 15-year follow-up results of the randomised nationwide Dutch D1D2 trial. *Lancet Oncol* 11:439-449.

[10] Degiuli M, Sasako M, Ponti A, Calvo F. (2004). Survival results of a multicentre phase II study to evaluate D2 gastrectomy for gastric cancer. *Br J Cancer* 90: 1727–32.

[11] Degiuli M, Sasako M, Calgaro M et al. (2004). Morbidity and mortality after D1 and D2 gastrectomy for cancer: interim analysis of the Italian Gastric Cancer Study Group (IGCSG) randomised surgical trial. *Eur J Surg Oncol* 30: 303–08.

[12] Wu CW, Hsiung CA, Lo SS, Hsieh MC, Chen JH, Li AF, et al. (2006). Nodal dissection for patients with gastric cancer: a randomised controlled trial. *Lancet Oncol* 7:309-315.

[13] Hundahl SA, Phillips JL, Menck HR. (2000). The National Cancer Data Base report on poor survival of U.S. gastric carcinoma patients treated with gastrectomy: fifth edition American Joint Committee on Cancer staging, proximal disease, and the "different disease" hypothesis. *Cancer* 88: 921-32.

[14] Nashimoto A, Nakajima T, Furukawa H, Kitamura M, Kinoshita T, Yamamura Y, et al. (2003). Gastric Cancer Surgical Study Group, Japan Clinical Oncology Group. Randomized trial of adjuvant chemotherapy with mitomycin, Fluorouracil, and Cytosine arabinoside followed by oral Fluorouracil in serosa-negative gastric cancer: Japan Clinical Oncology Group 9206- 1. *J Clin Oncol* 21:2282-2287.

[15] Miyashiro I, Furukawa H, Sasako M, et al. (2005). No survival benefit with adjuvant chemotherapy for serosa-positive gastric cancer: randomized trial of adjuvant chemotherapy with cisplatin followed by oral fluorouracil (UFT) in serosa-positive gastric cancer. Presented at the 2005 Gastrointestinal Cancers Symposium, Hollywood, FL, January 27-29, abstract.

[16] Kinoshita T, Nakajima T, Ohashi Y. (2005). Adjuvant chemotherapy with uracil-tegafur (UFT) for serosa negative advanced gastric cancer: results of a randomized trial by national surgical adjuvant study of gastric cancer. *Prog Proc Am Soc Clin Oncol* 23:Suppl:313s. Abstract.

[17] Sakuramoto S, Sasako M, Yamaguchi T, Kinoshita T, Fujii M, Nashimoto A, et al. (2007). ACTS-GC Group. Adjuvant chemotherapy for gastric cancer with S-1, an oral fluoropyrimidine. *N Engl J Med* 357:1810-1820.

[18] Janunger KG, Hafström L, Glimelius B. (2002). Chemotherapy in gastric cancer: a review and updated meta-analysis. *Eur J Surg* 168:597-608.

[19] Oba K, Morita S, Tsuburaya A, Kodera Y, Kobayashi M, Sakamoto J. (2006). Efficacy of adjuvant chemotherapy using oral fluorinated pyrimidines for curatively resected gastric cancer: a meta-analysis of centrally randomized controlled clinical trials in Japan. *J Chemother* 18:311-317.

[20] Mari E, Floriani I, Tinazzi A, Buda A, Belfiglio M, Valentini M, et al. (2000). Efficacy of adjuvant chemotherapy after curative resection for gastric cancer: a meta-analysis of published randomised trials. A study of the GISCAD (Gruppo Italiano per lo Studio dei Carcinomi dell'Apparato Digerente). *Ann Oncol* 11:837- 843.

[21] Hermans J, Bonenkamp JJ, Boon MC, Bunt AM, Ohyama S, Sasako M, et al. (1993) Adjuvant therapy after curative resection for gastric cancer: meta-analysis of randomized trials. *J Clin Oncol* 11:1441-1447.

[22] Liu TS, Wang Y, Chen SY, Sun YH. (2008). An updated meta-analysis of adjuvant chemotherapy after curative resection for gastric cancer. *Eur J Surg Oncol* 34:1208-1216.

[23] Earle CC, Maroun JA. (1999). Adjuvant chemotherapy after curative resection for gastric cancer in non-Asian patients: revisiting a meta-analysis of randomised trials. *Eur J Cancer* 35:1059- 1064.

[24] GASTRIC (Global Advanced/Adjuvant Stomach Tumor Research International Collaboration) Group, Paoletti X, Oba K, Burzykowski T, Michiels S, Ohashi Y, Pignon JP, et al. (2010) Benefit of adjuvant chemotherapy for resectable gastric cancer: a meta-analysis. *JAMA* 303:1729-1737.

[25] Nakajima T, Nashimoto A, Kitamura M, Kito T, Iwanaga T, Okabayashi K, et al. (1999). Adjuvant mitomycin and fluorouracil followed by oral uracil plus tegafur in serosa-negative gastric cancer: a randomised trial. Gastric Cancer Surgical Study Group. *Lancet* 354:273-277.

[26] Webb A, Cunningham D, Scarffe JH, et al. (1997). Randomized trial comparing epirubicin, cisplatin, and fluorouracil versus fluorouracil, doxorubicin, and methotrexate in advanced esophagogastric cancer. *J Clin Oncol* 15: 261-267.

[27] Ross P, Nicolson M, Cunningham D, et al. (2002). Prospective randomized trial comparing mitomycin, cisplatin, and protracted venous-infusion fluorouracil (PVI 5-FU) with epirubicin, cisplatin, and PVI 5-FU in advanced esophagogastric cancer. *J Clin Oncol* 20:1996-2004.

[28] Waters JS, Norman A, Cunningham D, et al. (1999) Long-term survival after epirubicin, cisplatin and fluorouracil for gastric cancer: results of a randomized trial. *Br J Cancer* 80:269-72.

[29] Wagner AD, Grothe W, Behl S, et al. (2005). Chemotherapy for advanced gastric cancer. *Cochrane Database Syst Rev* 2: CD004064.

[30] Cunningham D, Allum WH, Stenning SP, et al. (2006). Perioperative chemotherapy versus surgery alone for resectable gastroesophageal cancer. *N Engl J Med* 355:11-20,

[31] Hartgrink HH, van de Velde CJ, Putter H, et al. (2004). Neo-adjuvant chemotherapy for operable gastric cancer: long term results of the Dutch randomized FAMTX trial. *Eur J Surg Oncol* 30:643.

[32] Sakata Y, Ohtsu A, Horikoshi N, Sugimachi K, Mitachi Y, Taguchi T. (1998). Late phase II study of novel oral fluoropyrimidine anticancer drug S-1 (1 M tegafur-0.4 M

gimestat-1 M otastat potassium) in advanced gastric cancer patients. *Eur J Cancer* 34: 1715-20.

[33] Koizumi W, Kurihara M, Nakano S, Hasegawa K. (2000). Phase II study of S-1, a noveloral derivative of 5-fluorouracil, in advanced gastric cancer. *Oncology* 58:191-7.

[34] Kochi M, Fujii M, Kanamori N, et al. (2007). Effect of gastrectomy on the pharmacokinetics of S-1, an oral fluoropirimidine, in resectable gastric cancer patients. *Cancer Chemother Pharmacol* 60:693-701.

[35] Bang YJ, Kim YW, Yang HK, Chung HC, Park YK, Lee KH, et al. (2012). CLASSIC trial investigators. Adjuvant capecitabine and oxaliplatin for gastric cancer after D2 gastrectomy (CLASSIC): a phase 3 open-label, randomised controlled trial. *Lancet* 379:315-321.

[36] Deng J, Liang H, Wang D, Sun D, Pan Y, Liu Y. (2011). Investigation of the recurrence patterns of gastric cancer following a curative resection. *Surg Today* 41: 210–215.

[37] Macdonald JS, Smalley SR, Benedetti J, et al. (2001). Chemoradiotherapy after surgery compared with surgery alone for adenocarcinoma of the stomach or gastroesophageal junction. *N Engl J Med* 345:725-30.

[38] Waters JS, Norman A, Cunningham D, et al. (1998). Long-term survival after epirubicin, cisplatin and fluorouracil for gastric cancer: results of a randomized trial. *Br J Cancer* 80:269-72.

[39] McCulloch PG, Ochiai A, O'Dowd GM, Nash JR, Sasako M, Hirohashi S. (1995). Comparison of the molecular genetics of c-erb-B2 and p53 expression in stomach cancer in Britain and Japan. *Cancer* 75:920-5.

[40] Bang YJ, Van Cutsem E, Feyereislova A, et al., and the ToGA Trial Investigators. (2010). Trastuzumab in combination with chemotherapy versus chemotherapy alone for treatment of HER2-positive advanced gastric or gastro-oesophageal junction cancer (ToGA): a phase 3, open-label, randomised controlled trial. *Lancet* 2010; 376: 687–97.

[41] Landry J, Tepper JE, Wood WC, Moulton EO, Koerner F, Sullinger J. (1990). Patterns of failure following curative resection of gastric cancer. *Int J Radiat Oncol Biol Phys* 1990;191:1357-62.

[42] Gunderson LL, Sosin H. (1982). Adenocarcinoma of the stomach: Areas of failure in a reoperation series (second or symptomatic looks): Clinicopathologic correlation and implications for adjuvant therapy. *Int J Radiat Oncol Biol Phys* 8:1-11.

[43] Hallissey MT, Dunn JA, Ward LC, Allum WH. (1994). The second British Stomach Cancer Group trial of adjuvant radiotherapy or chemotherapy in resectable gastric cancer: five-year follow-up. *Lancet* 343:1309-1312.

[44] Zhang ZX, Gu XZ, Yin WB, et al. (1998). Randomized clinical trial on the combination of preoperative irradiation and surgery in the treatment of adenocarcinoma of gastric cardia (AGC)--report on 370 patients. *Int J Radiat Oncol Biol Phys* 42:929-934.

[45] Valentini V, Cellini F, Minsky BD, et al. (2009). Survival after radiotherapy in gastric cancer: systematic review and meta-analysis. *Radiother Oncol* 92:176-183.

[46] Wieland C, Hymmen U. (1970). Mega-volt therapy of malignant stomach neoplasms. *Strahlentherapie.* 140:20-26.

[47] Takahashi M, Abe M. (1986). Intra-operative radiotherapy for carcinoma of the stomach. *Eur J Surg Oncol.* 12:247-250.

[48] Smalley SR, Benedetti JK, Haller DG, Hundahl SA, Estes NC, Ajani JA et al. (2012). Updated analysis of SWOG-directed Intergroup study 0116: a phase III trial of adjuvant

radiochemotherapy versus observation after curative gastric cancer resection. *J Clin Oncol* 30: 2327-2333.

[49] Kim S, Lim DH, Lee J, et al. (2005). An observational study suggesting clinical benefit for adjuvant postoperative chemoradiation in a population of over 500 cases after gastric resection with D2 nodal dissection for adenocarcinoma of the stomach. *Int J Radiat Oncol Biol Phys* 63: 1279–1285.

[50] Lee HS, Choi Y, Hur WJ, et al. (2006). Pilot study of postoperative adjuvant chemoradiation for advanced gastric cancer: adjuvant 5-FU/cisplatin and chemoradiation with capecitabine. *World J Gastroenterol* 12:603-607.

[51] Park SH, Kim DY, Heo JS, Lim DH, Park CK, Lee KW, Choi SH, Sohn TS, Kim S, Noh JH. (2003). Postoperative chemoradiotherapy for gastric cancer. *Ann Oncol.* 14:1373-1377.

[52] Vanhoefer U, Rougier P, Wilke H, Ducreux MP, Lacave AJ, Van Cutsem E, Planker M, Santos JG, Piedbois P, Paillot B. (2000). Final results of a randomized phase III trial of sequential high-dose methotrexate, fluorouracil, and doxorubicin versus etoposide, leucovorin, and fluorouracil versus infusional fluorouracil and cisplatin in advanced gastric cancer: A trial of the European Organization for Research and Treatment of Cancer Gastrointestinal Tract Cancer Cooperative Group. *J Clin Oncol.* 18:2648-2657.

[53] Ohtsu A, Shimada Y, Shirao K, Boku N, Hyodo I, Saito H, Yamamichi N, Miyata Y, Ikeda N, Yamamoto S. (2003). Randomized phase III trial of fluorouracil alone versus fluorouracil plus cisplatin versus uracil and tegafur plus mitomycin in patients with unresectable, advanced gastric cancer: The Japan Clinical Oncology Group Study (JCOG9205). *J Clin Oncol.* 21:54-59.

[54] Leong T, Joon DL, Willis D, et al. (2011). Adjuvant chemoradiation for gastric cancer using epirubicin, cisplatin, and 5-fluorouracil before and after three-dimensional conformal radiotherapy with concurrent infusional 5-fluorouracil: a multicenter study of the Trans-Tasman Radiation Oncology Group. *Int J Radiat Oncol Biol Phys* 79:690-695.

[55] Fuchs CS, Tepper JE, Niedzwiecki D, et al. (2011). Postoperative adjuvant chemoradiation for gastric or gastroesophageal junction (GEJ) adenocarcinoma using epirubicin, cisplatin, and infusional (CI) 5-FU (ECF) before and after CI 5-FU and radiotherapy (CRT) compared with
bolus 5-FU/LV before and after CRT: Intergroup trial CALGB 80101[abstract]. *J Clin Oncol* 29 (Suppl 15):Abstract 4003.

[56] Kwon HC, Kim MC, Kim KH, et al. (2010). Adjuvant chemoradiation versus chemotherapy in completely resected advanced gastric cancer with D2 nodal dissection. *Asia Pac J Clin Oncol* 6:278-285.

[57] Kilic L, Ordu C, Ekenel M, Yildiz I, Keskin S, Sen F, Gural Z, Asoglu O, Kizir A, Aykan F. (2013). Comparison of two different adjuvant treatment modalities for pN3 gastric cancer patients after D2 lymph node dissection: can we avoid radiotherapy in a subgroup of patients? *Med Oncol* 30: 660.

[58] Jeeyun Lee, Do Hoon Lim, Sung Kim, Se Hoon Park, Joon Oh Park, Young Suk Park et al. (2012). Phase III trial comparing capecitabine plus cisplatin versus capecitabine plus cisplatin with concurrent capecitabine radiotherapy in completely resected gastric cancer with D2 lymph node dissection: The ARTIST trial. *J Clin Oncol* 30: 268-273.

[59] Leong T, Willis D, Joon DL, et al. (2005). 3D conformal radiotherapy for gastric cancer results of a comparative planning study. *Radiother Oncol* 74:301–306.

[60] Milano MT, Garofalo MC, Chmura SJ, et al. (2006). Intensity modulated radiation therapy in the treatment of gastric cancer: early clinical outcome and dosimetric comparison with conventional techniques. *Br J Radiol* 79:497–503.

[61] Ringash J, Perkins G, Brierley J, et al. (2005). IMRT for adjuvant radiation in gastric cancer: a preferred plan? *Int J Radiat Oncol Biol* Phys 63:732–8.

[62] Zhu WG, Xua DF, Pu J, Zong CD, Li T, Tao GZ, et al. (2012). A randomized, controlled, multicenter study comparing intensity-modulated radiotherapy plus concurrent chemotherapy with chemotherapy alone in gastric cancer patients with D2 resection. *Radiother Oncol* 104: 361-366.

[63] Dikken JL, van Sandick JW, Maurits Swellengrebel HA, Lind PA, Putter H, Jansen EP, Boot H, van Grieken NC, van de Velde CJ, Verheij M, Cats A. (2011). Neo-adjuvant chemotherapy followed by surgery and chemotherapy or by surgery and chemoradiotherapy for patients with resectable gastric cancer (CRITICS). *BMC Cancer* 11:329.

Reviewed by Ibrahim Yildiz M.D. from Istanbul University, Institute of Oncology, Department of Medical Oncology (Istanbul/TURKEY).

In: Gastric Cancer
Editor: Jasneet Singh Bhullar

ISBN: 978-1-63117-983-9
© 2014 Nova Science Publishers, Inc.

Chapter 7

Surgical Evaluation of Lymph Node Involvement in Gastric Cancer - Maruyama Computer Program and the Sentinel Lymph Node Biopsy

Dezső Tóth, M.D., Ph.D.[1], and Miklós Török, M.D.[2]*

[1]Department of General Surgery, Kenézy Teaching Hospital,
Debrecen, Hungary
[2]Department of Pathology, Kenézy Teaching Hospital,
Debrecen, Hungary

Abstract

Approximately, one-third of patients with gastric cancer have an unnecessarily extended lymph node dissection with a higher rate of morbidity and mortality. Preoperative diagnostic tools have a low sensitivity and specificity determining lymph node involvement. The Maruyama computer program (MCP) can estimate the lymph node involvement preoperatively and the sentinel lymph node (SLN) biopsy may help to reduce the number of redundant lymphadenectomy intraoperatively.

74 patients were investigated by the Maruyama computer program and 58 patients were labelled with blue dye for SLN mapping. All patients underwent open gastric resection and D2 lymphadenectomy. Twenty patients were marked submucosal by an endoscopist and in 38 patients injection was performed by the surgeon subserosal. The staining method and the lymphadenectomy were supervised by the same surgeon. To measure the probability calculations by MCP, we had to define a 'cut-off level', with using the calculation of the receiver-operating characteristics analysis.

The Maruyama computer program had a 90.2% of sensitivity, 63.3% of specificity and 78.4 % of accuracy. The positive predictive value was 75.5% and the negative predictive value was 84%. The false negative rate was 9.8%. The sensitivity of sentinel lymph node mapping was 96.6%, the false negative rate was 3.4% and the specificity was

---

* Phone:+36-309388867; Fax:+36-52511797; E-mail: detoth@gmail.com.

100%. The accuracy of SLN mapping was 98.2%. The positive predictive value was 100% and the negative predictive value was 96.6%.

The intraoperative sentinel lymph node examination is superior to the preoperative estimation by the Maruyama computer program. However, using these two methods in a parallel fashion could be useful in decision-making for determining the appropriate extent of lymphadenectomy. The individualized stage-adapted surgery can guarantees the best outcome for the patients with gastric cancer.

Introduction

The modern, optimal treatment of patients with different neoplasms can be achieved, in most cases, with the stage adapted, combined modality therapy according to international protocols. In case of solid tumors the presence and exact number, or the absence of lymph node metastases are among the most important prognostic factors. Adjuvant chemotherapy, as well as, prognosis of the patient is determined primarily by the TNM stage. Preoperative imaging techniques provide a much more accurate determination of the T and M stage than that of the N stage. The correct status of lymph node metastases can be obtained only by histology following an optimally extended node dissection. The removal of more lymph nodes, on the other hand, increases operative time, the rate of complications, and if negative may be considered unnecessary.

Presence of lymph node metastases is the most important predictive factor of survival in gastric cancer in cases of potentially curative resection [1, 2]. Approximately, one-third of patients with gastric adenocarcinoma have an unnecessarily extended lymph node dissection [3]. Several studies have shown an increased perioperative morbidity and mortality with D2 versus D1 lymph node dissection [4, 5, 6]. However, the 15-year follow-up results of Dutch trial revealed that cancer-related death rates were lower in the D2 lymphadenectomy group [7].

Successful estimation of lymph node involvement may help to define those patients who would and those who would not benefit from an extended lymph node dissection in association with gastrectomy. For this purpose, a computer program was developed by Keiichi Maruyama to estimate the incidence of lymph node metastases, the expected prognosis, and the percentage of curability at surgery, based on the most significant preoperative prognostic factors [8].

This program was later improved as the Windows-based program WinEstimate v. 2.5 using a database of 4302 primary gastric cancer patients treated at the National Cancer Center Hospital in Tokyo between 1968 and 1989. [9]. The first potentially affected lymph node, the sentinel lymph node (SLN), reflects reliably the status of the nodes in the second and third line, which is supported by data of numerous publications. If the SLN contains tumor deposit(s), extended dissection is warranted, while in case of negativity, the patient could be spared of additional complications associated with extended dissection. Sentinel lymph node biopsy (SNB) has become a standard procedure in breast cancer and malignant melanoma [10, 11]. A meta-analysis of SNB demonstrated a high detection rate (93.7%) and an accuracy of 92 percent in patients with gastric cancer [12]. However, the method of dye/tracer injection and selection of tracer(s) for SLN mapping in gastric cancer remain controversial. Accurate determination of the lymph node status, as well as, minimizing operative morbidity are the key objectives of sentinel node-based surgery. Keeping the well-known differences between Asian and European gastric cancer phenotypes in mind [13, 14, 15], authors applied and compared, for the first time, Maruyama computer program (MCP) and "dye only" labelling technique of sentinel lymph nodes in cases of gastric cancer in Hungary [16, 17].

Material and Methods

We evaluated the efficacy of MCP and the sentinel lymph node biopsy technique to predict the nodal status and localization of lymph node metastases in our patients from February 2008 to April 2013 at the Department of Surgery of the "Gyula Kenézy" Teaching County Hospital, Debrecen, Hungary. Exclusion criteria were gastric stump tumor, cardia cancer, distant metastases for MCP and SNB. Involvement of surrounding organs was an exclusion criteria only for SNB. Seventy-four consecutive patients were evaluated by MCP. The calculation required the following prognostic factors in every patient: age, gender, position of the tumor (upper, middle, and lower third of the stomach, anterior or posterior wall, lesser or greater curve), Bormann's classification or early gastric cancer classification according to the Japanese Endoscopy Society, estimated depth of infiltration and histological type. Based on these data, the computer model calculated the percentage likelihood of metastasis at each lymph node location (stations 1-16) (Figure 1.).

All the patients underwent open gastric resection and D2 lymph node dissection routinely. Sampling of station 10 and compartment 3 nodes (13 to 16) was optional and carried out if macroscopically suspicious. Therefore, these nodal stations were not routinely assessed using MCP.

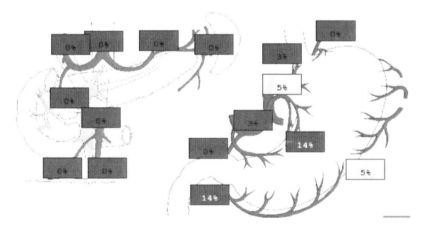

Figure 1. Prediction of lymph node involvement by the Maruyama computer program in a 65-year-old male patient. The tumor histology was well differentiated adenocarcinoma, showing muscular mucosa involvement (MM), early cancer type 2B. The lesion was found in the anterior wall in the lower third of the stomach and had a maximal diameter of 30 mm.

Sixty-four of 74 patients were labelled with blue dye only method for SNB. After laparotomy, the lesser sac was opened (if it was needed) and 4 X 0.5 mL blue dye (Bleu Patenté V Sodique Guerbet 2,5%, F-95943 Roissy CdG, Cedex, France) was injected in four quadrants around the tumor. Six patients were excluded based on pathological diagnosis of T4 tumor. Therefore, fifty-eight patients were enrolled. Of these, twenty patients were marked by submucosal injection of dye by an endoscopist (Figure 2.) and in the remaining 38 patients, subserosal dye injection was performed by the surgeon (Figure 3).

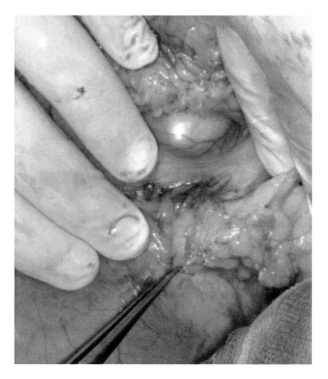

Figure 2. Sentinel lymph node mapping following submucosal marking by an endoscopist.

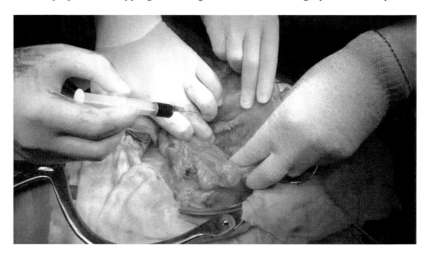

Figure 3. Subserosal marking by a surgeon.

Lymphatic drainage was observed for up to 10 minutes following injection. Blue stained lymph nodes were marked as sentinel lymph nodes and D2 lymph node dissection was performed after gastric resection or total gastrectomy. The staining procedure and the lymphadenectomy were supervised by the same surgeon. The position of lymph nodes was labelled according to the Japanese Classification of Gastric Carcinoma (JCGC) [18]. Only negative sentinel nodes based on standard microscopy were examined for micrometastases. This included sectioning at 0.2mm intervals and hematoxylin and eosin (HE) staining and in histologically ambiguous cases pan-Cytokeratin immunohistochemistry examinations were performed with DAKO Monoclonal Mouse Anti-Human Cytokeratin (clone AE1/AE3; dilution 1:30; Dakocytomation; Glostrup; Denmark).

To measure the probability calculations by MCP, we had to define a 'cut-off level', by using the calculation of the receiver-operating characteristics analysis (ROC) [19]. This logistic regression model indicates the probability of concordance between the predicted probability and the proven diagnosis of lymph node metastasis. We estimated the sensitivity and specificity with several cut-off points of MCP expected percentage values obtained by the ROC analysis for each of the 12 lymph node (LN) stations. We defined the best cut-off points for every LN station and the common critical cut-off point to maximize the test validity.

For each station, we declared positivity if its Maruyama value was greater than or equal to the cut-off specific to that station. Overall positivity was then declared based on the presence of station-specific positivity at any station included in the analysis. Thus, the only way for station elimination to produce a difference is if positive stations are eliminated such that all remaining stations are negative. Statistical analysis of equivalence between the results of submucosal and subserosal SLN mapping was based on calculating ratios of test performance indicators (those of the submucosal mapping method divided by those of the subserosal procedure). Equivalence was established when the 95% exact confidence interval around such a ratio was fully contained within the range 0.8 to 1.25.

Results

We investigated 74 consecutive patients, 35 females and 39 males with a mean age of 67 (range: 48 to 82) years for MCP. The average body mass index (BMI) was 22.6 (range: 17.1 to 27.9). Twenty-one patients had signet-ring cell carcinoma while 19 patients had poorly differentiated adenocarcinoma, 32 patients moderately differentiated adenocarcinoma and 2 patients well differentiated adenocarcinoma. The tumor was localized in the upper third of the stomach in 8 cases, middle third in 20 cases, and lower third in 46 cases. The depth of invasion - based on the 6th TNM Classification of Malignant Tumors - was T1 in 20, T2 in 13, T3 in 29 and T4 in 12 patients. Total gastrectomy was performed in 28 patients, and subtotal gastrectomy in 46. A total of 1424 lymph nodes were removed with an average of 19.2 per patient (range: 10 to 38).

Table 1. shows the data of patients with SNB. The mean number of sentinel lymph nodes was 5.0 per patient. The frequency of lymph node labelling in relation to the tumor's location was evaluated (Table 2).

Table 1. Characterization of patients with sentinel lymph node biopsy

Number of patients	58
Female	25
Male	33
Age	67.1 (48-82)

Table 1. (Continued)

Tumor sites	
Upper	8
Middle	16
Lower	34
Depth of invasion	
T1	20
T2	13
T3	25
Nodal involvement	
N0	29
N1	17
N2	10
N3	2
Total number of dissected lymph nodes	1109
Median number of dissected lymph nodes (range)	19.1 (10-38)
Total number of SLN	285
Mean number of SLN (range)	5.0 (1-16)

Based on TNM Classification of Malignant Tumours, 6th edition. Edited by L.H. Sobin and Ch. Wittekind, 2002.

Table 2. Frequency of lymph node labelling in relation to the tumor's location

LN station	Upper third N=8	Middle third N=15	Lower third N=34
1	2 (25%)	6 (40%)	4 (12%)
3	4 (50%)	6 (40%)	16 (48%)
4	0 (0%)	2 (13%)	8 (24%)
5	0 (0%)	0 (0%)	15 (44%)
6	1 (12.5%)	5 (33%)	22 (65%)
7	2 (25%)	4 (27%)	14 (41%)
8	2 (25%)	3 (20%)	6 (18%)
10	0 (0%)	0 (0%)	2 (6%)
11	0 (0%)	0 (0%)	2 (6%)
12	0 (0%)	0 (0%)	2 (6%)

Uncommonly, two patients in the cohort of lower third tumors had sentinel lymph nodes in lymph node station 10. Both patients had a circumferential tumor. One patient had a T3, grade 3, papillary adenocarcinoma with lymphatic invasion and five lymph nodes were labelled (LN no.3, no.6, no.7, no.8, no.10), while the other had a T3, grade 3, signet-ring cell carcinoma and twelve lymph nodes were stained (LN no.5, no.6, no.7, no.8, no.10, no.11 and no.12).

Based on the evaluation of area under the ROC curve we defined the best cut-off points station by station and the common critical cut-off point which maximized the test validity (cut-off point=18) (Table 3.). In 2 cases with metastases in LN station 9 and 12, the MCP calculated 0%, so the sensitivity was zero with any cut-off level, as in other 2 cases with metastases in LN station 10.

The sensitivity, specificity, negative predictive value, positive predictive value and accuracy of MCP were calculated with „18% cut-off point" and the „best cut-off point" (Table 4).

MCP with the „best cut-off point" (station by station) had equal statistical result as with „18% cut-off point".

In all except one out of 58 cases, sentinel lymph nodes were successfully identified, resulting in a detection rate of 98.3%. The sentinel lymph nodes were in the D1 compartment in 32 cases (56%), in 21 cases (37%) both in the D1 and D2 compartments and in four cases (7%) in the D2 compartment only.

Table 3. Estimated relation between given cut-off points (the best cut-off level and cut-off level of 18) of MCP's expected percentage of LN positivity, and the corresponding statistical data (area under the ROC curve, sensitivity and specificity) for each of 12 LN stations

LN station[a]	MCP's percent cut- off points	Area under the ROC curve	Sensitivity (%)	Specificity (%)
1	6	0.781	100	56.3
	18	0.591	40	78.1
2	18	0.472	0	94.2
3	18	0.642	84.6	43.8
4	18	0.702	70	70.4
5	18	0.814	75	87.9
6	18	0.613	64.7	57.9
7	12	0.588	68.4	49.1
	18	0.527	52.6	52.7
8	15	0.752	80	70.3
	18	0.602	50	70.3
9	18	0.361	0	72.2
10	18	0.486	0	97.2
11	9	0.623	33.3	91.2
	18	0.456	0	91.2
12	18	0.417	0	83.3

The cut-off point of the best results station by station is highlighted in bold
[a]JCGC [18] numbering system. LN: lymph node, MCP: Maruyama computer program, ROC: receiver operating characteristic.

In the group of T1 tumors (n=20), all the patient were node negative. In the T2 group (n=13), 10 patients had positive SLN while 8 also had metastasis among non-sentinel LNs. Only seven out of 25 (28%) patients with T3 tumor did not have any nodal metastasis.

Regarding lymph node involvement of the patients, exclusively SLN were positive in 8/29 cases (28%). Two of them could be found only in the D2 compartment. Twenty-nine patients (50%) were histologically node negative, in 28 patients both sentinel lymph nodes and non-sentinel lymph nodes were negative.

Table 4. Statistical features of MCP with the common and the best cut-off levels

	MCP (cut-off 18)	MCP (cut-off best)
Sensitivity	90.2	90.2
Specificity	63.3	63.3
ROC area	0.769	0.769
PPV	75.5	75.5
NPV	84.0	84.0
Accuracy	78.4	78.4

ROC: receiver operating characteristic, PPV: postive predictive value, NPV: negative predictive value, MCP: Maruyama computer program.

In one case there was not any sign of labelling, the BMI of this patient was 26.8. In the 28 SLN negative cases micrometastasis were not found in the sentinel lymph nodes.

In 28/29 cases at least one SLN showed tumor involvement, with a false negative rate of 1/29 (3.4 %). In this single false negative case the tumor was T3 in extension, and grade 3 with perineural invasion histopathologically and the macroscopically involved lymph nodes could be found during the operation. Results of the intraoperative frozen sections of the SLN correlated completely with the postoperative pathological findings. Sensitivity of SNB was 96.6%, and the specificity was 100%. Negative predictive value (NPV) was 96.6% and the positive predictive value (PPV) was 100%. The accuracy was 98.2%.

Submucosal and subserosal marking method was proven equivalent in detection rate, sensitivity and specificity based on 95% confidence interval (CI) of ratio of indicators (Table 5).

Sensitivity, specificity, negative predictive value, positive predictive value and accuracy with SNB method were superior to those of MCP. The difference was statistically significant (p=0.0008).

We evaluated the accuracy of MCP for the first tier lymph nodes, due to the low value of area under the ROC curve in stations 9, 10 and 12. However, the accuracy and the statistical features (sensitivity, specificity, PPV, NPV) did not change, because patients with false negative second tier lymph nodes had false negative lymph node in the first tier also. The accuracy of MCP in sentinel node positive patients was 85.7% and only 75% in the complete group of the fifty-eight patients.

Table 5. Sensitivity and specificity of SLN mapping procedure in correlation to the marking method (submucosal versus subserosal)

	Submucosal (n=20)	Subserosal (n=37)	Result (95% CI)
Mean number of SLN	4.3	5.4	
Detection rate (%)	100%	97.3%	equivalent
False negative rate (%)	0%	5.9%	
Sensitivity (%)	100%	94.1%	equivalent
Specificity (%)	100%	100%	equivalent

Criterion of equivalence: 95% of confidence interval (CI) should be fully within the range 0.8-1.25.

However, only the PPV of MCP and SNB was proven equivalent in the sentinel node positive group. In these patients the specificity and NPV could not be defined, due to the lack of negative cases.

There were no side-effects of blue dye mapping.

Conclusion

Dutch and British prospective randomized trials found a higher morbidity and mortality rate following extended lymph node dissection of patients with gastric cancer when compared to those undergoing D1 dissection only [4, 5]. Revision of Dutch trial revealed that cancer-related death rates were lower in the D2 lymphadenectomy group [7]. However, forty percent of Western European patients have an unnecessary extended lymph node dissection in cases of R0 resection [3]. Preoperative diagnostic tools have a low sensitivity and specificity defining the patient subpopulations which would and which would not benefit from an extended lymph node dissection. Sensitivity, specificity and accuracy of spiral computer tomography for detection of pathologic lymph node involvement are 73.1, 50.0 and 84.2%, respectively [20]. Endoscopic ultrasonography has an accuracy of 68.6%, with a sensitivity and specificity of 66.7% and 73.7 %, respectively [21]. The real problem of these imaging procedures is looking only at the size of lymph nodes (excepting endoscopic ultrasonography); however, metastases can be found in small nodes as well, and conversely, large nodes may be metastasis free.

For this purpose, the Maruyama computer model was developed and first described in the English literature in 1989 [8]. It calculates the probability (%) of lymph-node metastases for the different lymph-node positions 1–16, according to the JCGC. In Japanese patients, the program was able to predict lymph node involvement in 94% [22]. In the European region the accuracy of MCP was 91% in Slovenian patients [23]. In Italian patients the accuracy was 83.4% for stations 1 to 6 and 81.6% for stations 7 to 12 [24]. The sensitivity for lymph node detection was high (97–100%) in a German study of 222 patients, but a specificity, as low as, 20% was found for perigastric lymph nodes (stations 1 to 6) [25]. Similarly in an Italian study, where the sensitivity increased to 100% with a lower cut-off level, the specificity dropped to 26%. The false positive rate was close to that of the German study, but the false negative rate was higher [24]. Better prediction of lymph node metastases may be feasible with the artificial neural network (ANN) using the following parameters: Bormann classification, depth of tumor infiltration, size, location of tumor, and lymph node metastases in station 3. The accuracy increased from 66% to 93% [26]. These studies demonstrate, that even if the sensitivity and the negative predictive value are high, the specificity and the positive predictive value of the Maruyama model may be low. Nevertheless, the results of the computerized prediction of LN metastases are superior to those of the standard pre-operative imaging techniques.

We demonstrated a similar degree of reliability of MCP to the above cited studies, with 90.2% of sensitivity, 63.3% of specificity and 78.4% of accuracy. The false negative rate was 9.8%.

Recent studies have shown that SLN mapping in gastric cancer has a high detection rate (> 95%) and a sensitivity of 90-95% [27-31]. The latest meta-analysis of SLN mapping has shown a high detection rate (93.7%) and an accuracy of 92% therefore, SLN mapping may help in avoiding unnecessarily radical dissections [12]. Based on the results of the largest prospective multicenter trial from Japan [32], a phase III multi-center trial for individualized surgery for early gastric cancer based on SLN mapping has been started in Japan and in South Korea.

Various mapping techniques have been described in the literature. The injection method and selection of tracers for SLN mapping remain controversial. Some authors use dye alone [30, 33, 34], others apply 99m Tc tin colloid imaging [27], while others use these two techniques in a parallel fashion [35]. Yaguchi et al. and Lee et al. have compared the subserosal with the submucosal labeling method without any significant differences [36, 37]. We have had an excellent outcome of SLN mapping with blue dye only method in breast cancer [38]. So, we tried to adopt this method for SNB in gastric cancer. This chapter represents our experience using the blue dye only (submucosal versus subserosal) SNB method for patients with gastric cancer from the Central-Eastern European region. Although it is difficult to draw definitive conclusions due to the small size of the series; however, we have detected SLNs in 98.3% of patients with gastric cancer with a 96.6% sensitivity, and a 100% specificity using the blue dye alone technique. The false negative rate was 3.4%. Although, in our series this means only one patient, (stage T3, perineural and lymphovascular invasion) mandates the necessity of a more extended lymph node removal in advanced cases even if labeling is negative. The two cases of positive SLNs in the D2 compartment only are calling attention to the possibility of skip metastases. Using this marking method we can avoid an inadequate surgical procedure applying a limited lymph node dissection. The sensitivity of SNB was 100 % in the cohort of patients with T1 and T2 tumors in our study.

We investigated only the negative sentinel lymph nodes for micrometastasis, because of the widely recognized concept that lymphatic micrometastasis spread first to sentinel nodes in gastric cancer [39]. The equivalence between the submucosal marking and the subserosal injection was proven in this chapter. Identification of sentinel lymph nodes in obese patients can be difficult with subserosal injection due to the feathering of blue dye in the fatty tissues. It has been shown that BMI affects the sentinel lymph node detection rate [40]. In our investigation, the single non marking patient's BMI was higher than average (26.8 versus 22.8). In cases of non-palpable tumors, we preferred the endoscopically injection.

In conclusion, sentinel lymph node mapping with blue dye only seemed to be a safe and feasible procedure in our hands for non-obese patients during open surgical procedure. Validation of this single agent method and the subserosal injection of the tracer requires further evaluation.

We are planning a reduced lymphadenectomy in SLN negative patients with early gastric cancer (T1) in the near future, according to the results of the international phase III trials of sentinel lymph node biopsy tailored surgery.

A single comparative study (SNB versus MCP) from Germany has proven SNB to be of higher clinical relevance than the MCP for predicting nodal status and compartmental involvement [31]. We have confirmed that the sensitivity, specificity, negative predictive value, positive predictive value and accuracy were higher with SNB, than with MCP.

It is generally accepted, that metastases in the SLNs warrant a D2 lymphadenectomy. We analyzed the relevance of MCP in sentinel node positive patients. The accuracy of MCP in sentinel node positive patients was higher by 10% in the group of our fifty-eight patients. The positive predictive value of MCP and SNB was proven equivalent in the sentinel node positive group. Unfortunately, the accuracy of MCP was low in prediction of lymph node involvement in station 7 to 12 in this cohort of patients. So, it would be interesting in the future to find the appropriate combined technique the sentinel node status and the results of MCP, determining the adequate extension of lymphadenectomy.

In summary, this chapter showed a lower clinical impact of the Maruyama computer program compared to SNB; however we suggest to use these two methods in a parallel fashion in operating room. It could be useful in preoperative and intraoperative decision making for appropriate extent of lymphadenectomy and individualized stage-adapted surgery in gastric cancer.

Chapter was reviewed by Sebastianus Kwon MBBS FRACS

Northern Oesophago-Gastric Cancer Unit, Royal Victoria Infirmary, Newcastle Upon Tyne, UK

References

[1] Siewert, J. R.; Bottcher, K.; Stein, H. J.; Roder, J. D. Relevant prognostic factors in gastric cancer: ten-year results of the German Gastric Cancer Study. *Ann. Surg.*, 1998;228,449–461.

[2] Kim, J. P.; Kim, Y. W.; Yang, H. K.; Noh, D. Y. Significant prognostic factors by multivariate analysis of 3926 gastric cancer patients. *World J. Surg.*, 1994;18,872–877.

[3] Kooby, D. A.; Suriawinata, A.; Klimstra, D. S.; Brennan M. F.; Karpeh, M. S. Biologic Predictors of Survival in Node-Negative Gastric Cancer. *Ann. Surg.*, 2003;237,828–837.

[4] Bonenkamp, J. J.; Songun, I.; Hermans, J.; Sasako, M.; Welvaart, K.; Plukker, J. T. Randomised comparison of morbidity after D1 and D2 dissection for gastric cancer in 996 Dutch patients. *Lancet,* 1995;345,745–748.

[5] Cuschieri, A.; Weeden, S.; Fielding, J.; Bancewicz, J.; Craven, J.; Joypaul, V. Patient survival after D1 and D2 resections for gastric cancer: long-term results of the MRC randomized surgical trial. Surgical Co-operative Group. *Br. J. Cancer*, 1999;79,1522–1530.

[6] Dent, D. M.; Madden, M. V.; Price, S. K. Randomized comparison of R1 and R2 gastrectomy for gastric carcinoma. *Br. J. Surg.,* 1988;75,110–112.

[7] Songun, I.; Putter, H.; Kranenbarg, E. M.; Sasako, M.; van de Velde, C. J. Surgical treatment *Lancet Oncol.*, 2010;11, 439-49.

[8] Kampschöer, G. H.; Maruyama, K.; van de Velde, C. J.; Sasako, M.; Kinoshita, T.; Okabayashi, K. Computer analysis in making preoperative decisions: a rational approach to lymph node dissection in gastric cancer patients. *Br. J. Surg.,* 1989;76,905-8.

[9] Siewert, Jr.; Kelsen, D.; Maruyama, K.; Feussner, H.; Omote, K.; Etter, M.; Hoos, A. Gastric cancer diagnosis and treatment. An interactive training program. Windows Version. CD-ROM. Berlin Heidelberg. Springer-Verlag 2000.

[10] Nieweg, O. E.; Bartelink, H. Implications of lymphatic mapping for staging and adjuvant treatment of patients with breast cancer. *Eur. J. Cancer*, 2004;40,179-181.

[11] Kretschmer, L.; Hilgers, R.; Mohrle, M.; Balda, B. R.; Breuninger, H.; Konz, B. Patients with lymphatic metastasis of cutaneous malignant melanoma benefit from sentinel lymphonodectomy and early excision of their nodal disease. *Eur. J. Cancer*, 2004;40,212-218.

[12] Wang, Z.; Dong, Z. Y.; Chen, J. Q.; Liu, J. L. Diagnostic Value of Sentinel Lymph Node Biopsy in Gastric Cancer: A Meta-Analysis. *Ann. Surg. Oncol.*, 2012;19,1541-50.

[13] Hohenberger, P.; Gretschel, S. Gastric cancer. *Lancet,* 2003;362, 305–315.

[14] La Vecchia, C. L.; Negri, E.; Franceschi, S.; Gentile, A. Family history and the risk of stomach and colorectal cancer. *Cancer,* 1992;70,50–55.

[15] Lauren, P. The two histological main types of gastric carcinoma: diffuse and so-called intestinal-type carcinoma. An attempt at histo-clinical classification. *Acta. Pathol. Microbiol. Scand.*, 1965;64,31–39.

[16] Tóth, D.; Kincses, Zs.; Plósz, J.; Török, M.; Kovács, I.; Kiss, Cs.; Damjanovich, L. Value of sentinel lymph node mapping using a blue dye-only method in gastric cancer: a single-center experience from North-East Hungary. *Gastric. Cancer*, 2011;14,360-364.

[17] Tóth, D.; Török, M.; Kincses, Zs.; Damjanovich, L. Prospective, comparative study for the evaluation of lymph node involvement in gastric cancer. Maruyama computer program versus sentinel lymph node biopsy. *Gastric Cancer*, 2013;16,201-7.

[18] Japanese Gastric Cancer Association Japanese Classification of Gastric Carcinoma -2nd English Edition-. *Gastric Cancer*, 1998;1,10-24.

[19] Swets, J. A. Measuring the accuracy of diagnostic systems. *Science,* 1988;240,1285–93.

[20] Chamadol, N.; Wongwiwatchai, J.; Bhudhisawasd, V.; Pairojkul, C. Accuracy of spiral CT in preoperative staging of gastric carcinoma: correlation with surgical and pathological findings. *J. Med. Assoc. Thai.*, 2008;3,356-363.

[21] Xi, W. D.; Zhao, C.; Ren, G. S. Endoscopic ultrasonography in preoperative staging of gastric cancer: determination of tumor invasion depth, nodal involvement and surgical resectability. *World J. Gastroenterol.*, 2003;9,254-257.

[22] Maruyama, K.; Gunven, P.; Okabayashi, K. Lymph node metastases of gastric cancer. General pattern in 1931 patients. *Ann. Surg.*, 1989;210,596–902.

[23] Omejc, M.; Mekicar, J. Role of computer *World J. Surg.*, 2004;28,59-62.

[24] Guadagni, S.; de Manzoni, G.; Catarci, M.; Valenti, M.; Amicucci, G.; De Bernardinis, G.; Cordiano, C.; Carboni, M.; Maruyama, K. Evaluation of the Maruyama computer *World J. Surg.*, 2000;24,1550-8.

[25] Bollschweiler, E.; Boettcher, K.; Hoelscher, A. H.; Sasako, M.; Kinoshita, T.; Maruyama, K.; Siewert, J. R. Preoperative assessment *Br. J. Surg.*, 1992;79,156-60.

[26] Bollschweiler, E. H.; Mönig, S. P.; Hensler, K.; Baldus, S. E.; Maruyama, K.; Hölscher, A. H. Artificial neural network *Ann. Surg. Oncol.*, 2004;11,506-11.

[27] Kitagawa, Y.; Fujii, H.; Mukai, M.; Kubota, T.; Otani, Y.; Kitajima, M. Radio-guided sentinel node detection for gastric cancer. *Br. J. Surg.*, 2002;89,604–608.

[28] Ichikura, T.; Morita, D.; Uchida, T.; Okura, E.; Majima, T.; Ogawa, T. Sentinel node concept in gastric carcinoma. *World J. Surg.*, 2002;26,318–322.

[29] Hiratsuka, M.; Miyashiro, I.; Ishikawa, O.; Furukawa, H.; Motomura, K.; Ohigashi, H. Application of sentinel node biopsy to gastric cancer surgery. *Surgery,* 2001;129,335–340.

[30] Rino, Y.; Takanashi, Y.; Hasuo, K.; Kawamoto, M.; Ashida, A.; Harada, H. The validity of sentinel lymph node biopsy using dye technique alone in patients with gastric cancer. *Hepatogastroenterology,* 2007;54,1882-1886.

[31] Gretschel, S.; Bembenek, A.; Ulmer, Ch.; Hünerbein, M.; Markwardt, J.; Schneider, U. Prediction of gastric cancer lymph node status by sentinel lymph node biopsy and the Maruyama computer model. *Eur. J. Surg. Oncol.,* 2005;31,393-400.

[32] Kitagawa, Y.; Takeuchi, H.; Takagi, Y.; Natsugoe, S.; Terashima, M.; Murakami, N.; Fujimura, T.; Tsujimoto, H.; Hayashi, H.; Yoshimizu, N.; Takagane, A.; Mohri, Y.; Nabeshima, K.; Uenosono, Y.; Kinami, S.;Sakamoto, J.; Morita, S.; Aikou, T.; Miwa, K.; Kitajima, M. Sentinel node mapping for gastric cancer: a prospective multicenter trial in Japan. *J. Clin. Oncol.,* 2013;31,3704-10.

[33] Rabin, I.; Chikman, B.; Halpern, Z.; Wassermann, I.; Lavy, R.; Gold-Deutch, R. Sentinel node mapping for gastric cancer. *IMAJ,* 2006;8, 40-43.

[34] Tajima, Y.; Yamazaki, K.; Masuda, Y.; Kato, M.; Yasuda, D.; Aoki, T. Sentinel node mapping guided by indocyanine green fluorescence imaging in gastric cancer. *Ann. Surg.,* 2009;249,58-62.

[35] Aikou, T.; Higashi, H.; Natsugoe, S.; Hokita, S.; Baba, M.; Takao, S. Can sentinel node navigation surgery reduce the extent of lymph node dissection in gastric cancer? *Ann. Surg. Oncol.,* 2001;9,90-93.

[36] Yaguchi, Y.; Ichikura, T.; Ono, S.; Tsujimoto, H.; Sugasawa, H.; Sakamoto, N. How should tracers be injected to detect for sentinel nodes in gastric cancer – submucosally from inside or subserosally from outside of the stomach? *J. Exp. Clin. Cancer Res.,* 2008;27,79.

[37] Lee, J. H.; Ryu, K. W.; Kim, C. G.; Kim, S. K.; Choi, I. J.; Kim, Y. W. Comparative study of the subserosal versus submucosal dye injection method for sentinel node biopsy in gastric cancer. *Eur. J. Surg. Oncol.,* 2005;31,965-8.

[38] Tóth, D.; Kathy, S.; Bokor, L.; Kincses, Zs.; Sebő, É.; Kovács, I. Treatment of non-palpable breast cancer and the single-agent sentinel lymph node biopsy. Paper presented at the 59th Congress of Hungarian Surgical Society, Debrecen, 2008.

[39] Ishii, K.; Kinami, S.; Funaki, K.; Fujita, H.; Ninomiya, I.; Fushida, S. Detection of sentinel and non-sentinel lymph node micrometastases by complete serial sectioning and immunohistochemical analysis for gastric cancer. *J. Exp. Clin. Cancer Res.,* 2008;27,7.

[40] Nakahara, T.; Kitagawa, Y.; Yakeuchi, H.; Fujii, H.; Suzuki, T.; Mukai, M. Preoperative lymphoscintigraphy for detection of sentinel lymph node in patients with gastric cancer—initial experience. *Ann. Surg. Oncol.,* 2008;15,1447-53.

In: Gastric Cancer
Editor: Jasneet Singh Bhullar

ISBN: 978-1-63117-983-9
© 2014 Nova Science Publishers, Inc.

Chapter 8

Clinical and Surgical Management of Gastric Cancer: Principles of Treatment

Stefano Rausei, M.D., Ph.D., Sebastiano Spampatti, M.D., Federica Galli, M.D., Laura Ruspi, M.D., Francesca Rovera, M.D., Luigi Boni, M.D., FACS and Gianlorenzo Dionigi, M.D., FACS
Department of Surgery, University of Insubria, Varese, Italy

Abstract

Nowadays gastric cancer is less common, but still remains a global phenomenon representing the second leading cause of cancer-related deaths worldwide, with 5-year survival rates of 20-25%.

This chapter aims to discuss open issues in the surgical management of gastric malignancies in order to define the current principles of gastric cancer therapy.

The validity and usefulness of the 7th edition of the AJCC/UICC tumor node metastases classification in the context of clinical management of gastric cancer are discussed.

Despite considerable improvements in the management of gastric cancer over the past decades, surgery remains the mainstay of treatment, provided that the patient is medically fit. Aim of curative surgery is the complete primary tumor excision with a wide surgical dissection field that allows to obtain a safe "circumferential" margin and a lymphnode dissection larger than positive stations. In fact, long-term benefit of systematic D2 lymphadenectomy has now been shown in randomized trials. Further extension of lymphadenectomy, including para-aortic nodal dissection, should be restricted to selected high risk patients.

Additionally, a hot topic in gastric cancer treatment debate is represented by the role of laparoscopy. The laparoscopic approach is strongly recommended for staging, whereas the use of minimally invasive surgery for resection and lymphadenectomy is still to be demonstrated. In locally advanced gastric cancer (as commonly diagnosed gastric cancer in Western countries) the multimodal treatment, in comparison to surgery alone, can improve survival with a better local and regional tumor control and with a reduction of systemic metastases rate.

Multimodal treatment strategies, including perioperative chemotherapy and/or radiotherapy options, are analyzed in order to clarify their indications and results.

Standardization of staging system, with accurate identification of prognostic factors, and multimodal approach are needed to achieve tailored therapeutic approaches, improving survival results in gastric cancer patients.

Overview on Risk Factors, Staging and Priciples of Treatment

Epidemiology

Worldwide gastric cancer represents the 2nd leading cause of cancer-related death [1]. Despite incidence and mortality are decreasing, gastric cancer remains the 5th most common malignancy diagnosed in developed countries in both men and women, with more than 270,000 new diagnoses in 2011. More than 180,000 gastric cancer deaths were reported for the same year [2].

Throughout the world the incidence of gastric cancer varies tremendously: the highest incidence is reported in South Korea (66.5–72.5 per 100,000 males and 19.5–30.4 per 100,000 females) [3]. Other high incidence countries for gastric cancer are located in China and Japan and, less diffusely, in Eastern Europe and in the Andean regions of South America.

In contrast in Western countries gastric cancer is decreasing: in 2010 in the USA the estimated number of new gastric cancer cases was 21,000 with 10,570 deaths [2]. This declining incidence of gastric cancer is due to a decrease in tumors of the stomach body and antrum, whereas the incidence of proximal and esophagogastric junction tumors is slowly increasing since the 1980s [4]. Consistently there is also a corresponding increase in the number of adenocarcinomas of the distal esophagus. Natural history, response to treatment and prognosis of cancer of gastric proximal third, esophagogastric junction, and distal third of the esophagus are very similar, suggesting a common pathogenesis. The possible causes include infectious pathogens (Helicobacter Pylori), Barrett metaplasia and obesity [5].

Generally in gastric cancer patients the age of presentation is between 60 and 70 years and males are affected twice as frequently as females. About 95% of gastric cancer cases have an histology of adenocarcinoma. Risk factors for gastric adenocarcinoma include Helicobacter pylori infection, prior gastric surgery, chronic atrophic gastritis, intestinal metaplasia, pernicious anemia and high consumption of salty or smoked foods [6]. Moreover there are some known cancer syndromes that increase the risk of develop gastric cancer: hereditary diffuse gastric cancer (HDGC), hereditary nonpolyposis colon cancer (HNPCC), Li–Fraumeni syndrome and Peutz–Jeghers syndrome [7].

Clinical and Pathological Features

Gastric adenocarcinoma arises from the gastric mucosa in the epithelial cell layer and grows deeper into the wall of the stomach. Gastric cancer cells spread via lymphatics to regional lymphnodes and hematogenously to distant sites; the liver is the most frequent organ interested by metastases [6]. If for mucosal tumors lymphnodal metastases are rare, for tumors invading the submucosa this possibility is in about 20% of patients, while for tumors invading the muscularis propria the lymphnode metastases rate increases to over 50% [8] (Figure 1). Tumors that penetrate the subserosa or serosa of the stomach have a high incidence of positive nodes and furthermore can progress to invade adjacent organs (such as the pancreas, spleen, and colon) or disseminate through the peritoneal cavity causing the so called peritoneal carcinomatosis. Gastric adenocarcinoma in early stages presents only few symptoms and more frequently only in later stages causes weight loss, epigastric pain, gastrointestinal bleeding, vomiting, and/or anorexia [6]. In East Asia, especially in Japan and South Korea, common endoscopic screening, justified from the high rates of incidence, has led to obtain early diagnosis in a lot of patients: 50% of cases are now presenting with early gastric cancer (mucosal tumors) [9, 10].

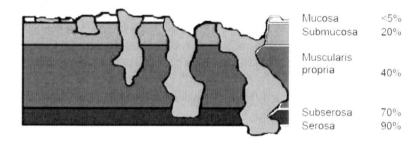

Figure 1. Probability of lymphnode metastases according to tumor depth invasion [8].

Unfortunately, in most other countries, including Europe and the USA, gastric cancer is found most frequently in advanced stages: in these countries only 10-15% of gastric cancer are diagnosed in early stages and more than 50% have already metastasized to regional nodes [11]. Despite many modern advances in diagnosis, surgical techniques, chemo- and radiation therapy, gastric cancer remains a highly fatal disease (even more for Western countries). The 5-year relative survival for gastric cancer (all stages) is 20% to 25% with a median survival of about 24 months [12, 13].

Introduction to Treatment

In gastric cancer setting the main factors determining the treatment plan (with multimodal possibility) and consequently the extent of resection and lymphadenectomy are tumor stage, tumor site and growth patterns [14, 15], details hopefully detectable by pretreatment staging. Pretherapeutic staging includes endoscopy with biopsy, CT scan of the thorax, abdomen and pelvis [16, 17], while the clinical value of endoscopic ultrasound is still to be confirmed. Fluorodeoxyglucose positron emission tomography scan (FDG-PET) is not recommended for gastric cancer because more than 50% of the diffuse type gastric cancer is not avid for FDG [18-20]. In locally advanced gastric cancers, about 20% occult peritoneal carcinomatosis can be detected by laparoscopy [21], therefore for patients undergoing neoadjuvant chemotherapy, pretreatment laparoscopy helps for risk stratification; finally a staging laparoscopy may add important information to conventional staging even in early stages [22].

It has been demonstrated how surgical treatment's radicality and the level of lymphnode involvement independently influence survival rates [11]. Hence, provided that the patient is medically fit, as detailed below, surgery alone or surgery included in a multimodal treatment plan, remains the mainstay of treatment in gastric cancer.

Gastric Cancer Staging

TNM: A Critical View

From January 1st 2010, according to the WHO, newly diagnosed gastric cancers are staged using the 7th edition of the AJCC/UICC TNM staging system [23]. Staging of gastric cancer considers depth of invasion (T stage), number of lymphnode metastases (N stage), and presence of distant disease (M stage). The T and N categories of gastric cancers have been further modified in order to likely ensure a better correlation to the prognostic outcome. Major changes are the subclassifications of the T categories (Table 1).

T1 changed to T1a and T1b to delineate mucosal versus submucosal lesions;
T2a and T2b changed to T2 and T3 to represent muscularis propria and subserosa invasion, respectively;
T3 and T4 changed to T4a and T4b to represent serosal perforation and invasion of adjacent structures, respectively.

The new N categorization now considers the number of lymphnodes involved within four categories, instead of three (Table 1); moreover, for the classification of pN status, the number of lymphnodes to remove has been adjusted to 16. Patients with a positive peritoneal cytological lavage are now included in the M+ category.

Whether the new classification provides a more detailed stratification for both local tumor invasion (T) and lymphnode involvement (N), compared with the previous editions, is not well demonstrated. Many studies confirmed the validity of the new classification system in its prognostic efficacy compared to the previous edition, even if the changes included in the last edition seem to respond to statistical considerations more than to clinical practice suggestions [24-30]. For example, a study from Korea with a large series of patients proved a more detailed prognostic assessment for the new TNM system, especially between T2 and T3 and N1 and N2 tumors, although authors concluded that further studies are needed for the N3a and N3b classification [24].

**Table 1. Sixth and seventh editions of the AJCC staging system
for gastric adenocarcinoma**

Sixth edition AJCC staging system		Seventh edition AJCC staging system	
Tis	Carcinoma in situ	Tis	Carcinoma in situ
T1	Invades lamina propria or submucosa	T1	Invades lamina propria (T1a) or submucosa (T1b)

Sixth edition AJCC staging system		Seventh edition AJCC staging system	
T2	Invades muscularis propria or subserosa	T2[a]	Invades muscularis propria[a]
T3	Invades serosa	T3[a]	Invades subserosa[a]
T4	Invades adjacent organs	T4a[a]	Invades serosa[a]
		T4b[a]	Invades adjacent organs[a]
TX	Primary tumor cannot be assessed	TX	Primary tumor cannot be assessed
N0	No lymph node metastasis	N0	No lymph node metastasis
N1	Metastasis in 1-6 regional lymph nodes	N1[a]	Metastasis in 1-2 regional lymph nodes[a]
N2	Metastasis in 7-15 regional lymph nodes	N2[a]	Metastasis in 3-6 regional lymph nodes[a]
N3	Metastasis in more than 15 regional lymph nodes	N3a[a]	Metastasis in 7-15 regional lymph nodes[a]
		N3b[a]	Metastasis in more than 15 regional lymph nodes[a]
NX	Regional lymph node(s) cannot be assessed	NX	Regional lymph node(s) cannot be assessed
M0	No distant metastasis	M0	No distant metastasis
M1	Distant metastasis	M1	Distant metastasis
Stage 0	Tis, N0	Stage 0	Tis, N0
Stage IA	T1, N0	Stage IA	T1, N0
Stage IB	T1, N1; T2, N0	Stage IB	T1, N1; T2, N0
Stage II	T1, N2; T2, N1; T3, N0	Stage IIA	T1, N2; T2, N1; T3, N0
		Stage IIB	T1, N3; T2, N2; T3, N1; T4a, N0
Stage IIIA	T2, N2; T3, N1; T4, N0	Stage IIIA	T2, N3; T3, N2; T4a, N1
Stage IIIB	T3, N2	Stage IIIB	T3, N3; T4a, N2; T4b, N0-1
		Stage IIIC	T4aN3; T4b, N2-3
Stage IV	T4, N1-3; T1-3, N3; any T, any N, M1	Stage IV	Any T, any N, M1

[a] Changes in T and N definitions between sixth and seventh editions.

Regarding the description of tumors with origin in the esophagus the new classification has been simplified and includes tumors of the esophagogastric junction as well as gastric tumors extending to the proximal 5 cm of the stomach. Historically the Siewert criteria, published in 1998, have been used to classify adenocarcinomas arising at, or near to, the esophagogastric
junction [31]:

- Type I: lesion of the distal esophagus, 1–5 cm proximal to the esophagogastric junction;
- Type II: lesion arising within the esophagogastric junction, within 1 cm proximal and 2 cm distal to the esophagogastric junction;
- Type III: Lesion arising 2 cm to 5 cm distal to the esophagogastric junction with invasion into the esophagus.

In the 7th edition of the TNM staging system esophagogastric junction adenocarcinomas are reclassified (in some cases not without confusion):

- A lesion with epicenter within 5 cm of the esophagogastric junction, and with extension into the esophagus, is staged using esophageal carcinoma criteria.
- A lesion with epicenter within 5 cm of the esophagogastric junction, but without extension into the esophagus, and a lesion with epicenter greater than 5 cm away from the esophagogastric junction, are staged using gastric carcinoma criteria.

To evaluate the clinical effects of the new TNM staging system, in regard to esophagogastric junction cancers, Suh and colleagues [32] retrospectively reviewed 497 adenocarcinomas of the esophagogastric junction in patients operated with curative intent, based on Siewert classification. Analyzing the stage, 11 of 230 (4.6%) lesions that before would have been classified as TNM stage I under gastric guidelines, were upstaged to TNM stage II esophageal lesions. The 5-year survival rates of gastric TNM stage I and esophageal TNM stage II in this study were 92.1% and 90.6%, respectively. Twenty of 125 (16.0%) gastric TNM stage II cancers were upstaged to esophageal TNM stage III cancers. Five-year survival rates of gastric TNM stage II and esophageal TNM stage III were 84.6% and 51.4%, respectively. The investigators argued that the new guidelines did not adequately distinguish EGJ tumors, because upstaging did not correlate with clinical outcomes.

The lymphnode ratio (number of metastatic lymphnodes related to the total number of dissected lymphnodes) is considered with increasingly interest by many authors who are proposing it as an alternative lymphnode staging system for its important additional prognostic value in patients with gastric cancer [33]. The perspective of a "T-R (lymphnode ratio)-M" classification seems to offer a more reliable pathological staging and might obviate the open problem of minimum number of lymphnodes to be retrieved [33]. However, the extent of lymphnode retrieval during surgery largely varies among different countries and even among different centers; therefore it is still unclear whether "20 positive nodes out of 60 examined nodes" and "2 positive nodes out of 6 examined nodes" could be considered the same metastatic grade [34].

Some authors proposed different staging systems that include not only anatomical factors, like in the current TNM system, but also patient- and treatment-related variables [35]. When compared to the TNM system, these systems showed to be more accurate in defining overall survival and risk of recurrence, allowing more precise stratification between different prognostic groups, even among patients in the same TNM stage with no residual disease after surgery. In fact, recent evidences may suggest that also a revision of the definition of residual disease after surgery (R) may be necessary. Indeed, some discrepancies have been shown in survival rates between patients who underwent resection classified as curative (R0) [34,36-38].

Surgical Staging

In Western countries almost two-thirds of patients with gastric cancer present at diagnosis with advanced disease, and most of them show no significant findings on physical examination. For many years in the past, laparotomy was the standard approach for staging:

the decision between a resection with curative intent versus a non-curative procedure was taken based on macroscopic evaluation of nodal disease, adjacent organs involvement or distant metastases.

Today clinical staging is achieved before any therapeutic approach. The pretherapeutic staging aims to define not only tumor stage but also the patient's prognosis, identifying at the same time patients who may benefit from preoperative treatment [39]. In fact, although the radical tumor resection (R0) plays an important role among the independent prognostic factors in gastric cancer [40, 41], an accurate estimation of real local tumor infiltration (T) and nodal involvement (N) are also essential in order to obtain an appropriate patients selection for treatment. While patients with cT1a could be treated endoscopically and cT1b tumors (without lymphnodes metastases) by primary resection and lymphnode dissection, patients with more advanced cancers should be addressed to surgery in a multimodal treatment setting [42]. However, even the definition of locally advanced gastric cancer, requiring multimodal approach, is still to be definitely codified [43].

Surgical Treatment

Extent of Gastric Resection

Worldwide surgeons are still widening the surgical dissection field in order to obtain a safe "circumferential" resection margin and a lymphnode dissection larger than metastatic lymphnode stations [34, 44].

The type and the extent of resection is mainly based on the localization of the tumor (Table 2), provided that the stomach is divided into two "surgical" parts: the proximal one (a cumulative category for fundus and esophagogastric junction) and the middle-distal one.

Distal Disease

After the well known publication of the Bozzetti trial [45], other retrospective studies [46, 47] confirmed the oncologic adequacy of subtotal gastrectomy for distal tumors. The aim of achieving adequate gastric resection, through 5-cm negative margins, contributed to the worldwide spread of the concept of limited gastrectomy, regardless of the histological type of tumor.

Table 2. Recommendations for the extent of resection depending on tumor location and clinical staging. From Rausei S et al. [34]

Location	Clinical staging	Extent of gastrectomy
Proximal third	cT1cN0	Proximal gastrectomy[a]
(cardia/fundus)	> cT1cN0	Total gastrectomy
Mediun third (body)	cT1cN0	Pylorus preserving gastrectomy[b]
	>cT1cN0	Distal gastrectomy[a]
Distal third (antrum)	Any cT, any cN	Distal gastrectomy

[a] Only if a 5-cm free resection margin can be achieved.
[b] Only if the distal tumor border is at least 4 cm proximal to the pylorus.

From 1982 to 1993 Bozzetti and colleagues [45] conducted a large randomized controlled trial to compare results after subtotal gastrectomy with those obtained after total gastrectomy. Six-hundred-twenty-four patients were included, 320 in the subtotal gastrectomy group and 306 in the total gastrectomy group. All patients underwent D2 dissection, splenectomy was optional, and 6-cm margins were obtained when possible. Although perioperative mortality was similar between the two groups (1.3% vs 2.3%, p= 0.27), morbidity was greater in the total gastrectomy group (15.5% vs 10.3%, p= 0.05). Mean length of stay was improved in the subtotal gastrectomy group (13.8 days vs 15.4 days, p < 0.001). Five-year survival rates between subtotal gastrectomy and total gastrectomy were similar (65.3% vs 62.4%).

One of the main issues in favor of subtotal gastrectomy, over total gastrectomy, is the influence of gastrectomies on quality of life. Karanicolas [48] prospectively analyzed 134 patients undergoing gastrectomy (82 distal-, 16 proximal-, and 36 total-gastrectomy); participants completed the European Organization for Research and Treatment of Cancer cancer (QLQ-C30) and gastric (QLQ-STO22) questionnaires preoperatively and at 5 postoperative intervals up to 18 months. In the immediate postoperative period, 55% of patients suffered from significant impairment in their global quality of life, particularly after proximal gastrectomy and (less frequently) total gastrectomy. Davies and colleagues [49] evaluated 47 consecutive patients who underwent potential R0 resection for gastric cancer. Total gastrectomy was performed for lesions of the proximal and middle thirds of the stomach (n = 26), and subtotal gastrectomy was performed for those of the distal third (n = 21). D2 lymphadenectomy was performed in all patients, whereas spleen and pancreas were preserved whenever possible. Quality of life was assessed preoperatively and at 1, 3, 6, and 12 months postoperatively, using 5 validated questionnaires: authors revealed better quality of life in the subtotal gastrectomy group, when compared to the total gastrectomy group. The over mentioned data show that the comparison between subtotal gastrectomy and total gastrectomy for distal gastric cancer generally resulted in higher perioperative morbidity and mortality in patients undergoing total gastrectomy, and quality of life is improved for patients undergoing subtotal-gastrectomy. For these reasons, provided that adequate proximal margins of 5 cm to 6 cm are obtained, for distal gastric cancer the procedure of choice is subtotal-gastrectomy.

Analyzing the optimal reconstruction after distal or subtotal gastrectomy there are only few good studies. Western surgeons usually perform a Roux-en-Y or Billroth II reconstruction, while in East Asia generally a Billroth I reconstruction is preferred. It has been observed that Roux-en-Y reconstruction results in less bile reflux into the residual stomach, but can also often cause a Roux stasis syndrome. Ishikawa randomized 50 patients, who underwent distal gastrectomy for cancer, to Billroth I or to Roux-en-Y reconstruction [50]. Gastrojejunal stasis in the early postoperative period, causing a longer mean hospital stay, was observed in 5 of 24 patients in the Roux group, however patients of the Billroth I group had a higher incidence of bile reflux gastritis at 6 months after surgery (62% vs. 30%). Another randomized study compared Billroth I or II reconstructions to Roux-en-Y reconstruction: patients with Roux-en-Y reconstructions had less gastroesophageal reflux and faster and more complete gastric emptying; however no improvement in gastrointestinal quality of life was observed [51].

In a metanalysis by Zong and Chen [52], 15 studies where included comparing Billroth I vs. Billroth II vs. Roux-en-Y reconstructions following distal gastrectomy. The results show that Roux-en-Y reconstruction significantly reduces the reflux symptoms and the rates of postoperative gastritis/esophagitis. Quality of life was significantly improved in patients with Roux-en-Y, compared with patients with Billroth I or Billroth II.

Proximal Disease

There are few high quality studies examining the best surgical resective approach (proximal gastrectomy versus total gastrectomy) for cancers of the proximal third of the stomach. Despite the promising results of some small eastern prospective studies [53,54], several retrospective analyses [55-57] demonstrated a high frequency of complications (anastomotic stenosis and reflux esophagitis) and cancer recurrences after proximal gastrectomy. This results significantly affected the diffusion of this procedure.

A nonrandomized norwegian study, with 763 patients enrolled [58], obtained higher complication and mortality rates for patients who underwent proximal gastrectomy (52% and 16%), compared to those submitted to total gastrectomy (38% and 8%). Also An et al. observed that perioperative complications were markedly higher in a proximal gastrectomy group in comparison to a total gastrectomy group (61.8% vs. 12.6%). Main differences were found regarding anastomotic stenosis rate (6.9% vs. 1.8%) and reflux esophagitis (38.2% vs. 29.2%) [59].

Additionally, proximal gastrectomy is not justified from any quality of life result in comparison with total gastrectomy [48]. Hence, although some groups advocate proximal gastrectomies for proximal gastric cancers [60,61], considering the higher perioperative morbidity, as well as the more challenging D2 dissection, proximal gastrectomy could not be recommended as the gold standard.

Surgical reconstruction after total gastrectomy is generally performed worldwide with a Roux-en-Y esophagojejunostomy.

Esophagogastric Junction Tumors

The management of patients with esophagogastric junction tumors continues to be a matter of debate. Despite their rising incidence, there are still marked discrepancies in the classification of such tumors (as above detailed) and in the selection of appropriate surgical approach. According to the tumor origin, localization and stage, some open problems for the surgeons are addressed with particular attention to the extent and type of resection. The classification of esophagogastric junction tumors according to Siewert (approximately, type I: esophagus; type II: cardia; type III: subcardia) is helpful for a correct selection of the surgical strategy. While type I tumors need to be treated by a transthoracic en bloc esophagectomy, including a two-field lymphadenectomy, type II and III tumors can be treated by an extended total gastrectomy, with a transhiatal resection of the distal esophagus.

The National Cancer Center (NCC) group in Tokyo randomized 167 patients with gastroesophageal junction cancers submitted to total extended gastrectomy and D2 lymphadenectomy, via a laparotomy with transhyatal esophageal access, or via a left thoraco-abdominal incision. The results were in favor of the abdominal transhyatal approach with 5-year survival rate of 52% versus 38%, perioperative complication rate of 34% versus 49% (p=0.06), and mortality of 0% versus 4% [62].

Conversely, a retrospective analysis on 505 patients with gastroesophageal junction cancer from the Sloan Kettering Cancer Center of New York shows that in patients with gastroesophageal junction cancer primarily resected, a safety margin of at least 5 cm in situ and a dissection of at least 15 lymphnodes are necessary to improve prognosis [41,63]. Based on these data, an abdomino-thoracic approach (Ivor Lewis procedure) should be discussed for Seewert II and III esophagogastric junction cancer, in order to guarantee adequate safety margin and more radical lymphnode dissection [64].

In a recent review Uzunoglu [65] concluded that in type III esophagogastric junction carcinomas, the transhiatal extended gastrectomy is the standard of care, and the minimally invasive approach should be performed only in specialized centers. However, up to now no relevant randomized clinical trial was conducted comparing the transhiatal extended gastrectomy with the right abdominothoracic approach.

Resection of Adjacent Organs

Although direct tumor involvement of the spleen or distal pancreas needs resection to achieve potential R0 resection, routine splenectomy and distal pancreatectomy, as part of a standard D2 dissection, adds early morbidity without a proven long-term survival benefit. Particularly the postoperative morbidity is represented by infection and pancreatic fistula [66-68]. Good evidence has discouraged prophylactic splenectomy in cardia tumors [69-71]. Against routine splenectomy one of the most significant studies was published by Yu and colleagues [71]. Between 1995 and 1999 two-hundred-seven patients, submitted to total gastrectomy for proximal gastric adenocarcinoma, were randomized to undergo either splenic resection or preservation. The resection and preservation groups had similar perioperative morbidity (15.4% vs 8.7%) and mortality (1.9% vs 1.0%), median hospital stay (11 days in each group), median number of harvested lymphnodes (40 in each group), and 5-year overall survival (54.8% vs 48.8%, p=0.503). The authors concluded that, without any survival benefit nor improved lymphnodes count, routine splenectomy should not be recommended.

Differently, retrospective analyses by many authors recommend the aggressive combined resection of adjacent organs for patients with T4b carcinoma [72,73], even if in the presence of a supposed T4b cancer a curative resection is not always achievable. Multiorgan resection interests spleen, pancreas, colon and left liver [66-68,72]. Histopathological examination reveals that multi-organ resections are often performed for pT4a tumors, because only a relatively small proportion of tumors really invades adjacent organs [74]. Carboni and colleagues [75] performed a retrospective review analyzing data from 65 patients with T4b gastric adenocarcinoma undergoing surgery. In this series extended resections included spleen (n=31), pancreas (n= 28), colon (n=16), and other (n= 24): desmoplastic reaction instead of tumor invasion was confirmed in 13 (20%) patients.

Martin and colleagues [72] demonstrated that, with an appropriate identification of T4a or T4b tumors, additional organ resection is recommended, due to its potential benefit and low additional morbidity and mortality.

Several subsequent series have supported the role of extended organ resection for patients who have potentially curable disease [67,68,75,76]. Particularly, in a recent study from Italy, Pacelli et al. indicates that after extended combined resections patients have acceptable postoperative morbidity and mortality rates, but multivisceral resections could be effective only when complete resection is achievable (R0) and when nodal involvement is not evident (N0) [76].

Extent of Lymphadenectomy

Generally, in the surgical oncology the lymphadenectomy has three main purposes: staging of disease, prevention of loco-regional recurrence, and improvement in overall survival. More extensive lymphadenectomies for gastric cancer can lead to better staging of disease. The 7th edition of the AJCC/UICC TNM staging system for gastric adenocarcinoma recommends that at least 16 lymphnodes should be examined to obtain a correct assessment of the N category [23]. However, an analysis of the Surveillance, Epidemiology, and End Results (SEER) database found that only 29% of 10,807 resected gastric cancer patients had 15 or more lymphnodes examined [77]. According to this data many patients should be considered understaged, due to inadequate lymphnodes retrieval. When fewer than 10 lymphnodes are examined, it is difficult to be confident that a gastric cancer is truly node negative [78,79]; similarly N1 patients can be upstaged to N2 or even to N3 if more lymphnodes are harvested [79,80] and it is impossible to categorize a patient as N3b if less than 16 lymphnodes are harvested.

Moreover, an adequate lymphadenectomy is very important in gastric cancer treatment because, although the pT grade is directly associated with the probability of lymphnode metastases, already in early pT categories the risk of nodal involvement is high (Figure 1).

Lymphnode stations surrounding the stomach have been classified by the Japanese Research Society for Gastric Cancer (JRSGC) [81]. According to the old JRSGC classification there were four levels of lymphnode stations: from N1 to N4. The designation of N1–N4 nodes varied in correlation to the site of the primary tumor (upper, middle, or lower third of the stomach). The D level represented the extent of lymphadenectomy and was based on the JRSGC definitions of lymphnode station level [82]. A D1 lymphadenectomy was defined as removal of all N1 level nodes, while a D2 dissection as removal of all N1 and N2 level nodes. It is well known how the localization of the primary tumor influences the lymphatic spread; therefore the Japanese Gastric Cancer Association used to recommend the removal of specific lymphnode stations, based on the location of the primary tumor, in order to obtain a D1 or a D2 lymphadenectomy [83]. Given the low reproducibility of this complex approach to nodal dissection (in fact in Western countries the respect of Japanese rules has been often dissatisfied), and in order to compare worldwide surgical results, today the new Japanese Guidelines simplified the lymphnode dissection technique, depending on different types of gastric resection [84] (Figure 2).

In the last decades the extent of lymphadenectomy has been controversially discussed in the management of gastric cancer. The D2 lymphadenectomy is standard in Japan and in Western centers [85], despite first negative data from two European randomized trials comparing D1 versus D2 lymphadenectomy [86,87]. These randomized controlled trials revealed no survival benefit for D2 nodal dissection with spleno-pancreatectomy and confirmed an increase in morbidity related to this procedure. However, a reanalysis of the Dutch study data, after a long-term follow-up, revealed an improved survival trend for selected patients who had D2 dissection [88]. This finding was later confirmed in other two studies showing that D2 gastrectomy without routine spleno-pancreatectomy could improve survival for gastric cancer patients, without any significant increase in morbidity or mortality, compared to D1 gastrectomy [89,90].

The last randomized controlled trial concerning the efficacy of D2 lymphadenectomy without spleno-pancreasectomy, confirmed that compared with D1 nodal dissection, D2 dissection offers a survival benefit, if performed by well-trained, experienced surgeons [91]. This conclusion was derived from the knowledge that an extended nodal dissection could be associated with a potential increase of morbidity rates.

To assess whether an even more extensive lymphnode dissection than D2 could provide any survival benefit, a large Japanese prospective randomized study was conducted on 523 patients, comparing a D2 lymphadenectomy to a D2 lymphadenectomy with additional paraaortic (station 16) lymphadenectomy (PAND) [92].

Morbidity was higher in the PAND group, but did not achieve statistical significance (28.1% vs 20.9%, p=0.07). Comparing standard D2 dissection with D2+PAND, overall survival rates (69.2% vs 70.3%) and recurrence-free survival rates (62.6% vs 61.7%) were similar between the two groups. Therefore, the investigators concluded that there is no recommendation for routine para-aortic node dissection as part of resection of potentially curable gastric malignancies. Nevertheless, according to some authors, para-aortic node dissection should remain as option only for patients with high risk of metastasis to station 16. This patients could be identified preoperatively on the basis of cancer site (upper third), depht of tumor invasion (T3-T4) and histology (mixed or diffuse type) [93].

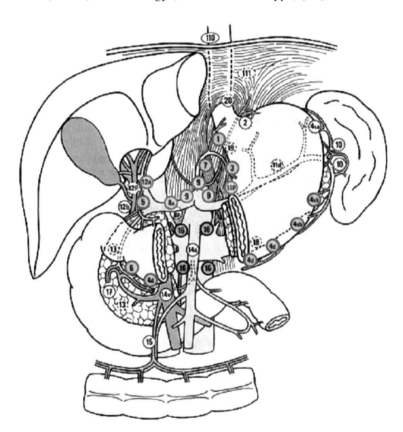

Figure 2. The circles show the lymph nodal stations as classified by the Japanese Gastric Cancer Association [81]. The colored circles represent the stations to be removed by nodal dissection for gastric cancer; the different colors indicate the different dissection levels, and the dashed circles represent the nodal stations to be removed only in case of total gastrectomy [84]. The red stations are included in a D1 dissection, the green stations are included in a D2 dissection, and the blue stations are to be removed for a para-aortic nodal dissection. From Rausei et al. [34].

Role of Laparoscopic Surgery

Laparoscopy has a main role in the management of gastric cancer: in fact staging laparoscopy is a crucial point in the staging algorithm of gastric cancer patients. The potential purposes of a staging laparoscopy are the detection of serosal involvement, the assessment of lymphnode enlargement and the evaluation of liver and/or peritoneal metastases. All this aspects are defined more accurately with a staging laparoscopy than after a CT scan [94]. In addition, during laparoscopy a peritoneal washing is performed for cytological examination: this should be considered mandatory to exclude metastatic disease for free peritoneal tumor cells, according to the new TNM edition [22,23,95].

Laparoscopic staging in gastric cancer has very high accuracy and laparoscopic assessment of TNM parameters (lapTNM) modifies clinical staging (cTNM) in almost 60% of patients, with treatment consequences in almost half of the cases [96].

The clinical application of staging laparoscopy and restaging laparoscopy (after neoadjuvant chemotherapy), are still very low, although their routine application could significantly reduce useless laparotomies in patients with metastatic disease.

Differently, with regard to the use of laparoscopy to perform gastrectomy, these technique was adopted since the beginning of the 1990s in Eastern countries [97], and presented encouraging results in terms of feasibility and safety. Laparoscopic gastrectomy has mainly been applied to the management of early gastric cancer (T1/T2, N0 tumors), however technical difficulties and oncological concerns delayed the widespread use of this approach. Concerns were expressed about adequacy of resection/lymphadenectomy, increased risk of peritoneal and port site recurrence and adequacy of surgical training.

In the literature there are six prospective, randomized trials comparing laparoscopic versus open distal gastrectomy for gastric adenocarcinoma [98-103]. All but one of this trials focused on early gastric cancer (T1/T2, N0); four trials had less than 60 patients, while two had 164 and 340 patients respectively.

A recent meta-analysis of the six trials showed an increase in the operating time, decrease in estimated blood loss, decrease in morbidity and similar low rates of mortality [104]; this study observed a decrease in the number of lymph nodes retrieved in the laparoscopic group.

Only one of the randomized trials, comparing open gastrectomy with laparoscopic gastrectomy analyzed also long-term outcomes: no significant difference was observed in overall survival and disease-free survival between the two groups, however only 59 patients were studied [99]. Many large retrospective series showed long-term survival rates similar to historical controls [105,106]. Moreover long-term oncological outcomes of laparoscopic gastrectomy are under examination in ongoing randomized clinical trials (JCOG 0912 and KLASS trials) [107,103].

Multimodal Treatment

As above specified, in the Western world more than half of patients with gastric cancers are diagnosed in locally advanced stages, and for these patients surgery should not be the first step in the management of their disease. In fact, although extended lymphadenectomy improved results of gastric cancer surgery [91,92], and new effective postoperative chemotherapeutic schedules have been introduced [108,109], the prognosis still remains unacceptable for patients with advanced disease (T3-T4 or N+ gastric cancers) [91,108,109]. Today there is current evidence supporting the use of systemic chemotherapy in the perioperative setting, and the role of chemotherapy in gastric cancer is constantly evolving to improve outcomes and lessen the toxicity associated with therapy. Worldwide there are many different multimodal approaches and treatment options vary geographically [110]: in the United States most patients are treated initially with surgery followed by adjuvant chemoradiotherapy based on the results of the Intergroup 0116 trial [108]; in Japan the preferred option is adjuvant chemotherapy alone [109]; the European approach is in favor of a perioperative or neoadjuvant chemotherapy based on the result of the MAGIC trial [42] and French FNCLCC trial [36].

Chronologically the SWOG/Intergroup 0116 trial was the first prospective, randomized trial demonstrating a survival benefit of postoperative chemoradiation over surgery alone [108]. The three-year overall survival was increased from 41% to 50% with chemoradiation (p=0.005). However, in this trial, 54% of patients received less than a D1 lymphadenectomy, only 10% of patients received a D2 lymphadenectomy, and therefore the chemoradiation seemed to primarily reduce loco-regional recurrence, improving survival by adjusting inadequate surgery [111]. Moreover, in the subgroup of patients with D2 lymphadenectomy, there was no survival difference between the two treatment arms. Therefore, it seems not appropriate to validate the trial's conclusions also in Europe and the adjuvant chemoradiotherapy should only be offered as an individual decision, due to an inadequate lymphadenectomy, and not as a standard concept. In contrast a large randomized Japanese trial [109], comparing adjuvant oral chemotherapy with S-1 to surgery alone, obtained excellent results. Five-hundred-twenty-nine patients received an oral chemotherapy (fluoropyrimidine S-1) over 1 year after surgery, and 530 patients were treated only with surgery (in both arms a D2 lymphadenectomy was performed). The 3-year survival was significantly higher in the chemotherapy group (p=0.003) and, particularly, the adjuvant treatment reduced the risk of nodal and peritoneal recurrences. The FLAGS study was conducted in order to evaluate whether these data could be transferred into the Western population, however the first satisfactory results were not confirmed [112].

Hence, Western clinician are more available to a preoperative chemotherapy. Theoretical advantages supporting the neoadjuvant approach include:

- Possibility to apply a more intensive medical treatment, thanks to a better general condition of the patient before surgery;
- No surgical alteration of blood and lymphatic vessels (important for the chemotherapy-induced cell kill);
- Higher complete resection rates (R0), thanks to the induced downsizing and downstaging of the tumor;
- Earlier treatment of micrometastases;
- Reduced free tumor cells contamination of the abdominal cavity;
- Possibility to test the applied therapy, and consequently to modify the postoperative therapy, according to the individual pathological response [113].

In fact, with this regard, it must be considered that prognosis is clearly influenced by response to chemotherapy: responding patients have a significantly improved prognosis compared to non-responding patients [114]. The percentage of responding patients varies among 20–45% [16,17,115,116] and depends on the used chemotherapeutic regimen. However, pathological response is a late parameter and, according to some reports, an earlier evaluation could be achievable by the analysis of the metabolic response to chemotherapy. The possibility of a reliable early response evaluation and a response prediction seems to represent a very challenging issue [20,117-122].

Even if some questions remain open, perioperative chemotherapy is standard at the moment in Europe for locally advanced gastric cancer and all advantages of preoperative chemotherapy have been proposed after the publication of the results of several European randomized phase-III clinical trials: MAGIC, FFCD9703, EORTC 40954 and SWS-SAKK 43/99 [36-38,42].

Particularly, effectiveness and superiority of perioperative chemotherapy followed by surgery, compared to surgery alone, was proven by two randomized phase-III studies (MAGIC and FFCD9703), where early tumor stages (low rate of serosal invasion and nodal involvement), R0 resections and even survival rates increased after neoadjuvant therapy. Between the two treatment groups, no significant difference in morbidity, mortality, and hospital stay was documented. Nevertheless both studies have been criticized, due to the long recruitment period (8 years each), the insufficient preoperative staging, the low surgical quality (questionable lymphadenectomy), and the high dropout rate in the postoperative treatment arm. Moreover, in both studies neither a clinical, nor a histopathological response evaluation was performed.

To answer open questions and to obviate to those criticism of the previous trials, a new study, the EORTC 40954, has been designed. This study was stopped for slow patients recruitment, but it confirmed the same short-term results as the other two trials, failing to show a survival benefit for the neoadjuvant treatment arm. The lack of survival benefit after neoadjuvant chemotherapy might be caused by the excellent results in the surgery alone arm and by the low sample size of this trial. The last, before cited, trial (SAKK trial) still does not present any survival data. Anyhow, in the multimodal treatment of advanced gastric cancer, the topic of a neoadjuvant approach still remains "hot". Therefore, many phase-III randomized clinical trials are ongoing focusing on this issue: MAGIC B (United Kingdom National Cancer Research Institute ST03 trial – started in 2007) [123], JCOG 0501 (Japan Clinical Oncology Group Study trial- started in 2005) [124] and CRITICS (Dutch Colorectal Cancer Group trial- started in 2006) [125]. Interestingly, the CRITICS multicenter trial is currently comparing perioperative chemotherapy to preoperative chemotherapy followed by postoperative chemoradiation. All these trials are expected to provide further data related to the open problems in the management of advanced gastric cancer.

Finally, biologic agents have been tested also in gastric cancer. These include monoclonal antibodies and small molecule tyrosine kinase inhibitors: in particular agents that target Her2/neu (trastuzumab, lapatinib), epidermal growth factor receptor (cetuximab, gefitinib, erlotiniib) and vascular-endothelial growth factor (bevacizumab, sunitinib, sorafenib). Most promising results are obtained with anti-Her2 therapy. Her2/neu (type II EFGR) is overexpressed in around 25% of gastric cancers and it is more frequent with intestinal-type than diffuse type (32% vs 6%) [126]. A randomized phase-III trial (ToGA trial) demonstrated the efficacy of the addition of anti-Her2 therapy in patients with metastatic gastric and esophagogastric cancers, with overexpression of Her2 [127]. Patients were either randomized to six cycles of infusional 5-FU/capecitabine and cisplatin versus the same regimen with trastuzumab. Response rate (47% vs 35%) and median overall survival (13.8 vs 11.1 months) were improved with trastuzumab. This trial could demonstrate the efficacy of biologic agents in advanced gastric cancer treatment. Also the, before mentioned, ongoing MAGIC-B trial is already investigating the efficacy of bevacizumab, a different biologic agent that acts as anti-angiogenic molecule.

There is great interest for these agents that hopefully may represent the new way to achieve more and more better results in the complex management of gastric cancer patients.

References

[1] Cancer. World Health Organization fact sheet No 297. 2009 http://www.who.int/mediacentre/factsheets/fs297/en/index.html. Last access Nov 2013.

[2] Jemal A, Bray F, Center MM, et al. Global cancer statistics. *CA Cancer J. Clin.* 2011;61(2):69–90.

[3] Lee J, Demissie K, Lu SE, et al. Cancer incidence among Korean-American immigrants in the United States and native Koreans in South Korea. *Cancer Control.* 2007;14:78–85.

[4] Crew KD, Neugut AI. Epidemiology of gastric cancer. *World J. Gastroenterol.* 2006;12:354–362.

[5] Wijnhoven BP, Siersema PD, Hop WC, et al. Adenocarcinomas of the distal esophagus and gastric cardia are one clinical entity. Rotterdam Esophageal Tumor Group. *Br. J. Surg.* 1999;86:529.

[6] Pisters PWT, Kelsen DP, Teper JE. Cancer of the stomach. In: DeVita VT, Lawrence TS, Rosenberg SA, eds. Cancer: Principles & Practice of Oncology. 9th edition. Philadelphia: Lippincott Williams & Wilkins; 2008;1741–1794.

[7] Pandalai PK, Yoon SS. Hereditary diffuse gastric cancer. In: Chung DC, Haber DA, eds. *Principals of Clinical Cancer Genetics*. New York: Springer; 2010;97–107.

[8] Gotoda T, Yanagisawa A, Sasako M et al. Incidence of lymph node metastasis from early gastric cancer: estimation with a large number of cases at two large centers. *Gastric. Cancer.* 2000;3:219–225.

[9] Suzuki H, Gotoda T, Sasako M, et al. Detection of early gastric cancer: misunderstanding the role of mass screening. *Gastric. Cancer.* 2006;9:315–319.

[10] Ahn HS, Lee HJ, Yoo MW et al. Changes in clinicopathological features and survival after gastrectomy for gastric cancer over a 20-year period. *Br. J. Surg.* 2011 Feb;98(2):255-60.

[11] Klein Kranenbarg E, Hermans J, van Krieken JH, et al. Evaluation of the 5th edition of the TNM classification for gastric cancer: improved prognostic value. *Br. J. Cancer* 2001;84:64.

[12] SEER Cancer Statistics. Available at: http://www.seer.cancer.gov/statistics/. Last access Nov 2013.

[13] Hartgrink HH, Jansen EPM, von Grieken NCT, et al. Gastric Cancer. *Lancet* 2009; 374: 477–90.

[14] Monig SP, Schroder W, Baldus SE, et al. Preoperative lymph-node staging in gastrointestinal cancer—correlation between size and tumor stage. *Onkologie.* 2002; 25(4):342–344.

[15] Kitagawa Y, Kitajima M. Gastroesophageal carcinoma: individualized surgical therapy. *Surg. Oncol. Clin. N. Am.* 2006;15(4):793–802.

[16] Schuhmacher CP, Fink U, Becker K, et al. Neoadjuvant therapy for patients with locally advanced gastric carcinoma with etoposide, doxorubicin, and cisplatinum. Closing results after 5 years of follow-up. *Cancer.* 2001;91 (5):918–927.

[17] Ott K, Sendler A, Becker K, et al. Neoadjuvant chemotherapy with cisplatin, 5-FU, and leucovorin (PLF) in locally advanced gastric cancer: a prospective phase II study. *Gastric. Cancer.* 2003;6(3):159–167.

[18] Stahl A, Ott K, Weber WA, et al. FDG PET imaging of locally advanced gastric carcinomas: correlation with endoscopic and histopathological findings. *Eur. J. Nucl. Med. Mol. Imaging.* 2003;30 (2):288–295.

[19] Herrmann K, Ott K, Buck AK, et al. Imaging gastric cancer with PET and the radiotracers 18 F-FLT and 18 F-FDG: a comparative analysis. *J. Nucl. Med.* 2007;48(12):1945–1950.

[20] Ott K, Herrmann K, Lordick F, et al. Early metabolic response evaluation by fluorine-18 fluorodeoxyglucose positron emission tomography allows in vivo testing of chemosensitivity in gastric cancer: longterm results of a prospective study. *Clin. Cancer Res.* 2008;14(7):2012–2018.

[21] Feussner H, Hartl F. Staging laparoscopy in oncology. *Chirurg.* 2006;77(11):971–980.

[22] Rosenberg R, Nekarda H, Bauer P, et al. Free peritoneal tumour cells are an independent prognostic factor in curatively resected stage IB gastric carcinoma. *Br. J. Surg.* 2006;93(3):325–331.

[23] Stomach. In: Edge SB, Byrd DR, Compton CC, et al., eds.: AJCC Cancer Staging Manual. 7th ed. New York, NY: *Springer*, 2010, pp 117-26.

[24] Ahn HS, Lee HJ, Hahn S, et al. Evaluation of the seventh American Joint Committee on Cancer / International Union Against Cancer Classification of gastric adenocarcinoma in comparison with the sixth classification. *Cancer.* 2010;116:5592–8.

[25] Chae S, Lee A, Lee JH. The effectiveness of the new (7th) UICC N classification in the prognosis evaluation of gastric cancer patients: a comparative study between the 5th / 6th and 7thUICC N classification. *Gastric Cancer.* 2011;14:166–71.

[26] Hayashi T, Yoshikawa T, Bonam K, et al. The superiority of the seventh edition of the TNM classification depends on the overall survival of the patient cohort: comparative analysis of the sixth and seventh TNM editions in patients with gastric cancer from Japan and the United Kingdom. *Cancer.* 2013;119(7):1330-7.

[27] Graziosi L, Marino E, Cavazzoni E, et al. Prognostic value of the seventh AJCC/UICC TNM classification of non-cardia gastric cancer. *World J. Surg. Oncol.* 2013;20;11:103.

[28] Reim D, Loos M, Vogl F, et al. Prognostic implications of the seventh edition of the international union against cancer classification for patients with gastric cancer: the Western experience of patients treated in a single-center European institution. *J. Clin. Oncol.* 2013;10;31(2):263-71.

[29] Zhang J, Niu Z, Zhou Y, et al. A comparison between the seventh and sixth editions of the American Joint Committee on Cancer/International Union Against classification of gastric cancer. *Ann. Surg.* 2013;257(1):81-6.

[30] Sun Z, Wang ZN, Zhu Z, et al. Evaluation of the seventh edition of American Joint Committee on Cancer TNM staging system for gastric cancer: results from a Chinese monoinstitutional study. *Ann. Surg.* Oncol. 2012;19(6):1918-27.

[31] Siewert JR, Stein HJ. Classification of adenocarcinoma of the oesophagogastric junction. *Br. J. Surg.* 1998;85(11):1457–9.

[32] Suh YS, Han DS, Kong SH, et al. Should adenocarcinoma of the esophagogastric junction be classified as esophageal cancer? A comparative analysis according to the seventh AJCC TNM classification. *Ann. Surg.* 2012;255(5):908–15.

[33] Wang W, Xu DZ, Li YF, et al. Tumor-ratio-metastasis staging system as an alternative to the 7th edition UICC TNM system in gastric cancer after D2 resection– results of a single-institution study of 1343 Chinese patients. *Ann. Oncol.* 2011;22:2049–56.

[34] Rausei S, Dionigi G, Sano T, et al. Updates on surgical management of advanced gastric cancer: new evidence and trends. Insights from the First International Course on Upper Gastrointestinal Surgery--Varese (Italy), December 2, 2011. *Ann. Surg. Oncol.* 2013;20(12):3942-7.

[35] Novotny AR, Schuhmacher C, Busch R, et al. Predicting individual survival after gastric cancer resection: validation of a US-derived nomogram at a single high-volume center in Europe. *Ann. Surg.* 2006;243:74–81.

[36] Ychou M, Boige V, Pignon JP, et al. Perioperative chemotherapy compared with surgery alone for resectable gastroesophageal adenocarcinoma: an FNCLCC and FFCD multicenter phase III trial. *J. Clin. Oncol.* 2011;29:1715–21.

[37] Schuhmacher C, Gretschel S, Lordick F, et al. Neoadjuvant chemotherapy compared with surgery alone for locally advanced cancer of the stomach and cardia: European Organisation for Research and Treatment of Cancer randomized trial 40954. *J. Clin. Oncol.* 2010;28:5210–8.

[38] Biffi R, Fazio N, Luca F, et al. Surgical outcome after docetaxel-based neoadjuvant chemotherapy in locally-advanced gastric cancer. *World J. Gastroenterol.* 2010;16:868–74.

[39] Barbour AP, Rizk NP, Gerdes H, et al. Endoscopic ultrasound predicts outcomes for patients with adenocarcinoma of the gastroesophageal junction. *J. Am. Coll. Surg.* 2007;205(4):593–601.

[40] Roder JD, Bottcher K, Siewert JR, et al. Prognostic factors in gastric carcinoma. Results of the German Gastric Carcinoma Study 1992. *Cancer.* 1993;72(7):2089–2097.

[41] Barbour AP, Rizk NP, Gonen M, et al. Adenocarcinoma of the gastroesophageal junction: influence of esophageal resection margin and operative approach on outcome. *Ann. Surg.* 2007;246(1):1–8.

[42] Cunningham D, Allum WH, Stenning SP, et al. MAGIC Trial Participants. Perioperative chemotherapy versus surgery alone for resectable gastroesophageal cancer. *N. Engl. J. Med.* 2006;355:11–20.

[43] Rausei S, Boni L, Rovera F, et al. Locally advanced gastric cancer: a new definition to standardise. *J. Clin. Pathol.* 2013;66(2):164-5.

[44] Brennan MF. Current status of surgery for gastric cancer: a review. *Gastric. Cancer.* 2005;8(2):64-70.

[45] Bozzetti F, Marubini E, Bonfanti G, et al. Total versus subtotal gastrectomy: surgical morbidity and mortality rates in a multicenter Italian randomized trial. The Italian Gastrointestinal Tumor Study Group. *Ann. Surg.* 1997;226(5):613–20.

[46] De Manzoni G, Verlato G, Roviello F, et al. Subtotal versus total gastrectomy for T3 adenocarcinoma of the antrum. *Gastric Cancer*. 2003; 6: 237-242.

[47] Gockel I, Pietzka S, Gönner U, et al. Subtotal or total gastrectomy for gastric cancer: impact of the surgical procedure on morbidity and prognosis—analysis of a 10-year experience. *Langenbecks Arch Surg*. 2005; 390:148-155.

[48] Karanicolas PJ, Graham D, Gönen M, et al. Quality of life after gastrectomy for adenocarcinoma: a prospective cohort study. *Ann. Surg*. 2013 Jun;257(6):1039-46.

[49] Davies J, Johnston D, Sue-Ling H, et al. Total or subtotal gastrectomy for gastric carcinoma? A study of quality of life. *World J. Surg*. 1998;22(10):1048–55.

[50] Ishikawa M, Kitayama J, Kaizaki S, et al. Prospective randomized trial comparing Billroth I and Roux-en-Y procedures after distal gastrectomy for gastric carcinoma. *World J. Surg*. 2005;29:1415–1420.

[51] Montesani C, D'Amato A, Santella S, et al. Billroth I versus Billroth II versus Roux-en-Y after subtotal gastrectomy. Prospective [correction of prespective] randomized study. *Hepatogastroenterology*. 2002;49:1469–1473.

[52] Zong L, Chen P. Billroth I vs. Billroth II vs. Roux-en-Y following distal gastrectomy: a meta-analysis based on 15 studies. *Hepatogastroenterology*. 2011;58(109):1413-24.

[53] Katai H, Sano T, Fukagawa T, et al. Prospective study of proximal gastrectomy for early gastric cancer in the upper third of the stomach. *Br. J. Surg*. 2003; 90:850-853.

[54] Yoo CH, Sohn BH, Han WK, et al. Proximal gastrectomy reconstructed by jejunal pouch interposition for upper third gastric cancer: prospective randomized study. *World J. Surg*. 2005; 29: 1592-1599.

[55] Kim JH, Park SS, Kim J, et al. Surgical outcomes for gastric cancer in the upper third of the stomach. *World J. Surg*. 2006; 30: 1870-1886; discussion 1870-1886.

[56] Nozaki I, Kurita A, Nasu J, et al. Higher incidence of gastric remnant cancer after proximal than distal gastrectomy. *Hepatogastroenterology*. 2007; 54: 1604-1608.

[57] An JY, Youn HG, Ha TK, et al. Clinical significance of tumor location in remnant gastric cancers developed after partial gastrectomy for primary gastric cancer. J. *Gastrointest Surg*. 2008; 12: 689-694.

[58] Viste A, Haugstvedt T, Eide GE, et al. Postoperative complications and mortality after surgery for gastric cancer. *Ann. Surg*. 1988; 207(1):7–13.

[59] An JY, Youn HG, Choi MG, et al. The difficult choice between total and proximal gastrectomy in proximal early gastric cancer. *Am. J. Surg*. 2008;196:587–591.

[60] Harrison LE, Karpeh MS, Brennan MF. Total gastrectomy is not necessary for proximal gastric cancer. *Surgery*. 1998;123:127–130.

[61] Katai H, Morita S, Saka M, et al. Long-term outcome after proximal gastrectomy with jejunal interposition for suspected early cancer in the upper third of the stomach. *Br. J. Surg*. 2010;97:558–562.

[62] Sasako M, Sano T, Yamamoto S, et al. Left thoracoabdominal approach versus abdominal-transhiatal approach for gastric cancer of the cardia or subcardia: a randomised controlled trial. *Lancet Oncol*. 2006;7(8):644–651.

[63] Barbour AP, Rizk NP, Gonen M, et al. Lymphadenectomy for adenocarcinoma of the gastroesophageal junction (GEJ): impact of adequate staging on outcome. *Ann. Surg. Oncol*. 2007;14(2):306–316.

[64] Ott K, Bader FG, Lordick F, et al. Surgical factors influence the outcome after Ivor-Lewis esophagectomy with intrathoracic anastomosis for adenocarcinoma of the

esophagogastric junction: a consecutive series of 240 patients at an experienced center. *Ann. Surg. Oncol.* 2009;16(4):1017–1025.

[65] Uzunoglu FG, Reeh M, Kutup A, et al. Surgery of esophageal cancer. *Langenbecks Arch. Surg.* 2013;398(2):189-93.

[66] Shchepotin IB, Chorny VA, Nauta RJ, et al. Extended surgical resection in T4 gastric cancer. *Am. J. Surg.* 1998;175(2):123–6.

[67] Kobayashi A, Nakagohri T, Konishi M, et al. Aggressive surgical treatment for T4 gastric cancer. *J. Gastrointest. Surg.* 2004;8(4):464–70.

[68] Kunisaki C, Akiyama H, Nomura M, et al. Surgical outcomes in patients with T4 gastric carcinoma. *J. Am. Coll. Surg.* 2006;202(2):223–30.

[69] Csendes A, Burdiles P, Rojas J, et al. A prospective randomized study comparing D2 total gastrectomy versus D2 total gastrectomy plus splenectomy in 187 patients with gastric carcinoma. *Surgery.* 2002; 131: 401-407.

[70] Fatouros M, Roukos DH, Lorenz M, et al. Impact of spleen preservation in patients with gastric cancer. *Anticancer Res.* 2005; 25:3023-3030.

[71] Yu W, Choi GS, Chung HY. Randomized clinical trial of splenectomy versus splenic preservation in patients with proximal gastric cancer. *Br. J. Surg.* 2006; 93: 559-563

[72] Martin RC, Jaques DP, Brennan MF, et al. Extended local resection for advanced gastric cancer: increate survival versus increased morbidity. *Ann. Surg.* 2002; 236: 159-165.

[73] Jeong O, Choi WY, Park YK. Appropriate selection of patients for combined organ resection in cases of gastric carcinoma invading adjacent organs. *J. Surg. Oncol.* 2009; 100:115-120.

[74] Colen KL, Marcus SG, Newman E, et al. Multiorgan resection for gastric cancer: intraoperative and computed tomography assessment of locally advanced disease is inaccurate. *J. Gastrointest. Surg.* 2004; 8: 899-902.

[75] Carboni F, Lepiane P, Santoro R, et al. Extended multiorgan resection for T4 gastric carcinoma: 25-year experience. *J. Surg. Oncol.* 2005;90(2):95–100.

[76] Pacelli F, Cusumano G, Rosa F, et al. for the Italian Research Group for Gastric Cancer (IRGGC). Multivisceral Resection for Locally Advanced Gastric Cancer: An Italian Multicenter Observational Study. *JAMA Surg.* 2013;148(4):353-360.

[77] Coburn NG, Swallow CJ, Kiss A, et al. Significant regional variation in adequacy of lymph node assessment and survival in gastric cancer. *Cancer.* 2006;107:2143–2151.

[78] Bouvier AM, Haas O, Piard F, et al. How many nodes must be examined to accurately stage gastric carcinomas? Results from a population based study. *Cancer.* 2002;94:2862–2866.

[79] Smith DD, Schwarz RR, Schwarz RE. Impact of total lymph node count on staging and survival after gastrectomy for gastric cancer: data from a large US-population database. *J. Clin. Oncol.* 2005;23:7114–7124.

[80] Estes NC, Macdonald JS, Touijer K, et al. Inadequate documentation and resection for gastric cancer in the United States: a preliminary report. *Am. Surg.* 1998;64:680–685.

[81] Japanese Research Society for Gastric Cancer. The general rules for the gastric cancer study in surgery. *Jpn. J. Surg.* 1973;3:61.

[82] Nishi M, Omori Y, Miwa K. Japanese Classification of Gastric Carcinoma. Kanehara & Co., Ltd; 1995.

[83] Japanese Gastric Cancer Association. Japanese classification of gastric carcinoma-2nd English edition-response assessment of chemotherapy and radiotherapy for gastric carcinoma: clinical criteria. *Gastric. Cancer.* 2001;4:1–8.

[84] Japanese Gastric Cancer Association. Japanese gastric cancer treatment guidelines 2010 (ver. 3). *Gastric Cancer.* 2011 Jun;14(2):113-23.

[85] Siewert JR, Bottcher K, Stein HJ, et al. Relevant prognostic factors in gastric cancer: ten-year results of the German Gastric Cancer Study. *Ann. Surg.* 1998;228(4):449–461.

[86] Bonenkamp JJ, Songun I, Hermans J, et al. Randomised comparison of morbidity after D1 and D2 dissection for gastric cancer in 996 Dutch patients. *Lancet.* 1995;345 (8952):745–748.

[87] Cuschieri A, Weeden S, Fielding J, et al. Patient survival after D1 and D2 resections for gastric cancer: long-term results of the MRC randomized surgical trial. Surgical Cooperative Group. *Br. J. Cancer.* 1999;79(9–10):1522–1530.

[88] Hartgrink HH, van de Velde CJ, Putter H, et al. Extended lymph node dissection for gastric cancer: who may benefit? Final results of the randomized Dutch gastric cancer group trial. *J. Clin. Oncol.* 2004;22(11):2069–2077.

[89] Degiuli M, Sasako M, Ponti A, et al. Survival results of a multicentre phase II study to evaluate D2 gastrectomy for gastric cancer. *Br. J. Cancer.* 2004; 90: 1727-1732.

[90] Edwards P, Blackshaw GR, Lewis WG, et al. Prospective comparison of D1 vs modified D2 gastrectomy for carcinoma. *Br. J. Cancer.* 2004; 90:1888-1892.

[91] Wu CW, Hsiung CA, Lo SS, et al. Nodal dissection for patients with gastric cancer: a randomised controlled trial. *Lancet Oncol.* 2006;7(4):309–315.

[92] Sasako M, Sano T, Yamamoto S,et al. D2 lymphadenectomy alone or with para-aortic nodal dissection for gastric cancer. *N. Engl. J. Med.* 2008;359(5):453–462.

[93] De Manzoni G, Di Leo A, Roviello F, et al. Tumor Site and Perigastric Nodal Status are the Most Important Predictors of Para-Aortic Nodal Involvement in Advanced Gastric Cancer. *Ann Surg Oncol.* 2011;18:2273–2280.

[94] Burke EC, Karpeh MS, Conlon KC, et al. Laparoscopy in the management of gastric adenocarcinoma. *Ann. Surg.* 1997;225(3):262–7.

[95] Bonenkamp JJ, Songun I, Hermans J, et al. Prognostic value of positive cytology findings from abdominal washings in patients with gastric cancer. *Br. J. Surg.*1996; 83(5):672–674.

[96] Karanicolas PJ, Elkin EB, Jacks LM, et al. Staging laparoscopy in the management of gastric cancer: a population-based analysis. *J. Am. Coll. Surg.* 2011; 213(5):644–51, 651 e1.

[97] Kitano S, Iso Y, Moriyama M, et al. Laparoscopyassisted Billroth I gastrectomy. *Surg. Laparosc. Endosc.* 1994;4:146–148.

[98] Kitano S, Shiraishi N, Kakisako K, et al. Laparoscopy-assisted Billroth-I gastrectomy (LADG) for cancer: our 10 years' experience. Surg Laparosc. *Endosc. Percutan Tech.* 2002;12:204–207.

[99] Huscher CG, Mingoli A, Sgarzini G, et al. Laparoscopic versus open subtotal gastrectomy for distal gastric cancer: five-year results of a randomized prospective trial. *Ann. Surg.* 2005;241:232–237.

[100] Lee JH, Han HS, Lee JH. A prospective randomized study comparing open vs laparoscopy-assisted distal gastrectomy in early gastric cancer: early results. *Surg. Endosc.* 2005;19:168–173.

[101] Kitano S, Shiraishi N, Fujii K, et al. A randomized controlled trial comparing open vs laparoscopyassisted distal gastrectomy for the treatment of early gastric cancer: an interim report. *Surgery* 2002;131:S306–S311.

[102] Hayashi H, Ochiai T, Shimada H, et al. Prospective randomized study of open versus laparoscopy-assisted distal gastrectomy with extraperigastric lymph node dissection for early gastric cancer. *Surg. Endosc.* 2005;19:1172–1176.

[103] Kim HH, Hyung WJ, Cho GS et al. Morbidity and mortality of laparoscopic gastrectomy versus open gastrectomy for gastric cancer: an interim report–a phase III multicenter, prospective, randomized Trial (KLASS Trial). *Ann. Surg.* 2010;251:417–420.

[104] Kodera Y, Fujiwara M, Ohashi N et al. Laparoscopic surgery for gastric cancer: a collective review with meta-analysis of randomized trials. *J. Am. Coll. Surg.* 2010;211:677–686.

[105] Kitano S, Shiraishi N, Uyama I, et al. A multicenter study on oncologic outcome of laparoscopic gastrectomy for early cancer in Japan. *Ann. Surg.* 2007;245:68–72.

[106] Lee SW, Nomura E, Bouras G, et al. Long-term oncologic outcomes from laparoscopic gastrectomy for gastric cancer: a single-center experience of 601 consecutive resections. *J. Am. Coll. Surg.* 2010;211:33–40.

[107] Katai H, Sasako M, Fukuda H, et al. JCOG Gastric Cancer Surgical Study Group. Safety and feasibility of laparoscopy-assisted distal gastrectomy with suprapancreatic nodal dissection for clinical stage I gastric cancer: a multicenter phase II trial (JCOG 0703). *Gastric. Cancer.* 2010 Nov;13(4):238-44.

[108] Macdonald JS, Smalley SR, Benedetti J, et al. Chemoradiotherapy after surgery compared with surgery alone for adenocarcinoma of the stomach or gastroesophageal junction. *N. Engl. J. Med.* 2001;345(10):725–730.

[109] Sakuramoto S, Sasako M, Yamaguchi T, et al. Adjuvant chemotherapy for gastric cancer with S-1, an oral fluoropyrimidine. *N. Engl. J. Med.* 2007;357(18):1810–1820.

[110] Van de Velde CJ, Koen CMJ, et al. The gastric cancer treatment controversy. *J. Clin. Oncol.* 2003;21:2234.

[111] Lordick F, Siewert JR. Recent advances in multimodal treatment for gastric cancer: a review. *Gastric. Cancer* 2005;8:78–85.

[112] Ajani JA, Rodriguez W, Bodoky G, et al. Multicenter phase III comparison of cisplatin/S-1 with cisplatin/ infusional fluorouracil in advanced gastric or gastroesophageal adenocarcinoma study: the FLAGS trial. *J. Clin. Oncol.* 2010;28 (9):1547–1553.

[113] Becker K, Langer R, Reim D, et al. Significance of histopathological tumor regression after neoadjuvant chemotherapy in gastric adenocarcinomas: a summary of 480 cases. *Ann. Surg.* 2011;253(5):934-9.

[114] Lowy AM, Mansfield PF, Leach SD, et al. Response to neoadjuvant chemotherapy best predicts survival after curative resection of gastric cancer. *Ann. Surg.* 1999;229 (3):303–308

[115] Fink U, Schuhmacher C, Stein HJ, et al.(Preoperative chemotherapy for stage III–IV gastric carcinoma: feasibility, response and outcome after complete resection. *Br. J. Surg.* 1995;82 (9):1248–1252

[116] Shah MA, Ramanathan RK, Ilson DH, et al. Multicenter phase II study of irinotecan, cisplatin, and bevacizumab in patients with metastatic gastric or gastroesophageal junction adenocarcinoma. *J. Clin. Oncol*. 2006;24 (33):5201–5206.

[117] Becker K, Fink U, Ott K, et al. How can the effectiveness of multimodality therapy concepts be evaluated? From the viewpoint of the pathologist. *Kongressbd Dtsch Ges Chir. Kongr*. 2001;118:58–62

[118] Fink U, Ott K, Weber W, et al. Neoadjuvant therapeutic principles guided by response prediction and evaluation. *Kongressbd Dtsch. Ges* Chir Kongr. 2002;119:829–833

[119] Ott K, Fink U, Becker K, et al. Prediction of response to preoperative chemotherapy in gastric carcinoma by metabolic imaging: results of a prospective trial. *J. Clin. Oncol*. 2003;21(24):4604–4610.

[120] Grundei T, Vogelsang H, Ott K, et al. Loss of heterozygosity and microsatellite instability as predictive markers for neoadjuvant treatment in gastric carcinoma. *Clin. Cancer Res*. 6 (12):4782–4788.

[121] Mutze K, Langer R, Becker K, et al. Histone deacetylase (HDAC) 1 and 2 expression and chemotherapy in gastric cancer. *Ann. Surg. Oncol*. 2010;17:3336–3343.

[122] Napieralski R, Ott K, Kremer M, et al. Methylation of tumor-related genes in neoadjuvant-treated gastric cancer: relation to therapy response and clinicopathologic and molecular features. *Clin. Cancer Res*. 2007;13(17):5095–5102.

[123] US National Institutes of Health. A Randomised Phase II/III Trial of Peri-Operative Chemotherapy With or Without Bevacizumab in Operable Oesophagogastric Adenocarcinoma and A Feasibility Study Evaluating Lapatinib in HER-2 Positive Oesophagogastric Adenocarcinomas.

[124] Available from: http://clinicaltrials.gov/show/NCT00450203. Last access Nov 2013.

[125] US National Institutes of Health. Randomized Phase III Trial of Surgery Plus Neoadjuvant TS-1 and Cisplatin Compared With Surgery Alone for Type 4 and Large Type 3 Gastric Cancer: Japan Clinical Oncology Group Study (JCOG 0501) Available from: http://clinicaltrials.gov/show/NCT00252161. Last access Nov 2013.

[126] US National Institutes of Health. A Multicenter Randomized Phase III Trial of Neo-adjuvant Chemotherapy Followed by Surgery and Chemotherapy or by Surgery and Chemoradiotherapy in Resectable Gastric Cancer (CRITICS Study). Available from: http://clinicaltrials.gov/show/NCT00407186. Last access Nov 2013.

[127] Takehana T, Kunitomo K, Kono K, et al. Status of c-erbB-2 in gastric adenocarcinoma: a comparative study of immunohistochemistry, fluorescence in situ hybridization and enzyme-linked immunosorbent assay. *Int. J. Cancer* 2002;98:833.

[128] Bang YJ, Van Cutsem E, Feyereislova A, et al. Trastuzumab in combination with chemotherapy versus chemotherapy alone for treatment of HER2-positive advanced gastric or gastro-esophageal junction cancer (ToGA): a phase 3, openlabel, randomized controlled trial. *Lancet* 2010;376:687.

In: Gastric Cancer
Editor: Jasneet Singh Bhullar

ISBN: 978-1-63117-983-9
© 2014 Nova Science Publishers, Inc.

Chapter 9

Bursectomy in Gastric Cancer Surgery

Konstantinos Blouhos,[1,*] M.D., MSc, Ph.D.,
Konstantinos Tsalis,[2,#] M.D., Ph.D.,
Konstantinos A. Boulas,[3,†] M.D., MSc.
and Anestis Hatzigeorgiadis,[4,‡] M.D., MSc.

[1]HPB-GI Surgeon - Staff Surgeon, Department of General Surgery,
General Hospital of Drama, Drama, Greece
[2]HPB Surgeon - Professor of Surgery and Chairman,
D' Surgical Department, "G. Papanikolaou" Hospital, Medical School,
Aristotle University of Thessaloniki, Thessaloniki, Greece
[3]Surgical Trainee - Department of General Surgery,
General Hospital of Drama, Drama, Greece
[4]Chairman - Department of General Surgery, General Hospital of Drama, Drama, Greece

Abstract

The continued practice of bursectomy over the years stems from its utility in facilitating: (a) elimination of microscopic tumor deposits in the greater omentum and lesser sac; (b) complete resection of disease from the head of the pancreas; (c) complete clearance of the high-risk No 6 lymph nodes; (d) an aesthetic, clean, celiac-based lymph node dissection (No 9, 10, 11p, 11d lymph nodes); and (e) direct access to the "difficult" No 14v, 14a, 15, 17, 18 lymph nodes. Although the Japanese gastric cancer treatment guidelines (2010) suggest performance of bursectomy for tumors penetrating the serosa of the posterior gastric wall, several surgeons, considering the balance between the risk and benefit, have remained skeptical about the procedure. The influence of bursectomy

---

* Corresponding author: Konstantinos Blouhos, MD, MSc, PhD. HPB-GI Surgeon. Staff Surgeon. Department of General Surgery, General Hospital of Drama. End of Hippokratous Street, 66100 Drama, Greece. Tel: +306946330417, Fax: +302521350412. E-mail: kostasblu@hotmail.com.
\# E-mail: ctsalis@yahoo.gr.
† E-mail: katerinantwna@hotmail.com.
‡ E-mail: ahatz@otenet.gr.

on operative mortality and morbidity, especially the risk of pancreatic fistula formation, is low; however, the risk of bowel obstruction due to adhesions formation to the skeletalised mesocolon and pancreas should always be taken into account when perfoming bursectomy. Although, there is little evidence that bursectomy has clinical benefit, it should not be abandoned as a futile procedure until more definitive data will be obtained.

Introduction

The continued practice of bursectomy stems from its utility in facilitating: (a) elimination of microscopic tumor deposits in the greater omentum and lesser sac; (b) complete resection of disease from the head of the pancreas; (c) complete clearance of the high-risk subpyloric station lymph nodes (LNs); (d) an aesthetic, clean, celiac based node dissection (No 9, 10, 11p, 11d LNs); and (e) direct access to the "difficult" No 14v, 14a, 15, 17, 18 LNs [1]. D2 gastrectomy plus bursectomy can be safely performed in high volume experience centers or by experienced surgeons with mortality rates of < 1 % and morbidity rates of around 14–24 % [2]. Although there is little evidence supporting the clinical benefit of bursectomy, the Japanese gastric cancer treatment guidelines suggest performance of bursectomy for tumors penetrating the serosa of the posterior gastric wall [3].

The Surgical Plane of Bursectomy

The surgical plane of bursectomy is the plane between the posterior aspect of the fused layers of the greater omentum lying anteriorly and the anterior layer of the peritoneum of the mesocolon lying posteriorly.

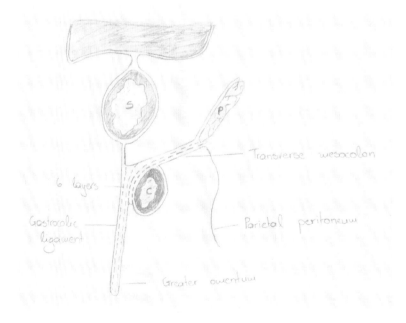

Figure 1. The surgical plane of omental bursectomy lies between the posterior aspect of the fused layers of the greater omentum lying anteriorly and the anterior layer of the peritoneum of the mesocolon.

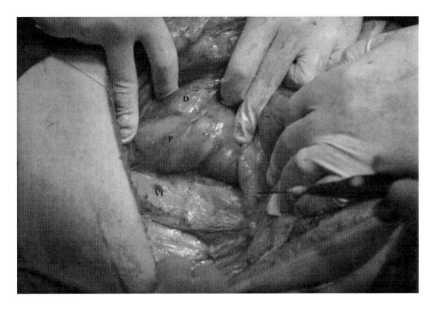

Figure 2. A very extensive Kocher's maneuver facilitates dissection of the No.13, 16a2, 16b1 LNs. D: Duodenum, P: Pancreas, VC: Inferior Vena Cava.

More thoroughly, the double layer of peritoneum, which forms the anterior layer of the greater omentum, descends across the transverse colon and passes inferiorly for a variable distance to the lower end of this apronlike fold; the posterior layer of the greater omentum then ascends, passes superiorly to the transverse colon, lies against the superior layer of the peritoneum of the transverse mesocolon, with which it fuses to a variable degree, and then attaches to the anterior aspect of the head and body of the pancreas. The surgeon uses this special anatomic relationship to enter the plane of bursectomy and to secure a bloodless route to the lesser sac and the pancreas (Figure 1) [4].

The Surgical Technique

Mobilize the Hepatic Flexure, the Duodenum and the Splenic Flexure

The hepatic flexure of the colon is mobilized from the underlying duodenum. Next, a very extensive Kocher's maneuver (Figure 2) is performed; incision of the lateral peritoneal attachment to the duodenum and sharp dissection of duodenum and head of pancreas from the inferior vena cava exposes the posterior aspect of the pancreas (No. 13 LNs). Sharp dissection is continued to expose not only the vena cava but also the left renal vein, the aorta and the left para-aortic area below the renal vein, as far as the gonadal vein. When paraaortic dissection is required, it is carried out at this stage (No. 16a2, 16b1 LNs). The splenic flexure of the colon is also mobilized. The splenic flexure is released from the left upper quadrant by incising the lateral peritoneal attachments. As the splenic flexure is released medially, the dissection turns toward the pancreas, and the attachments of the splenic flexure to the undersurface of the tail of the pancreas are incised.

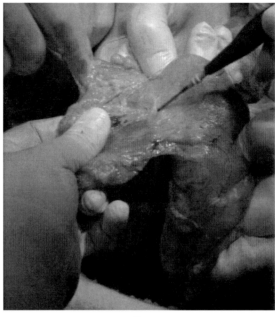

a

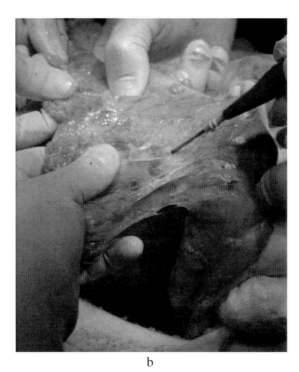

b

Figure 3. The omentum and the transverse colon is lifted up in order to expose the posterior surface of the greater omentum (a) a variable number of adhesions to the transverse colon are divided, and (b) the plane of omental bursectomy is entered.

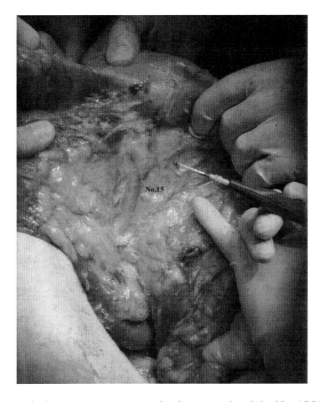

Figure 4. The anterior leaf of the transverse mesocolon is removed and the No. 15 LNs along the middle colic vessels are dissected.

Enter the Plane and Dissect the Greater Omentum from the Transverse Colon and Mesocolon

It is helpful to lift up the omentum and transverse colon to expose its posterior surface and to have the assistant apply gentle traction on the colon. A variable number of adhesions to the transverse colon are divided, and the plane between the posterior aspect of the fused layers of the greater omentum lying anteriorly and the anterior layer of the peritoneum of the mesocolon is entered (Figure 3). The usual site of entry into the plane is the midline. It is important to ensure that the correct plane is entered at the beginning of the dissection. The dissection of the omentum should be practically bloodless to the right and left of the midline. The dissection is continued on to the transverse mesocolon; the anterior layer of the mesocolon is taken with the omentum (Figure 4).
The dissection is guided by the middle colic vessels; care should be taken not to damage the colonic vasculature (No. 15 LNs). To the right of the middle colic vein is the accessory right colic vein, a very constant structure, which shares a common drainage route to the superior mesenteric vein (gastrocolic trunk) with the right gastroepiploic vein; there is, therefore, an inevitable vascular connection at this point between the mesocolon and the gastric vasculature [4]. The anterior leaf of the mesocolon is followed to the base of the transverse mesocolon at the lower border of the pancreas (No. 18, 14v LNs) (Figure 5).

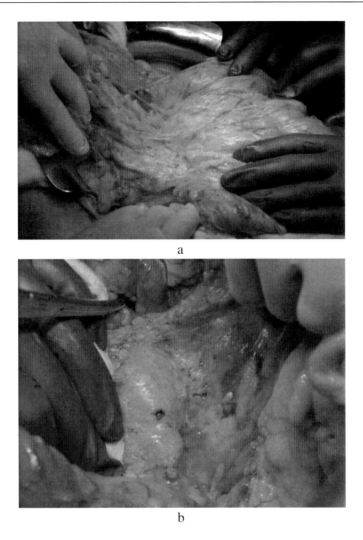

Figure 5. Dissection is continued towards the base of the transverse mesocolon and the No. 18 LNs along the inferior border of the pancreatic border are dissected.

Dissect the Peritoneal Sheet Overlying the Pancreas off the Gland

Care must be taken to enter the correct plane between the pancreatic capsule and the pancreas in order not to damage the pancreas. Elevation of the peritoneum is continued working from the neck of the gland cranially and to the right and left (Figure 6). Hydrodissection may be a useful manipulation in troublesome cases [5]. Working to the right towards the first part of the duodenum, one comes upon the gastroduodenal artery. The artery is followed distally until it branches into the superior pancreaticoduodenal and the right gastroepiploic and centrally to its origin from the common hepatic artery (No. 17 and 6 LNs). Visualization of this junction completes the right phase of dissection. Working to the left of the pancreatic neck the dissection is carried out to the tail of the pancreas. As complete removal of the left side of the bursa omentalis does not allow a subtotal gastrectomy, the pancreatic serosa is removed up to the proximal half of the splenic artery. Visualization of the splenic artery on the upper border of the pancreas to the tail of the pancreas completes the left phase of dissection (Figure 7).

Remove the Caudal Area of the Bursa Omentalis

The caudal area of the bursa omentalis is removed at latter phases of gastrectomy; lymph node dissection along the celiac artery (No. 9 LNs), the common hepatic artery (No. 8a, 8p LNs), the splenic artery (No. 11p, 11d LNs), the left gastric artery (No. 7 LNs) and the hepatoduodenal ligament (No. 12a, 12b, 12p LNs) facilitates complete removal of the caudal area of the bursa omentalis. At the end of this dissection the pancreas is skeletalised as are the celiac artery, the hepatic and splenic arteries (Figure 8).

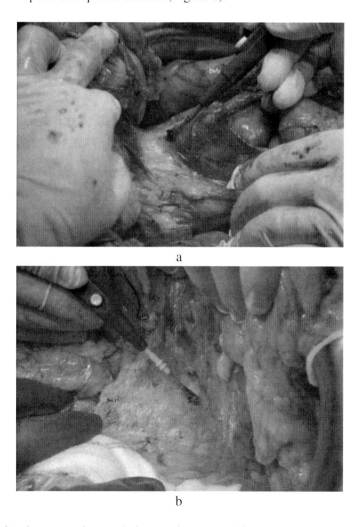

Figure 6. Removing the pancreatic capsule is a continuous work from (a) the inferior towards (b) the superior border of the pancreas. The No. 17 LNs along the anterior surface of the pancreatic head beneath the pancreatic sheath are dissected.

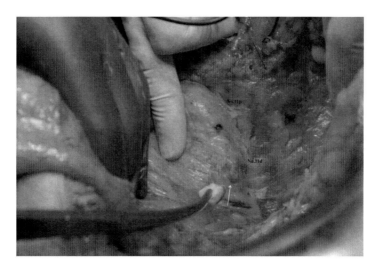

Figure 7. Visualization of the splenic artery (white arrow) at the upper border of the pancreas (No. 11 p, d) completes dissection of the caudal area (black arrow) of the bursa omentalis, which is removed en block with the surgical specimen a latter phases of gastrectomy.

Discussion

Bursectomy has been originally recommended in extended surgery for gastric cancer to facilitate elimination of microscopic tumor deposits in the lesser sac. However, several surgeons now discard the procedure since there is little evidence to support that bursectomy has oncologic benefit. A need to go over this procedure is cumbersome especially for laparoscopic surgeons. As bursectomy is still debatable, further clinical trials are needed to provide more definitive data regarding its role in gastric cancer surgery.

Does Bursectomy Provide an Easy, Safe and Bloodless Access to the Lesser Sac and the Pancreas?

In our study [6], the performance of bursectomy was associated with a median operative time of 41 min (range, 29-63 min) and with a median blood loss of 65 ml (range, 20-155 ml). These results, which are in parallel with results reported by high-volume centers in the East, show that bursectomy provides an easy and bloodless route to the lesser sac and the pancreas.

Removal of the pancreatic capsule and the anterior leaf of the transverse mesocolon is physically detrimental to patients and increases the risk of complications. In Imamura et al. [7] randomized controlled study, 210 patients were assigned to the bursectomy group (104 patients) and nonbursectomy group (106 patients). The hospital mortality rate was 0.95% and the overall morbidity rate was 14.3%, the same for the two groups. Interestingly, the incidence of major postoperative complications, including pancreatic fistula and bowel obstruction, were not significant different between the two groups. Fujita et al. [8] reported the same overall mortality (0.95%) and morbidity (14.3%) in the bursectomy and nonbursectomy group. Kochi et al. [9], in their retrospective cohort study of 254 gastric cancer patients, found an overall incidence of surgery-related complications of 24% in the bursectomy group and 25.6% in the nonbursectomy group.

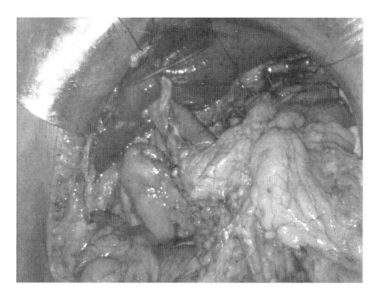

Figure 8. The surgical field after completion of bursectomy.

Among various adverse events of bursectomy, the most feared cause of morbidity is a leak from an injury site to the anterior surface of the pancreas with consequent development of a pancreatic fistula and its associated complications. Another concern is the possibility of adhesions formation to the skeletonized mesocolon and pancreas, which may cause specific local symptoms, such as delayed gastric emptying, afferent loop syndrome, or intestinal obstruction. In our series [6], pancreatic fistula was observed in three patients (4.2%). Kung et al. [10] reported that bursectomy is not a risk factor for postoperative pancreatic fistula among 83 gastric cancer patients submitted to D2 gastrectomy. The low incidence of pancreatic fistula that we reported, in combination with the 2.9% incidence of pancreatic fistula reported by Imamura et al. [7], suggest that resection of the pancreatic capsule can rarely induce injury to the pancreas. Moreover, in our study [6], eight patients (11.1%) suffered from bowel obstruction including two cases of delayed gastric emptying, one case of afferent loop syndrome, one case of early postoperative adhesions and four cases of prolonged postoperative ileus. According to our opinion, the high incidence of bowel obstruction that we reported is suggestive of an increased risk of adhesions formation to the skeletonized mesocolon and pancreas after D2 gastrectomy plus bursectomy; however, this finding is in contrast to the 4.8% incidence of such complications reported by Imamura et al. [7].

Does Bursectomy Provide Extended Lymphadenectomy?

When performed by experienced surgeons in high-volume centers, bursectomy has no impact on the extension of lymphadenectomy. Fujita et al. [8], reported that the total number of dissected lymph nodes were similar in the two groups, with a median of 38 (range 11-98) in the bursectomy group and 37 (range 7-97) in the non-bursectomy group. Even those lymph nodes dissected in the operative field of bursectomy, such as No 6, 14v and 8a LNs, were similar in the two groups. However, the lymphatic stream of the stomach is complicated and multidirectional. While operating in the surgical field of omental bursectomy, LNs along various anastomotic lymphatic channels, such as channels crossing the pancreatic surface toward the colonic vasculature and the gastrocolic trunk (Figure 9) are aesthetically dissected in the correct surgical plane. Consequently, bursectomy provides not only complete dissection of LNs along the standard LNs stations, but also provides dissection of LNs along their anastomotic channels.

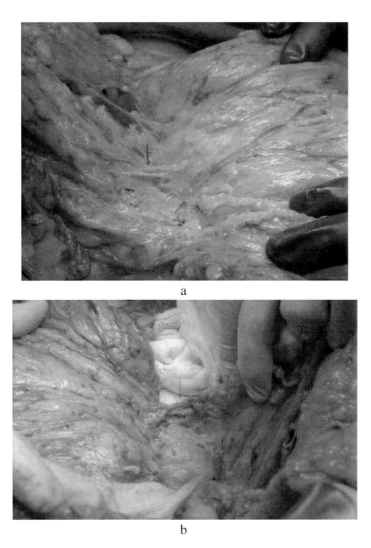

Figure 9. (a) Anastomotic channels originating from the right gastroepiploic, the left gastroepiploic artery, the posterior gastric artery and crossing the pancreatic surface towards the middle colic vessels can be seen (black arrow), (b) the gastrocolic trunk (arrow), a very constant structure connecting the right gastroepiploic vein and the superior mesenteric vein can be seen; after division of the accessory right colic vein, the superior mesenteric vein (No. 14v) can be easily reached with minimal dissection. Bursectomy provides not only complete dissection of LNs along the standard LNs stations, but also

provides dissection of LNs along their anastomotic channels, which is very important for an aesthetic lymph node dissection.

Although no confirmatory data exist supporting survival benefit of dissecting the above LNs stations, I still routinely perform bursectomy as a standard step in extended surgery for gastric cancer in order to achieve an aesthetic clean.

Does Bursectomy Reduce Peritoneal Recurrence?

It is generally accepted that peritoneal metastasis is completed by implantation of peritoneal free cancer cells exfoliated from serosa-invasive tumors through the process of fixation and progression of cancer cells on the peritoneum. The situation of CY+/P- could possibly mean a condition where the implantation of cancer cells to the peritoneal wall has not yet occurred; therefore, it is thought that there are apparent differences between the condition of CY+/P- and peritoneal metastasis. From this point of view, the situation of CY+/P- might be the last opportunity for the surgeons to undertake some countermeasures for the peritoneal metastasis [11]. Bursectomy is suggested as a standard prophylactic technique to achieve elimination of tumor deposits in the lesser sac for tumors penetrating the serosa of the posterior gastric wall. However, there are few reports which studied the efficacy of bursectomy for reduction of peritoneal recurrence.

Yamamura et al. [12] performed RT-PCR analysis of the peritoneal washes obtained from the Douglas pouch, left subphrenic cavity, and inside the omental bursa for 136 patients who underwent potentially curative surgery for gastric cancer. In 14 patients, CEA or CK20 mRNA were detected in samples obtained from the bursa omentalis (32.6% of patients with positive RT-PCR results). In 12 of these 14 patients, the mRNAs were also detected in samples taken from either or both of the remaining two sites. In the 2 other patients, only the samples obtained from the inside the omental bursa was positive for CEA. The authors concluded that it is unlike that viable cancer cells disseminated into the bursa remain restricted to this cavity without migrating into the free abdominal cavity, and that routine bursectomy may not be an essential procedure for resecting gastric cancer, from the viewpoint of eliminating microscopic peritoneal deposits within the omental bursa.

Zhao et al. [13] performed RT-PCR for tumor detection in pancreatic capsule samples collected from 83 patients who underwent radical gastrectomy for gastric cancer. RT-PCR detected CK20 mRNAs in 42 patients (50.6%). Metastasis in the pancreatic capsule was correlated mainly with the invasive serous membrane, lymph node metastasis and tumor stage. The authors concluded that for T1 and T2 stage, there was no evidence of pancreatic capsule metastasis, which may facilitate the decision making of the pancreatic capsule resection; however the number of cases with T3 and T4 cancer were few and therefore conclusions cannot be withdrawn.

Yoshikawa et al. [14], studied 134 serosa-positive pT4 patients submitted to D2 gastrectomy plus bursectomy; these patients were divided into patients with tumors invaded only the posterior wall, and patients with serosa-positive tumors in other locations. Based on the results on tumor recurrence, the authors concluded that bursectomy did not inhibit spreading of tumor cells into the retro-stomach space. Fujita et al. [8], in their randomized controlled trial of 210 patients with gastric adenocarcinoma submitted to D2 gastrectomy, reported a decreased frequency of peritoneal recurrence in the bursectomy group, although not statistical significant; 9 patients (8.7%) in the bursectomy group and 14 patients (13.2%) in the non-bursectomy group developed peritoneal recurrence, with an 11% overall incidence of peritoneal recurrence. Fujita et al. concluded that the non-statistical significant difference in the frequency of peritoneal metastasis and survival benefit were attributed to the en-bloc removal of free cancer cells or micrometastases contained in the bursa omentalis and not to the more accurate lymphadenectomy.

Does Bursectomy Offer a Better Survival Benefit?

There is little evidence that bursectomy has some clinical benefit. Yoshikawa et al. [14], in their retrospective study of 134 patients with T3-4 serosa-positive tumors who underwent curative D2 total gastrectomy found no survival benefit for bursectomy. Kochi et al. [9] in their retrospective study of 254 T2-4 gastric cancer patients reported no survival benefit for bursectomy plus D2 gastrectomy over D2 gastrectomy alone. Fujita et al., in their randomized controlled trial of 210 patients with T2-T4 gastric adenocarcinoma, found a survival benefit for bursectomy, although not statistically significant, among 48 patients with T3-4 serosa-positive tumors. The authors of the above article concluded that bursectomy should not be abandoned as a futile procedure until more definitive data can be obtained. The Japan Clinical Oncology Group is now embarking on a 1000 patient multi-institutional randomized controlled trial (JCOG 1001) of D2 gastrectomy plus bursectomy versus D2 gastrectomy without bursectomy among cT3 and cT4 cases [15]. Indeed, the Japanese gastric cancer treatment guidelines refer to the JCOG 1001 as a clinical trial that will prospectively provide more definitive data regarding this issue.

Chapter reviewed by Botsios D. MD, PhD, Professor of Surgery, Medical School, Aristotle University of Thessaloniki, Thessaloniki, Greece and Anestis Hatzigeorgiadis MD, MSc - Chairman - Department of General Surgery, General Hospital of Drama, Drama, Greece.

References

[1]   Hundahl SA (2012) The potential value of bursectomy in operations for trans-serosal gastric adenocarcinoma. *Gastric Cancer* 15:3-4.

[2]   Kurokawa Y, Fujiwara Y, Takiguchi S, et al. (2011) Randomized controlled trial of omental bursectomy for resectable cT2-3 gastric cancer. *J. Clin. Oncol.* (Meeting Abstracts) 29(4_suppl):72.

[3]   Japanese Gastric Cancer Association (2011) Japanese gastric cancer treatment guidelines (ver. 3). *Gastric Cancer* 14:113-123.

[4]   Skandalakis JE, Colborn GL, Weidman TA, et al. (2004) Skandalakis' Surgical Anatomy. AccessSurgery. http://accesssurgery.com/resourceToc.aspx?resourceID= 203. Accessed 16 June 2012

[5] Blouhos K, Boulas KA, Hatzigeorgiadis A. (2013) Making omental bursectomy, a routine in extended gastrectomy; a step-by-step guide. *Hellenic Journal of Surgery* 85:269-273.

[6] Blouhos K, Boulas KA, Hatzigeorgiadis A (2013) Bursectomy in gastric cancer surgery: surgical technique and operative safety. *Updates Surg.* 65:95-101.

[7] Imamura H, Kurokawa Y, Kawada J, et al. (2011) Influence of bursectomy on operative morbidity and mortality after radical gastrectomy for gastric cancer: results of a randomized controlled trial. *World J. Surg.* 35:625-630.

[8] Fujita J, Kurokawa Y, Sugimoto T, et al. (2012) Survival benefit of bursectomy in patients with resectable gastric cancer: interim analysis results of a randomized controlled trial. *Gastric Cancer* 15:42-48.

[9] Kochi M, Fujii M, Kanamori N, et al. (2012) D2 Gastrectomy With Versus Without Bursectomy for Gastric Cancer. *Am. J. Clin. Oncol.* [Epub ahead of print].

[10] Kung CH, Lindblad M, Nilsson M, et al. (2013) Postoperative pancreatic fistula formation according to ISGPF criteria after D2 gastrectomy in Western patients. *Gastric Cancer* [Epub ahead of print].

[11] Ikeshima S, Kuramoto M, Shimada S, et al. (2013) Standard Prophylactic Strategy against Peritoneal Dissemination Metastasis in Gastric Cancer. *Journal of Cancer Therapy* 4:99-103.

[12] Yamamura Y, Ito S, Mochizuki Y, et al. (2007) Distribution of free cancer cells in the abdominal cavity suggests limitation of bursectomy as an essential component of radical surgery for gastric carcinoma. *Gastric Cancer* 10:24-28.

[13] Zhao L, Wang Z, Xu J, et al. (2012) Radical distal gastrectomy in laparoscopic and open surgery: is it necessary for pancreatic capsule resection? *Hepatogastroenterology* 59:616-619.

[14] Yoshikawa T, Tsuburaya A, Kobayashi O, et al. (2004) Is bursectomy necessary for patients with gastric cancer invading the serosa? *Hepatogastroenterology* 51:1524-1526.

[15] Lee JH, Kim KM, Cheong JH, Noh SH (2012) Current management and future strategies of gastric cancer. *Yonsei Med. J.* 53:248-257.

Index

#

20th century, 8
21st century, 25

A

Abraham, v, 57
access, x, 8, 110, 179, 186, 193, 195, 196
accountability, 8
acetic acid, 115
acid, 27, 54, 104, 109, 112, 121
AD, 53, 138, 153
adenoma, 96, 115, 118
adhesion(s), 4, 31, 40, 131, 132, 195, 198, 199, 203
adjustment, 4
adjuvant treatment, viii, ix, 24, 38, 40, 141, 143, 144, 146, 147, 148, 149, 151, 155, 167, 184
adrenaline, 104, 106
adults, 112
advancements, vii, 71, 137
adverse event, 150, 203
aesthetic, x, 195, 196, 204, 205
Africa, 7
age, 2, 3, 4, 6, 7, 11, 27, 31, 33, 128, 159, 161, 172
aggressive behavior, 3, 16
AJCC, vii, ix, 2, 4, 11, 33, 34, 50, 58, 60, 61, 62, 64, 79, 81, 171, 174, 175, 181, 187, 188
algorithm, 79, 183
allergy, 110, 127
alopecia, 42
American Joint Committee on Cancer, vii, 2, 11, 33, 51, 58, 81, 82, 152, 187, 188
amines, 6
ammonia, 7
anaphylaxis, 65
anastomosis, 35, 147, 149, 189

anatomic site, 129
anatomy, 135
anemia, 27
angiogenesis, viii, 24, 46, 99
annotation, 111
anorexia, 145, 173
anthracycline, viii, 24
antibiotic, 94
antibody, 18, 93, 114, 136, 140
anti-cancer, 42, 43
anticancer drug, 138, 153
anticoagulant, 110
antigen, 40, 112, 113
antigen-presenting cell, 40
antitumor, 135, 136, 137
antrum, 7, 25, 66, 132, 134, 172, 177, 189
aorta, 197
APC, 31, 106
aplasia, 126
apoptosis, 4
arabinoside, 152
Aristotle, 195, 206
arteries, 201
artery, 35, 109, 200, 201, 202, 204
ARTIST, ix, 12, 14, 21, 38, 39, 52, 142, 150, 155
asbestos, 6
ascites, 61, 65, 67, 72, 73, 74, 75, 136
Asia, 1, 2, 6, 12, 35, 40, 42, 50, 64, 116, 141, 155
Asian countries, vii, 1, 6, 11
Asian patients, vii, 1, 14, 153
aspiration, 77, 110
assessment, 5, 34, 60, 71, 74, 76, 77, 79, 85, 96, 100, 104, 116, 168, 174, 181, 183, 190, 191
asthma, 110
asymptomatic, 17, 32, 74, 84
atrophy, 7, 18, 93, 116
attachment, 197
audits, 10

autoflourescent endoscopy, viii, 90
autosomal dominant, 4, 31
avoidance, 82, 132

B

barium, 32, 33, 92
basal layer, 104
base, 199, 200
basement membrane, 58
behaviors, 5
beneficial effect, 150
benefits, viii, 37, 57, 78, 146, 148
benign, 5, 32, 67, 74, 85
bias, 5, 71
bile, 178
biomarkers, 47, 128, 147
biopsy, viii, ix, 5, 33, 50, 57, 74, 77, 79, 80, 87, 92, 95, 96, 97, 101, 102, 105, 109, 111, 112, 116, 119, 122, 157, 158, 159, 161, 162, 166, 168, 169, 173
bismuth, 94
bladder cancer, 140
bleeding, 24, 47, 101, 107, 108, 109, 120, 132
blood, 99, 107, 108, 110, 131, 132, 135, 183, 184, 202
blood flow, 132
blood pressure, 110
blood supply, 108, 135
blood vessels, 99, 107, 108
body mass index (BMI), 5, 27, 161, 164, 166
body weight, 127
bone, 128
bowel, 72, 75, 133, 195, 202, 203
bowel obstruction, 195, 202, 203
bowel perforation, 133
brain, 68
breast cancer, 4, 9, 27, 29, 31, 43, 79, 135, 136, 140, 158, 166, 167, 169
breast carcinoma, 29
breathing, 72, 109, 110
Britain, 7, 154
burn, 106
bursa, 131, 200, 201, 202, 205, 206
bursectomy, x, 195, 196, 197, 198, 202, 203, 205, 206, 207

C

caliber, 99, 119
cancer care, 8, 9, 10, 11, 13, 18, 19

cancer cells, 68, 78, 79, 86, 102, 104, 130, 131, 139, 172, 205, 206, 207
cancer death, 172
cancer progression, 135
cancer screening, 50, 84, 114
cancer therapy, 135, 171
candidates, 42, 76, 77
capecitabine, viii, ix, 12, 21, 24, 38, 39, 40, 41, 42, 45, 52, 53, 55, 141, 142, 145, 147, 149, 150, 151, 154, 155, 186
capillary, 62, 63, 92, 99
capsule, 200, 201, 202, 203, 205, 207
carcinoembryonic antigen, 80, 86, 129, 130
carcinogen, 6, 93
carcinogenesis, ix, 7, 49, 125, 139
carcinoid tumor, 120
carcinoma, viii, 3, 5, 16, 17, 18, 20, 31, 32, 49, 50, 68, 72, 81, 82, 84, 85, 86, 87, 90, 95, 96, 101, 112, 116, 129, 132, 134, 137, 140, 152, 154, 161, 162, 167, 168, 176, 180, 187, 188, 189, 190, 191, 192, 193, 207
categorization, 174
catheter, 110, 132, 134
cauterization, 103, 109, 139
cecum, 127
cell biology, 4
cell culture, 136
cell line(s), 28, 127, 128, 129, 132, 135, 136, 137, 138
Central Asia, 90
chemical, 112, 126
chemical properties, 112
chemoprevention, 125, 127, 139
chemoradiation, viii, 24, 37, 40, 52, 55, 148, 149, 150, 151, 155, 184, 185
chemoradiotherapy, ix, 12, 21, 47, 52, 78, 141, 142, 146, 148, 149, 150, 151, 155, 156, 184
chemotherapeutic agent, 43, 132, 136
children, 18
Chile, 32
China, 2, 6, 7, 10, 13, 14, 16, 18, 20, 25, 49, 89, 93, 94, 103, 172
chromoscopy, viii, 90, 117
chromosomal instability, 7
cigarette smoking, 6
cisplatin, ix, 12, 14, 20, 21, 38, 39, 41, 42, 43, 44, 45, 52, 53, 54, 55, 142, 144, 149, 151, 152, 153, 154, 155, 186, 187, 192, 193
citizens, 2, 7
City, 89
classification, vii, ix, 1, 3, 16, 26, 28, 48, 51, 58, 60, 62, 63, 64, 81, 94, 95, 96, 100, 111, 114, 116,

117, 118, 159, 165, 168, 171, 174, 175, 176, 179, 181, 186, 187, 188, 191
clinical application, 87, 183
clinical diagnosis, 101, 108
clinical oncology, 19
clinical presentation, 2, 16, 131
clinical symptoms, 91
clinical trials, 10, 39, 41, 46, 126, 127, 139, 148, 183, 185, 202
clone, 161
closure, 122
clusters, 102
coal, 27
cognition, 110
colic, 199, 204
collagen, 129, 134
colon, 9, 59, 73, 114, 115, 117, 119, 126, 130, 132, 133, 135, 138, 139, 140, 172, 173, 180, 197, 198, 199
colon cancer, 9, 117, 126, 132, 133, 135, 138, 139, 140, 172
colon polyps, 117
color, 92, 94, 97, 101, 102, 114
colorectal cancer, 9, 10, 50, 83, 117, 134, 139, 168
combination therapy, 136
communication, 110
community(s), 9, 102
comparative analysis, 51, 187, 188
complexity, 34, 51, 57
compliance, 8, 9, 10
complications, 5, 16, 35, 79, 104, 107, 108, 110, 121, 127, 142, 145, 158, 179, 189, 202, 203
composition, 2
compounds, 127, 128
computed tomography, viii, 34, 57, 65, 85, 118, 190
computer, ix, 157, 158, 159, 163, 164, 165, 167, 168, 169
concordance, 161
conditioning, 128
confounding variables, 4
Congo, 117
Congress, 67, 82, 152, 169
connective tissue, 59
consensus, 10, 29, 32, 50, 77, 93, 94, 116
conservation, 80
consumers, 8
consumption, 7, 172
contact time, 134
contamination, 184
control group, 133
controlled trials, 11, 12, 94, 181
controversial, 2, 12, 30, 32, 34, 69, 158, 166
controversies, vii, viii, 24

cooperation, 110
coordination, 8
correlation, viii, 5, 6, 7, 29, 57, 61, 83, 84, 85, 112, 118, 130, 140, 154, 164, 168, 174, 181, 187
cost, 2, 7, 8, 33
Costa Rica, 7, 18, 25
counseling, 9
creep, 95
criticism, 12, 185
CT, 24, 34, 39, 46, 65, 66, 67, 68, 69, 70, 71, 72, 73, 83, 84, 85, 93, 94, 102, 118, 150, 168, 173, 183
CT scan, 65, 67, 68, 69, 70, 71, 93, 102, 173, 183
culture, 128
cure, viii, 23, 35, 90, 96, 102, 126
cycles, 38, 44, 145, 148, 150, 151, 186
cytology, viii, 57, 64, 78, 79, 86, 122, 191
cytotoxicity, 136, 138

D

damages, 150
data analysis, 114
database, 4, 15, 48, 81, 128, 158, 181, 190
death rate, 2, 11, 36, 90, 141, 143, 158, 165
deaths, vii, 2, 25, 90, 142, 171, 172
deficiency(s), 31, 126
delayed gastric emptying, 203
dendritic cell, 40
Denmark, 10, 19, 161
deposits, x, 195, 196, 202, 205
depression, 94, 95, 110
depth, viii, 5, 33, 34, 51, 58, 62, 63, 64, 68, 75, 76, 77, 90, 92, 100, 101, 102, 104, 111, 112, 159, 161, 165, 168, 174
derivatives, 41
dermatology, 127
detectable, 71, 104, 113, 173
detection, ix, 10, 24, 32, 33, 65, 68, 69, 72, 74, 79, 83, 85, 86, 90, 91, 92, 101, 112, 113, 115, 116, 117, 118, 119, 158, 163, 164, 165, 166, 168, 169, 183, 205
developed countries, 25, 90, 172
developing countries, 90, 91
diabetes, 110, 127
diagnostic criteria, 16, 96, 116
diaphragm, 72, 76, 77
diarrhea, 41, 42, 150
diet, vii, 1, 6, 9, 27, 29, 32, 125
dietary habits, vii, 23, 32, 135
differential diagnosis, 115, 118
diffusion, 179
digestion, 127, 134
dilation, 109

discomfort, 129
disease model, 125
disease progression, 42, 44, 145
diseases, 17, 25, 34, 85, 90, 96, 101, 143
distribution, 1, 2, 25
DNA, 8, 28, 40
docetaxel, 40, 41, 42, 43, 54, 137, 188
doctors, 101
DOI, 95
dosage, 133
downsizing, 184
drainage, 80, 142, 160, 199
drinking water, 27, 30
drug discovery, 127
drug resistance, 93, 127
drugs, 43, 94, 110, 127, 135, 137
duodenum, 3, 74, 197, 200
dyeing, viii, 90
dysplasia, 5, 18, 29, 96, 97, 104, 111, 117, 126

E

East Asia, 12, 37, 103, 173, 178
Eastern Europe, 90, 166, 172
E-cadherin, 4, 16, 27, 31, 50
edema, 72
electrocautery, 107, 108, 134
ELISA, 113
e-mail, 141
emission, 68
endocrinology, 127
endomicroscopy, viii, 90, 92, 101, 119
endoscope, viii, 90, 95, 99, 103, 104, 105, 120, 135
endoscopic diagnosis, viii, 90, 114, 117
endoscopic mucosal resection, viii, 5, 23, 47, 103, 114, 115, 119, 120, 121, 122, 135
endoscopic ultrasound, viii, 8, 34, 57, 65, 69, 71, 74, 85, 90, 118, 119, 173
endoscopy, viii, 33, 34, 50, 51, 74, 75, 83, 84, 85, 90, 91, 92, 93, 96, 97, 98, 99, 102, 103, 104, 115, 116, 117, 118, 173
energy, 68
enlargement, 183
enrollment, 65, 141
environment, 2, 8, 102, 112
environmental factors, 7
environmental influences, 15
enzyme(s), 113, 137, 193
enzyme-linked immunosorbent assay, 113, 193
epidemic, 32
epidemiologic, 7, 146
epidemiologic studies, 7
epidemiology, vii, 2, 25, 26, 49, 127, 137

epinephrine, 104, 105, 106, 107
epithelia, 99
epithelial cells, 102
epithelium, 97, 99
Epstein-Barr virus, 6
equipment, 103, 104
erosion, 94, 95, 134
ESD, ix, 90, 102, 103, 104, 105, 106, 107, 108, 109, 110, 111, 116, 119, 120, 121
esophageal cancer, 2, 12, 25, 34, 38, 105, 119, 188, 190
esophagitis, 179
esophagogastroduodenoscopy, viii, 57, 65, 74, 85
esophagus, 2, 5, 25, 30, 35, 48, 58, 74, 114, 117, 120, 122, 126, 135, 137, 145, 172, 175, 176, 179, 186
ethnicity, 15
etiology, 1, 6, 78, 91
Europe, 2, 5, 6, 7, 8, 10, 11, 13, 16, 25, 33, 36, 39, 40, 42, 143, 146, 147, 173, 184, 185, 188
evidence, 7, 8, 11, 47, 50, 58, 59, 61, 62, 65, 69, 77, 78, 128, 135, 147, 180, 184, 188, 196, 202, 205, 206
evolution, 11, 64
examinations, 60, 118, 161
excision, 112, 168, 171
exclusion, 159
expertise, 24, 35, 47
exposure, 6, 27, 31, 32, 65
extracellular matrix, 129, 134

F

false negative, 80, 92, 157, 164, 165, 166
false positive, 165
families, 4
family history, 6, 31, 33, 92
family members, 110
fasting, 109, 110
fat, 65, 71, 75, 133
F-FDG PET, 84
fibrinogen, 120
fibroblast growth factor, 129
fibrosis, 101
fibrous cap, 131
financial, 90
first degree relative, 31
first generation, 98
fish, 30
fixation, 111, 205
flank, 129
flex, 35
fluid, 104, 121

Index

fluorescence, 44, 101, 102, 119, 169, 193
fluorine, 187
Fluorodeoxyglucose-positron emission tomography, viii
fluoropyramidine, viii, 24
food, 6, 7
formaldehyde, 111
formation, 3, 6, 27, 131, 195, 203, 207
fovea, 99
France, 17, 48, 117, 151, 159
fructose, 104, 105, 106
fruits, 6

G

gadolinium, 83
gamma rays, 68
gastric cancer research, vii, 126
gastric lavage, 133
gastric mucosa, 7, 18, 29, 51, 92, 93, 97, 98, 116, 121, 122, 132, 134, 143, 172
gastric ulcer, 6, 30, 118, 120
gastrin, 30
gastritis, 3, 6, 7, 17, 27, 30, 33, 91, 98, 114, 123, 126, 172, 178, 179
gastroesophageal reflux, 178
gastrointestinal bleeding, 173
gastrointestinal tract, 84, 101, 103, 119, 122, 128, 133, 145
gel, 129, 134
gene amplification, 136
gene regulation, 127
genes, 31, 128, 193
genetic background, 128
genetic mutations, 7
genetic predisposition, 32
genetic syndromes, vii, 23, 33
genetic testing, 31
genetics, 127, 154
geography, 31
Germany, 166
gland, 3, 27, 28, 99, 200
glucose, 68, 83, 84
glue, 131, 132, 139
GLUT, 68
glutathione, 53
glycerin, 106, 121
glycerol, 104, 105, 109
Great Britain, 19, 67
Greece, 195, 206
growth, ix, 4, 12, 16, 27, 28, 46, 54, 62, 63, 68, 127, 128, 129, 130, 131, 132, 135, 136, 137, 139, 142, 147, 173, 185

growth factor, ix, 4, 12, 16, 46, 54, 135, 142, 147, 185
growth rate, 129
guidance, 38, 93, 100
guidelines, x, 8, 9, 10, 20, 35, 50, 51, 65, 67, 69, 72, 74, 77, 78, 79, 86, 114, 116, 119, 142, 176, 191, 195, 196, 206

H

H. pylori, vii, 3, 6, 7, 15, 18, 23, 29, 33, 91, 93, 94
Hawaii, 17
hazards, 6
HDAC, 193
HE, 161
healing, 109, 118, 120
health, 8, 10, 127, 141, 142, 151
health care, 8
health care system, 9
heart rate, 110
height, 99
Helicobacter pylori, vii, viii, 1, 3, 6, 17, 18, 24, 25, 49, 90, 91, 114, 116, 123, 126, 172
hematemesis, 108, 110
hemisphere, 41
hemoglobin, 102
hemorrhage, 56, 108
hemostasis, 109
heterogeneity, 67, 144
high risk patients, 171
high-risk populations, 91
histochemistry, 136
histogenesis, 3
histologic subtype, vii, 1
histological examination, 87, 93
histology, vii, viii, ix, 1, 3, 5, 16, 23, 28, 41, 122, 142, 158, 159, 172, 182
history, 6, 27, 33, 86, 110, 168, 172
HM, 18, 55
host, 7, 128
housing, 127, 129
human, ix, 6, 12, 43, 49, 54, 125, 126, 127, 128, 129, 130, 131, 132, 133, 135, 136, 137, 138, 139, 140, 142, 147
Hungary, 157, 159, 168
hybrid, 40
hydrogen, 106
hypermethylation, 123
hyperplasia, 93, 97, 102
hypersensitivity, 72
hypertension, 110
hypertonic saline, 105, 106
hypothesis, 5, 82, 128, 149, 152

I

iatrogenic, 121
ideal, 76, 102, 112, 131
identification, 72, 76, 77, 78, 79, 80, 101, 103, 113, 116, 131, 172, 180
image(s), 29, 49, 65, 67, 70, 71, 72, 73, 75, 78, 92, 98, 99, 101, 102
image analysis, 29, 49
imaging modalities, 67, 71, 137
immigrants, 186
immigration, 33
immune reaction, 29
immunocompromised, 130
immunoglobulins, 126
immunohistochemistry, 29, 112, 161, 193
immunotherapy, 126
improvements, 34, 78, 171
in situ hybridization, 44, 136, 193
in vitro, 28, 85, 127, 136, 137, 138, 139
in vivo, ix, 71, 119, 125, 132, 136, 137, 139, 187
incidence, vii, viii, 1, 2, 3, 5, 6, 7, 9, 10, 15, 23, 25, 29, 30, 31, 32, 33, 37, 42, 47, 67, 89, 90, 91, 93, 126, 138, 141, 142, 145, 158, 172, 173, 178, 179, 186, 189, 202, 203, 205
individuals, 32, 33, 84, 91, 126
INF, 63
infection, 3, 6, 7, 17, 18, 27, 29, 32, 49, 91, 93, 123, 126, 172, 180
inferior vena cava, 197
inferiority, 35, 41, 145
inflammation, 3, 7, 18, 72, 114
information technology, 8
infrared endoscopy, viii, 90
inheritance, 31
inhibition, 136
inhibitor, 46, 118, 120, 145
inhomogeneity, 102
injury, 109, 133, 134, 135, 203
inoculation, 128, 130
insertion, 134
institutions, 8, 10, 11, 60
interference, 75
intestinal obstruction, 203
intestine, 139
investment, 10
iodine, 65
ionizing radiation, 65, 70, 72
Ireland, 19, 67
irradiation, 55, 154
isotope, 68
issues, ix, 36, 171, 178
Italy, 10, 171, 180, 188

K

kidney, 128
kill, 184
Korea, 1, 2, 3, 6, 7, 10, 11, 12, 13, 14, 15, 19, 20, 25, 33, 39, 50, 93, 103, 108, 122, 142, 146, 174

L

labeling, 166
laparoscopic surgery, 77
laparoscopy, viii, ix, 57, 65, 76, 77, 78, 79, 86, 171, 173, 183, 187, 191, 192
laparotomy, 35, 58, 77, 78, 82, 108, 159, 176, 179
large intestine, 58
lead, 5, 29, 58, 65, 80, 91, 127, 181
learning, 80, 143
legs, 110
leiomyoma, 122
lesions, 2, 5, 15, 17, 18, 34, 50, 58, 59, 61, 62, 64, 71, 72, 75, 76, 91, 92, 95, 96, 97, 99, 101, 103, 104, 105, 106, 107, 109, 111, 114, 115, 117, 118, 119, 146, 148, 174, 176, 178
LIFE, 102
lifetime, 4
ligament, 85, 201
ligand, 4
light, 29, 49, 92, 96, 98, 102, 144, 147, 148
liver, 3, 61, 65, 66, 67, 69, 71, 72, 74, 75, 77, 130, 131, 135, 173, 180, 183
liver metastases, 61, 65, 66, 69, 74, 75
localization, 130, 159, 177, 179, 181
lockjaw, 110
lumen, 99, 106, 109, 112
luminescence, 113
lung cancer, 43
lung disease, 110
lung metastases, 67
lying, 196, 199
lymph node involvement, ix, 3, 33, 34, 91, 150, 151, 157, 158, 159, 163, 165, 167, 168
lymphadenopathy, 67, 85, 100
lymphatic system, 61, 82
lymphoid, 6, 7
lymphoid tissue, 7
lymphoma, 17

M

magnetic resonance, viii, 57, 65, 84
magnetic resonance imaging, viii, 57, 65, 84
majority, 79, 108, 148

Index

malabsorption, 117

malignancy, vii, 1, 2, 10, 38, 67, 74, 89, 126, 128, 172

malignant cells, 58

malignant melanoma, 158, 168

malignant tissues, 102

man, 129

management, viii, ix, 17, 19, 20, 35, 40, 50, 65, 69, 70, 77, 78, 79, 80, 82, 83, 85, 86, 90, 91, 92, 103, 105, 110, 111, 112, 115, 121, 122, 146, 171, 179, 181, 183, 185, 186, 188, 191, 207

manipulation, 131, 132, 200

mapping, ix, 80, 87, 157, 158, 160, 161, 164, 165, 166, 167, 168, 169

Maruyama computer program, ix, 157, 158, 159, 163, 164, 167, 168

mass, 5, 32, 48, 61, 63, 71, 75, 114, 161, 186

materials, 72, 104, 112

matter, 179

MB, 15, 18, 116, 117, 120

MCP, ix, 157, 159, 161, 162, 163, 164, 165, 166

media, 9, 129

median, 3, 37, 40, 41, 58, 78, 79, 130, 144, 145, 148, 149, 173, 180, 186, 202, 203

medical, 6, 9, 10, 11, 19, 20, 184

medicine, 15, 17

melanoma, 79, 139

melena, 108, 110

membranes, 136

meta-analysis, 7, 11, 12, 21, 29, 40, 43, 48, 49, 53, 54, 67, 81, 83, 84, 85, 100, 101, 114, 118, 120, 138, 139, 144, 146, 153, 154, 158, 165, 183, 189, 192

Metabolic, 28

metabolism, 68, 137

metabolites, 7, 40

metabolized, 68

metastases to the liver, 67

metastasis, viii, 3, 5, 20, 28, 35, 38, 58, 69, 78, 80, 83, 84, 87, 89, 91, 92, 103, 104, 113, 119, 127, 128, 129, 130, 131, 132, 133, 134, 135, 139, 147, 150, 151, 159, 161, 163, 165, 168, 175, 182, 186, 188, 205, 206

metastatic disease, viii, 24, 47, 61, 65, 67, 74, 77, 183

methylation, 8, 113

methylene blue, 117

mice, 125, 126, 127, 128, 129, 130, 131, 132, 133, 134, 135, 136, 138, 139

microscopy, 29, 49, 101, 161

migration, 4, 60, 143

miniature, 75

misunderstanding, 186

models, ix, 125, 126, 127, 128, 129, 130, 131, 132, 135, 136, 137, 138, 139, 140

modifications, 120

molecular pathology, 16, 48

molecules, 31

Mongolia, 2

monoclonal antibody, 12, 40, 43

Moon, 120, 121, 122

morbidity, ix, x, 11, 12, 13, 15, 36, 52, 78, 143, 149, 157, 158, 165, 167, 178, 179, 180, 181, 182, 183, 185, 188, 189, 190, 191, 195, 196, 202, 203, 207

morphology, 68, 71, 92, 94, 106, 127, 135

mortality, viii, ix, x, 9, 11, 12, 13, 15, 18, 25, 35, 36, 52, 65, 78, 82, 89, 90, 91, 93, 126, 131, 142, 144, 148, 152, 157, 158, 165, 172, 178, 179, 180, 181, 183, 185, 188, 189, 192, 195, 196, 202, 207

mortality rate, viii, x, 25, 52, 90, 91, 93, 126, 165, 179, 180, 188, 196, 202

mosaic, 8

MR, 35, 71, 72, 83, 84, 85

MRI, 65, 67, 69, 70, 71, 72, 73, 84, 93, 102

mRNA(s), 80, 136, 205

mucosa, viii, 3, 7, 18, 27, 35, 58, 59, 61, 63, 71, 90, 91, 93, 94, 95, 97, 98, 99, 100, 101, 102, 103, 106, 107, 109, 133, 135, 159

mucous membrane, 117

multiple factors, 15

multivariate, 4

multivariate analysis, 4, 167

murine models, ix, 125, 126, 128, 130, 132, 135, 137

mutagenesis, 126

mutant, 125

mutation(s), 4, 7, 27, 28, 31, 50, 113, 128

N

National Institutes of Health, 193

natural killer cell, 40

necrosis, 134

negativity, 158

nephropathy, 65

Netherlands, 10, 38

neural network, 165, 168

neurogenic shock, 109

neutral, 126

neutropenia, 41, 42, 150

nitrates, 6

nitroso compounds, 6

nodal involvement, 11, 60, 67, 168, 177, 180, 181, 185

nodes, 5, 35, 60, 64, 67, 74, 77, 79, 80, 81, 82, 85, 87, 142, 147, 148, 149, 151, 158, 159, 160, 162,

163, 164, 165, 166, 169, 173, 176, 181, 190, 195, 204
nodules, 94
North America, 7, 8, 16, 49
NSAIDs, 27
nucleolus, 102
nurses, 110

O

obesity, vii, 2, 5, 6, 16, 30, 32, 172
obstruction, 203
oesophageal, 21, 55, 82, 83, 85, 138, 154
ofloxacin, 94
OH, 89
omentum, x, 109, 195, 196, 198, 199
operations, 79, 206
opioids, 108
organ(s), 58, 69, 72, 76, 84, 100, 128, 130, 131, 132, 133, 147, 150, 159, 173, 175, 177, 180, 190
organism, 6
outreach, 94
ovaries, 67, 72, 77
overlap, 5
overtime, 134
oxaliplatin, viii, 12, 21, 24, 39, 40, 42, 43, 45, 53, 54, 55, 141, 145, 147, 154
oxygen, 110

P

p53, 113, 123, 154
Pacific, 15, 50, 116
paclitaxel, 40, 55
pain, 32, 47, 108, 110, 173
palliative, 24, 43, 47, 55, 65
pancreas, x, 56, 59, 66, 71, 84, 173, 178, 180, 195, 196, 197, 199, 200, 201, 202, 203
pancreatic cancer, 47
parallel, ix, 150, 158, 166, 167, 202
participants, 29, 178
pathogenesis, viii, ix, 6, 7, 15, 23, 25, 26, 30, 48, 125, 126, 127, 172
pathogens, 172
pathologist, 193
pathology, vii, viii, 1, 5, 12, 16, 18, 25, 48, 57, 58, 111, 114, 121, 127, 151
pathophysiological, 102
patient care, vii, 82
PCR, 80, 205
pelvis, 61, 67, 68, 173
penetrance, 4, 31

pepsin, 112
pepsinogen, viii, 18, 33, 90, 92, 93, 114
peptic ulcer, 6, 30, 49
peptic ulcer disease, 6
perforation, 106, 108, 109, 110, 120, 121, 122, 134, 174
performance indicator, 161
peripheral neuropathy, 42
peristalsis, 70, 71, 110
peritoneal carcinomatosis, 3, 72, 173
peritoneal cavity, 58, 86, 173
peritoneal lavage, 79, 87
peritoneum, 40, 59, 132, 196, 199, 200, 205
peritonitis, 109
permit, 75
pernicious anemia, 6, 30, 33, 172
PET, 24, 34, 51, 65, 68, 69, 83, 84, 173, 187
PET scan, 34, 68, 69
pharmacokinetics, 145, 154
phenotypes, 159
Philadelphia, 49, 186
phosphorylation, 145
physicians, viii, 9, 57
pilot study, 145, 149
placebo, 15, 29, 55
platinum, viii, 24, 40, 41, 42, 43
PM, 19
polymerase, 80
polymerase chain reaction, 80
polymorphism, 27
polypectomy, 105
polyps, 6, 93, 120
pools, 3
population, 2, 5, 8, 10, 11, 16, 17, 29, 32, 33, 38, 47, 78, 81, 82, 86, 123, 127, 144, 146, 155, 184, 190, 191
positive correlation, 130
positron, viii, 34, 57, 65, 68, 83, 84, 173, 187
positron emission tomography, viii, 34, 57, 65, 83, 84, 173, 187
potassium, 154
predictive accuracy, 34, 51
pregnancy, 72
preparation, 93, 105
preservation, 180, 190
prevention, 8, 10, 29, 120, 121, 125, 127, 138, 181
primary tumor, 4, 39, 58, 59, 62, 64, 68, 78, 147, 171, 181
principles, ix, 171, 193
probability, 11, 157, 161, 165, 181
probe, 87

Index

prognosis, viii, 3, 4, 5, 11, 16, 23, 28, 31, 32, 51, 60, 79, 85, 86, 90, 91, 107, 140, 144, 158, 172, 177, 179, 184, 185, 187, 189
prolapse, 110
proliferation, 4, 30
promoter, 113, 123
propagation, 128
prophylactic, 79, 87, 180, 205
prophylaxis, 9
protection, 134
prothrombin, 110
proton pump inhibitors, 108, 109, 120
prototype, 126
PTEN, 31
public health, 7, 8, 10
pyloric stenosis, 109
pylorus, 109, 177

Q

quality improvement, 8
quality of life, 35, 90, 145, 151, 178, 179, 189
quality of service, 10
questionnaire, 120

R

race, 6, 31
radiation, 9, 10, 12, 13, 24, 27, 31, 37, 38, 39, 40, 46, 55, 56, 126, 143, 148, 149, 150, 151, 155, 156, 173
radiation therapy, 9, 13, 37, 38, 39, 56, 148, 150, 156, 173
radio, 79, 80
radiography, 33
radiotherapy, ix, x, 21, 24, 34, 38, 47, 52, 55, 83, 141, 142, 146, 147, 148, 149, 150, 154, 155, 156, 172, 191
ramucirumab, viii, 24, 40, 46, 47
randomized controlled clinical trials, 153
RE, 49, 50, 52, 81, 116, 190
reactions, 94
reactive oxygen, 7
reactivity, 126
reality, 118
receptors, 54
recognition, 115
recommendations, 38, 65, 79, 82, 146
reconstruction, 35, 83, 178, 179
recovery, 132
rectum, 117

recurrence, 4, 11, 13, 36, 40, 46, 78, 79, 83, 87, 103, 110, 135, 141, 143, 146, 147, 148, 149, 150, 151, 154, 176, 181, 182, 183, 184, 205
reflux esophagitis, 5, 179
registries, 2
regression, 7, 161, 192
regression model, 161
relapses, 146
relatives, 4, 31
relevance, 146, 152, 166
reliability, 132, 165
relief, 35
repair, 7
requirements, 9
researchers, ix, 125, 128
residual disease, 35, 38, 103, 147, 176
resistance, 94
resolution, 18, 65, 71, 72, 75, 78, 117
resources, ix, 9, 47, 125
respiration, 68, 70, 110
response, 14, 28, 41, 42, 45, 83, 127, 144, 145, 147, 149, 151, 172, 184, 185, 187, 191, 192, 193
RFS, 148
RH, 16, 116
risk(s), viii, ix, x, 2, 4, 6, 7, 17, 18, 23, 25, 27, 29, 30, 31, 32, 33, 43, 49, 53, 61, 67, 74, 79, 93, 94, 103, 104, 109, 110, 126, 137, 144, 146, 147, 151, 168, 172, 174, 176, 181, 182, 183, 184, 195, 196, 202, 203
risk factors, viii, ix, 2, 6, 23, 25, 32, 33, 49, 137
rodents, 126, 127, 128
room temperature, 111
routes, 3
rubber, 6, 27
rules, 16, 142, 151, 181, 190

S

safety, 35, 37, 103, 108, 122, 179, 183, 206
saturation, 110
scattering, 116
science, vii, 127
scope, 101, 137
screening program, viii, 2, 23, 93, 126
second degree relative, 4
secretion, 110
seeding, 131
sensation, 134
sensitivity, viii, ix, 33, 34, 57, 67, 68, 71, 72, 73, 74, 80, 100, 136, 140, 144, 157, 161, 163, 164, 165, 166
sentinel lymph node, viii, ix, 57, 87, 157, 158, 159, 160, 161, 162, 163, 164, 166, 168, 169

sequencing, 7
serum, viii, 7, 17, 18, 30, 33, 90, 92, 93, 112, 113, 114, 123, 129, 130, 134, 139
services, 9
sex, 128
shape, 67, 74, 83, 99
showing, 7, 66, 73, 94, 129, 133, 135, 159, 181
side effects, 117, 150
signal transduction, 4
signals, 44, 71
signal-to-noise ratio, 71
signs, 32, 35, 94, 110, 134
Singapore, 28
skin, 131
SLN, ix, 79, 80, 157, 158, 161, 162, 163, 164, 165, 166
SLN mapping, ix, 80, 157, 158, 161, 164, 165, 166
small intestine, 58
smoking, 6, 110
SNP, 27
socioeconomic status, 6, 31
sodium, 119
solid tumors, 158
solution, 104, 105, 106, 107, 109, 111, 129, 134
somatic mutations, 7, 31
South America, 7, 90, 172
South Korea, 10, 11, 15, 33, 39, 141, 146, 166, 172, 173, 186
Soviet Union, 25
SP, 19, 20, 25, 41, 52, 81, 122, 138, 153, 187, 188
Spain, 10
species, 126
sphincter, 74
spleen, 84, 173, 178, 180, 190
squamous cell, 121
SS, 81, 152, 186, 189, 191
staging modalities, viii, 57, 77, 78
staging system(s), vii, viii, 2, 11, 33, 34, 51, 57, 58, 60, 61, 62, 63, 172, 174, 175, 176, 181, 188
standardization, 65, 121
stasis, 178
state(s), 7, 8, 47, 69, 74, 79, 93, 110, 116
statistics, 17, 19, 20, 49, 114, 186
stem cells, 28
stenosis, 24, 47, 108, 179
stent, 24, 47
stomatitis, 150
stratification, 9, 34, 174, 176
strictures, 75, 109
stroma, 3, 63
structure, 199, 204
subcutaneous emphysema, 110
subcutaneous injection, 128

subcutaneous tissue, 129
subgroups, 43
submucosa, viii, 28, 58, 59, 61, 71, 90, 91, 96, 100, 102, 103, 104, 106, 107, 109, 173, 174
subtraction, 84
success rate, 132
Sun, 15, 153, 154, 188
suppression, 18
surface area, 63
surface structure, 98, 118
surgical resection, vii, ix, 1, 8, 9, 10, 12, 34, 35, 47, 58, 78, 90, 141, 190
surgical technique, 11, 15, 24, 36, 132, 143, 146, 173, 206
surveillance, 8, 50
survival rate, viii, 3, 5, 11, 12, 19, 34, 35, 38, 40, 42, 60, 90, 91, 104, 126, 142, 143, 145, 146, 148, 171, 174, 176, 178, 179, 182, 183, 185
survivors, 148
susceptibility, 139
suspensions, 131
suture, 131, 132
symptomatic treatment, 24, 47
symptoms, 32, 55, 110, 144, 173, 178, 203
syndrome, 27, 31, 150, 172, 178, 203
synergistic effect, 137, 144

T

T lymphocytes, 40
Taiwan, 40, 141, 143, 146
target, 46, 106, 128, 140, 149, 150, 185
taxane, 24, 42
teams, 9, 10
techniques, viii, 10, 24, 35, 37, 80, 87, 103, 114, 116, 121, 125, 126, 132, 149, 151, 156, 158, 165, 166
technological advancement, 70
technology(s), 34, 35, 65, 93, 98, 101, 102, 103, 126
temperature, 129, 134
testing, 31, 33, 40, 127, 132, 187
texture, 95
therapeutic approaches, ix, 142, 172
therapeutic use, 125
therapeutics, 127
therapy, vii, viii, 1, 8, 9, 10, 11, 12, 15, 18, 24, 29, 30, 37, 38, 39, 41, 42, 45, 46, 47, 49, 53, 54, 55, 65, 77, 79, 83, 93, 94, 98, 103, 116, 126, 144, 145, 148, 150, 153, 154, 158, 184, 185, 187, 193
thorax, 67, 173
thrombosis, 9
thymus, 126
tin, 87, 166

Index

tissue, 7, 63, 68, 70, 71, 72, 77, 92, 95, 106, 111, 118, 123, 129, 130, 131, 132, 135, 139
tissue plasminogen activator, 129, 135
toxic effect, 145
toxicity, 42, 45, 55, 127, 148, 149, 150, 151, 184
toxin, 7, 32
TP53, 28, 31, 50, 128
training, 75, 91, 167, 183
transcription, 80, 87
transformation, 93, 99
transforming growth factor, 129, 135
transplant, 132
transplantation, 128, 130, 131, 139
transverse colon, 71, 72, 197, 198, 199
tremor, 35
tumor cells, 3, 28, 31, 40, 68, 86, 102, 107, 128, 129, 130, 131, 132, 133, 134, 183, 184, 205
tumor depth, 34, 64, 65, 173
tumor development, 127, 130
tumor growth, 128, 129, 130, 131, 132, 133, 135, 136, 140
tumor invasion, viii, 33, 34, 51, 58, 62, 64, 76, 77, 89, 92, 168, 174, 180, 182
tumours, 85
Turkey, 141
tyrosine, 4, 185

U

UL, 104
ulcer, 17, 30, 91, 95, 101, 103, 120, 134
ultrasonography, 51, 83, 85, 92, 102, 118, 119, 165, 168
ultrasound, viii, 8, 34, 57, 65, 67, 69, 71, 72, 73, 74, 75, 85, 90, 118, 119, 173, 188
uniform, 10, 15
United Kingdom (UK), 10, 13, 40, 142, 146, 167, 185, 187
United States (USA), 2, 6, 7, 8, 9, 11, 16, 19, 20, 25, 35, 36, 40, 45, 49, 50, 55, 89, 125, 126, 127, 137, 141, 143, 146, 147, 149, 172, 173, 184, 186, 190

V

validation, 87, 118, 188
variables, 128, 176
variations, 7

vascular endothelial growth factor (VEGF), 43
Vascular Endothelial Growth Factor Receptor, 25
vasculature, 199, 204
vegetables, 6
VEGFR, 24, 25, 44, 46
vein, 9, 102, 197, 199, 204
Venezuela, 32, 50
versatility, 70
vessels, 100, 184, 199, 204
videos, 121
virology, 127
viscera, 67
visualization, 71, 74, 75, 92
vomiting, 150, 173

W

Washington, 18, 50
water, 32, 66, 67, 104, 109
water quality, 32
web, 19, 49
weight loss, 32, 173
Western countries, 1, 5, 29, 31, 34, 96, 108, 126, 146, 171, 172, 173, 176, 181
Western Europe, 33, 143, 165
Western patients, vii, 1, 5, 207
wood, 6
workforce, 8
World Health Organization (WHO), 3, 25, 26, 93, 174, 186
worldwide, vii, ix, 1, 2, 6, 8, 15, 89, 90, 114, 142, 143, 171, 177, 179, 181

X

xenografts, 130

Y

yield, 60, 75, 78, 97, 98, 104, 119, 144

Z

zinc, 120